Canine and Feline Behavior for Veterinary Technicians and Nurses

Canine and Feline Behavior for Veterinary Technicians and Nurses

EDITED BY

Julie K. Shaw
RVT, VTS (Behavior)

Debbie Martin
RVT, VTS (Behavior)

WILEY Blackwell

This edition first published 2015 © 2015 by John Wiley & Sons, Inc.

Editorial offices: 1606 Golden Aspen Drive, Suites 103 and 104, Ames, Iowa 50010, USA
                      The Atrium, Southern Gate, Chichester, West Sussex, PO19 8SQ, UK
                      9600 Garsington Road, Oxford, OX4 2DQ, UK

For details of our global editorial offices, for customer services and for information about how to apply for permission to reuse the copyright material in this book please see our website at www.wiley.com/wiley-blackwell.

Library of Congress Cataloging-in-Publication Data

Canine and feline behavior for veterinary technicians and nurses / edited by Julie K. Shaw and Debbie Martin.
    p. ; cm.
  Includes bibliographical references and index.
  ISBN 978-0-8138-1318-9 (pbk.)
  I. Shaw, Julie K., 1963- editor. II. Martin, Debbie, 1970- editor.
  [DNLM: 1. Behavior, Animal. 2. Dogs–psychology. 3. Animal Technicians–psychology.
4. Cats–psychology. 5. Veterinary Medicine–methods. SF 433]
  SF433
  636.7'0887–dc23
                      2014017640

A catalogue record for this book is available from the British Library.

Wiley also publishes its books in a variety of electronic formats. Some content that appears in print may not be available in electronic books.

Typeset in 8.5/11pt MeridienLTStd by Laserwords Private Limited, Chennai, India
Printed and bound in Singapore by Markono Print Media Pte Ltd

1   2015

This text is dedicated to Dr. Andrew Luescher, DVM, Ph.D, DACVB. Dr. Luescher envisioned the role of a veterinary technician in animal behavior in 1998 and then developed and defined that role over the years. He believed pet owners were best served with a team approach to the treatment of behavior issues and he saw the importance of veterinary technicians on that team. He is our mentor, teacher, and friend and without him, it is unlikely this text would have ever come to fruition. Thank you Dr. Luescher for all you have done to promote, protect, and support the human–animal bond and veterinary technicians over the years. We hope we have made your proud.

Julie and Debbie

Contents

Appendix Section 1: Forms and Questionnaires

Appendix Section 2: Training Exercises

Appendix Section 3: Samples and Letters

Contributors

Sara L. Bennett, DVM, MS, DACVB

VCA Berwyn Animal Hospital, Berwyn, IL, USA

Dr. Bennett received her DVM degree in 2006 from Purdue University. She spent 3 years as an associate veterinarian in general practice in Evansville, IN before returning to Purdue to complete a residency in Animal Behavior with an emphasis in shelter behavior medicine and Master's of Science with support through the Maddie's Shelter Medicine Program®. She obtained certification as a diplomate of the American College of Veterinary Behaviorists in 2012.

Dr. Bennett addresses a variety of behavior problems and behavioral disorders including aggression, inappropriate elimination, compulsive disorder, fears and phobias and behavior problems associated with aging across a wide range of species. She particularly enjoys addressing problem behavior in shelter animals, helping to make these pets more adoptable, strengthen the budding human–animal bond and to keep these animals in their new homes.

Dr. Bennett can be found outside the clinic spending time with her husband, dogs, cats, horse or practicing yoga.

Linda M. Campbell, RVT, CPDT-KA, VTS (Behavior)

Humane Society of Missouri, St. Louis, MO, USA

Linda earned her AAS in veterinary technology from Jefferson College in 1990 and has worked for the Humane Society of Missouri (HSMO) since 1974. Over the years Linda developed an intense interest in how behavior impacts the surrender of animals to shelters.

Working at the HSMO provides Linda countless opportunities to expand her knowledge of animal behavior. Linda has assisted the HSMO Animal Cruelty Task Force over the years in disaster responses that include the 1999 E5 tornado that struck Moore City, Oklahoma and managed a field station in Mississippi during 2005 where she received animals displaced by Hurricane Katrina. Linda continues to assist HSMO throughout Missouri with large-scale rescues of animals suffering from abuse, neglect or living in substandard environments.

She has presented at veterinary conferences and animal control seminars, written articles on animal behavior, taught pet dog classes, developed a community-wide animal behavior helpline and implemented HSMO's highly successful Foster Program. During a widely publicized 2009 FBI confiscation of over 500 fighting dogs, Linda coordinated teams evaluating the behavior of each animal.

Currently Linda is the animal behavior manager overseeing training and enrichment programs emphasizing improving the lives and increasing adoptions of the shelter's animals.

Linda is the former secretary of the Society of Veterinary Behavior Technicians, a charter member of the Academy of Veterinary Behavior Technicians, belongs to the Association of Pet Dog Trainers, and a Certified Professional Dog Trainer-Knowledge Assessed, with the Certification Council of Professional Dog Trainers.

Lindsey M. Fourez, BS, RVT

Purdue Comparative Oncology Program, Purdue University, West Lafayette, IN, USA

Lindsey grew up in a small rural town in Illinois. After high school she attended Purdue University where she studied in animal science and veterinary technology. In 2004 she graduated with her AS in veterinary technology, and then in 2005 with a BS in veterinary technology. Currently Lindsey works with the Purdue Comparative Oncology Program.

Sarah Lahrman, RVT

Purdue Comparative Oncology Program, Purdue University, West Lafayette, IN, USA

Sarah Lahrman is a graduate of Purdue University and obtained her Associate's degree in Veterinary Technology in 1998. Following graduation she began work at a small animal practice in Fort Wayne, IN and later moved to another small animal practice in Columbia City, IN. In 2007, her family re-located to Lafayette, IN and Sarah was inspired to work at Purdue University's Small Animal Teaching Hospital. She currently works in the Purdue Comparative Oncology Program.

Andrew U. Luescher, DVM, PhD, DACVB, ECAWBM (BM)

Professor Emeritus, Purdue University, West Lafayette, IN, USA
Foundation Barry du Grand Saint Bernard, Martigny, Switzerland

Dr. Luescher was the Assistant Professor of Ethology at the University of Guelph (Ontario, Canada) from 1985–1997. From 1997–2011 Dr. Luescher was the assistant professor for Animal Behavior and the Director of the Animal Behavior Clinic at

Purdue University in West Lafayette, IN. Since 2011 to present he is the Professor Emeritus of Animal Behavior at Purdue University and the veterinarian responsible for animal behavior and control of genetic diseases for the Foundation Barry du Grand Saint Bernard in Martigny, Switzerland.

Debbie Martin, CPDT-KA, KPA CTP, RVT, VTS (Behavior)

TEAM Education in Animal Behavior, LLC, Spicewood, TX USA

Veterinary Behavior Consultations, LLC, Spicewood, TX, USA

Debbie is a registered veterinary technician and a Veterinary Technician Specialist (VTS) in Behavior. She is a Certified Professional Dog Trainer (Knowledge Assessed) and Karen Pryor Academy Certified Training Partner and Faculty. She has a Bachelor of Science degree from The Ohio State University in human ecology, and associate of applied science degree in veterinary technology from Columbus State Community College. She has been working as a registered veterinary technician since 1996 and has been actively involved in the field of animal behavior. Debbie was the president for the Academy of Veterinary Behavior Technicians (AVBT)from 2012–2014 and is the Treasurer. She is an active member and the previous recording secretary for the Society of Veterinary Behavior Technicians (SVBT). (Behavior) She is the co-author of Puppy Start Right: Foundation Training for the Companion Dog book and Puppy Start Right for Instructors Course.

Kenneth M. Martin, DVM, DACVB

TEAM Education in Animal Behavior, LLC, Spicewood, TX, USA

Veterinary Behavior Consultations, LLC, Spicewood, TX, USA

Dr. Martin completed a clinical behavioral medicine residency at Purdue University's Animal Behavior Clinic in 2004. He graduated from Louisiana State University – School of Veterinary Medicine in 1999. He is a licensed veterinarian in Texas. He practiced companion animal and exotic animal medicine and surgery, and emergency medicine and critical care prior to completing his behavioral medicine residency. His professional interests include conflict induced (owner directed) aggression, compulsive disorders, behavioral development, psychopharmacology, and alternative medicine. Dr. Martin is the co-author of Puppy Start Right: Foundation Training for the Companion Dog book and Puppy Start Right for Instructors Course. He is a member of the American Veterinary Medical Association, the Capital Area Veterinary Medical Association, and the recording secretary for the American Veterinary Society of Animal Behavior.

Virginia L. Price, MS, CVT, VTS (Behavior)

Saint Petersburg College, St Petersburg, FL, USA

Ginny Price is a professor at Saint Petersburg College where she teaches small animal behavior (in the AS and BAS programs) along with the entry level nursing laboratory, laboratory animal medicine and nursing one lecture. Between 2009 and 2011 she was the Critical Thinking Champion for the AS Veterinary Technology program. Ginny has served for the past year(2012–2013) as the Center of Excellence for Teaching and Learning representative for the St Petersburg College School of Veterinary Technology. From 2009 through 2011 she was privileged to serve on the board of directors for the Western Veterinary Conference as their Technician Director. She graduated from Saint Petersburg College Veterinary Technology program in 1981. She is certified in the state of Florida with the Florida Veterinary Technician Association. She has a master's degree in psychology earned in 2007 from Walden University. She is a founding member of the Society of Veterinary Behavior Technicians and the Academy of Veterinary Behavior Technicians. She earned her Veterinary Technician Specialist in Behavior in 2010.

Marcia R. Ritchie, LVT, CPDT-KA, VTS (Behavior)

The Family Companion, Springville, NY, USA

Marcia Rafter Ritchie graduated from SUNY Delhi with an AAS in Veterinary Science in 1977. She worked in private veterinary practices for 20 years where her passion for animal behavior was cultivated by the veterinarians she worked with.

She has been a professional pet obedience instructor since 1984 and was in the first group of 120 instructors to receive national certification through the Association of Pet Dog Trainers (APDT), of which she is a charter member. A past board member of the Society of Veterinary Behavior Technicians, she is currently serving on several committees. She is a founding member of the Academy of Veterinary Behavior Technicians, which was granted specialty status by National Association of Veterinary Technicians of America (NAVTA) in 2008.

Marcia is one of the co-authors of SVBT's "Building the Veterinary Behavior Team" manual. Her behavior articles have been published in both the SVBT newsletter and the Veterinary Technician magazine as well as local publications.

Marcia is the Director of Training and Behavior for "The Family Companion". She now supervises a training staff of 6 instructors who teach pet obedience classes in 7 different locations in the Buffalo New York area. Marcia teaches group classes, private instruction, assists veterinarians with behavior modification and does pet selection counseling. She is a consultant for the Erie County SPCA and a volunteer 4-H leader in the dog program.

Julie K. Shaw, KPA CTP, RVT, VTS (Behavior)

TEAM Education in Animal Behavior, LLC, Spicewood, TX, USA

Julie Shaw became a registered veterinary technician in 1983. After working in general veterinary practice for 17 years and starting her own successful dog training business. She became the Senior Animal Behavior Technologist at the Purdue Animal Behavior Clinic working with veterinary animal behaviorist, Dr. Andrew Luescher, PhD, DVM, DACVB. While at Purdue, Julie saw referral behavior cases with Dr. Luescher, organized and co-taught the acclaimed five-day DOGS! Behavior Modification course, taught many classes to veterinary and veterinary technician students, and instructed continuing education seminars for veterinary technicians, veterinarians, and trainers.

Julie is a charter member of the Society of Veterinary Behavior Technicians and the Academy of Veterinary Behavior Technicians. She is also a faculty member for the Karen Pryor Academy for Animal Training and Behavior.

Julie is a popular national and international speaker on problem prevention, practical applications of behavior modification techniques and other companion animal behavior related topics. She speaks extensively on the need for a TEAM approach that includes veterinarian, veterinary technician and qualified trainer to complete the companion animal mental health care TEAM.

Julie has received many awards including the North American Veterinary Conference Veterinary Technician Speaker of the Year Award, the Western Veterinary Conference speaker of the year and was named the 2007 NAVC Mara Memorial Lecturer of the year for her accomplishments and leadership in the veterinary technician profession.

Carissa D. Sparks, BS, RVT, VTS (Neurology)

Purdue University Veterinary Teaching Hospital, West Lafayette, IN, USA

Carissa Sparks obtained a bachelor's of science degree in animal science in 2002 and an associate's degree in Veterinary Technology in 2003 from the Purdue University College of Veterinary Medicine. She obtained her veterinary technician specialty in neurology from the Academy of Internal Medicine for Veterinary Technicians in 2011. Currently she is employed by the Purdue University College of Veterinary Medicine in West Lafayette, Indiana as the senior neurology veterinary technologist and serves as a committee member for the Academy of Internal Medicine for Veterinary Technicians in neurology.

Preface

The human–animal bond is a powerful and fragile union. Pets, dogs specifically, have evolved from being primarily for utilitarian purposes to taking on the role of a human companion and family member. Consequently, pet owners' expectations have changed and are continuing to change. As the stigma of human mental and emotional health begins to be shattered, so is the stigma of treating animals with behavioral issues. Pet owners are beginning to recognize their pet's emotional and mental needs and are reaching out to veterinary professionals for assistance.

We believe it takes a mental healthcare team that includes a veterinarian, veterinary technician, and a qualified trainer to most successfully prevent and treat behavior issues in companion animals.

The veterinary technician is in a unique position to be a pivotal and key component in that mental health care team. Technicians interact and educate pet owners on a daily basis about preventive and intervention medical treatments. Through behavioral preventive services and assisting the veterinarian with behavioral intervention, communicating and working closely with the qualified trainer, veterinary technicians can become the "case manager" of the team, in turn saving lives and enhancing the human–animal bond.

Many books have been published geared toward the role of the veterinarian in behavioral medicine. The purpose of this text is to provide the veterinary technician with a solid foundation in feline and canine behavioral medicine. All veterinary technicians must have a basic understanding of their patient's behavioral, mental,

and emotional needs. Companion animal behavior in this regard is not a specialty but the foundation for better understanding and treatment of our patients. General companion animal behavior healthcare should no longer be an "elective" in veterinary and veterinary technician curriculums but rather a core part of our education. How can we best administer quality healthcare if we do not understand our patient's behavioral needs?

The reader will learn about the roles of animal behavior professionals, normal development of dogs and cats and be provided with an in-depth and dynamic look at the human animal bond with a new perspective that includes correlations from human mental healthcare. Learning theory, preventive behavioral services, standardized behavior modification terms and techniques, and veterinary behavior pharmacology are also included.

There is vibrant change occurring in the world of animal behavior professionals. It is as though a snowball that took some work to get started has begun rolling and growing on its own. People like you are propelling that snowball forward and improving the lives of animals and the people who love them.

After the first moment you open this book we hope it becomes outdated – because you will continue to push the snowball forward with new ideas and techniques.

Thank you for improving the lives of animals.

Julie Shaw and Debbie Martin

Acknowledgments

Debbie Martin:

I would like to thank Julie Shaw, a wonderful teacher, mentor, and friend. It was her passion for educating others and initiative that brought this book to fruition. I was honored to have been invited to co-edit the book with her.

I would also like to acknowledge my husband, Kenneth Martin, DVM, DACVB, for his patience, guidance, and understanding as I spent countless hours, days, weeks, and months on this project. His insights and feedback provided much needed support and assistance throughout the process.

Julie Shaw:

Debbie Martin – my student, then my friend, then my colleague and now my sister and my teacher – thank you for putting up with me. You have enhanced my life in ways you will likely never fully understand.

Taylor, Dylan, and Skylar

Over the 5 years it took to complete this book you grew from strange pre-teen creatures into young productive and happy adults. I am very proud and grateful for each of you. For all the times you had to write notes to me because I had my headphones on while writing, for all the times I said, "No we can't, I have to work on the book" and for all the times you spoke and I didn't hear – thank you for believing in me and being patient.

I love you to the moon and back my sweet babies.

Rodney,

You are the highest reinforcement possible at the end of my very long and sometimes challenging learning curve. You are the best human being I've ever known and you help me to be the best person I can be. I adore you.

About the companion website

This book is accompanied by a companion website:

www.wiley.com/go/shaw/behavior

The website includes:

- Powerpoints of all figures from the book for downloading
- Appendices from the book for downloading
- Self-assessment quizzes

1 The role of the veterinary technician in animal behavior

Kenneth M. Martin[1,2] and Debbie Martin[1,2]

[1] TEAM Education in Animal Behavior, LLC, Spicewood, TX, USA
[2] Veterinary Behavior Consultations, LLC, Spicewood, TX, USA

The veterinary staff plays a significant role in preventing, identifying and treating behavioral disorders of pets. Inquiring about behavior at each veterinary visit, as well as, creating client awareness about behavior disorders and training problems, strengthens the client–hospital bond, the human–animal bond, and prevents pet relinquishment. The veterinary technician can excel and be fully utilized in the behavior technician role. The responsibilities of the veterinary technician in animal behavior begin with educating and building awareness regarding the normal behavior of animals. The veterinarian–veterinary technician partnership allows for prevention and treatment of behavioral disorders and training problems. Distinguishing and identifying behavior disorders, medical disorders, lack of training issues, and being able to provide prevention and early intervention allows for the maintenance and enhancement of the human–animal bond. Clearly defining the roles and responsibilities of the veterinary behavior team facilitates harmony within the team without misrepresentation. The veterinary technician's role as part of the behavior team is often that of "case manager"; the technician triages and guides the client to the appropriate resources for assistance. Before delving into the extensive role of the veterinary technician in the behavior team, the roles of the veterinarian and the dog trainer

Canine and Feline Behavior for Veterinary Technicians and Nurses, First Edition. Edited by Julie K. Shaw and Debbie Martin.
© 2015 John Wiley & Sons, Inc. Published 2015 by John Wiley & Sons, Inc.
Companion Website: www.wiley.com/go/shaw/behavior

will be explored. By understanding these roles first, the pivotal role of the technician will become evident.

> • The veterinary technician's role as part of the behavior team is often that of "case manager"; the technician triages and guides the client to the appropriate resources for assistance.

Veterinarian's roles and responsibilities

The veterinarian is responsible for the clinical assessment of all patients presented to the veterinary hospital. The veterinarian's role in behavior includes

1. setting the hospital's policy and procedures,
2. determining which behavioral services are offered and the corresponding fee structure,
3. developing the format of the behavior consultation history form for medical documentation,
4. establishing a behavioral diagnosis and list of differentials, as well as medical differentials,
5. providing the prognosis,
6. developing a treatment plan and making any changes to the plan,
7. prescribing medication and changing medication type or dosage, and
8. outlining the procedure and protocols for follow-up care.

> • The veterinarian is responsible for the clinical assessment of all patients presented to the veterinary hospital.

Only a licensed veterinarian can practice veterinary medicine. The practice of veterinary medicine means to diagnose, treat, correct, change, relieve, or prevent any animal disease, deformity, defect, injury, or other physical or mental conditions, including the prescribing of any drug or medicine (Modified from: Title 37 Professions and occupations Chapter 18. Veterinarians Louisiana Practice Act [La. R.S. 37:1511–1558]). The mental welfare of animals and the treatment of mental illness are included in many state veterinary practice acts. Only by evaluating the patient's physical and neurological health and obtaining and reviewing the medical and behavioral history, can the veterinarian

establish a diagnosis and prescribe appropriate treatment. When dealing with the behavior of animals, it must be determined whether the behavior is normal, abnormal, the manifestation of a medical condition, an inappropriately conditioned behavior, or simply related to lack of training.

The veterinarian, by establishing a diagnosis and prescribing behavioral treatment, is practicing veterinary behavioral medicine comparable to a medical doctor practicing human psychiatry; this medical specialty deals with the prevention, assessment, diagnosis, treatment, and rehabilitation of mental illness in humans. The goal of human psychiatry is the relief of mental suffering associated with behavioral disorder and the improvement of mental well-being. The focus of veterinary behavior is improving the welfare of pets and consequently enhancing the well-being of clients. This strengthens the human–animal bond. When addressing the behavior of animals, the mental well-being of the patient should be evaluated in direct relation to the patient's medical health. In this manner, the veterinarian is using a complete or holistic approach and treating the entire patient. This may be accomplished only by a visit to the veterinarian (Figure 1.1).

The veterinarian or veterinary technician should obtain behavioral information during every hospital visit. Many behavioral issues are overlooked in general veterinary practice without direct solicitation. Current pet management information regarding feeding, housing, exercising, training, and training aids should be documented in the medical record. Behavioral topics for puppy visits should include socialization, body language, house training, teaching bite inhibition, and methodology for basic training and problem solving. Behavioral

Figure 1.1 Veterinarian performing a physical examination of the patient at home.

topics for kitten visits should include teaching bite and claw inhibition, litter-box training and management, and handling and carrier training. All senior patients should be screened annually for cognitive dysfunction syndrome. Only through questioning clients regarding their pet's behavior will potential behavioral disorders or training problems be identified. The veterinary staff may then recommend suitable behavior services to address the specific issues. This may prompt scheduling an appointment with the appropriate staff member: the veterinarian, veterinary behavior technician, or a qualified professional trainer.

> • Many behavioral issues are overlooked in general veterinary practice without direct solicitation.

Figure 1.2 Boxer presenting for excoriation of the muzzle due to separation anxiety (barrier frustration) with frequent attempts to escape the crate.

When a behavioral disorder is suspected, interviewing the client and obtaining a thorough behavioral history is essential for the veterinarian to make a behavioral diagnosis. The behavioral history should include the signalment, the patient's early history, management, household dynamics and human interaction schedule, previous training, and a temperament profile. The temperament profile determines the pet's individual response to specific social and environmental stimuli. Triggers of the undesirable behaviors should be identified. Pet owners should describe the typical behavioral response of the pet. In addition, the chronological development of the behavior, including the age of onset, the historical progression, and whether the behavior has worsened, improved, or remained the same, must be documented. Discussing a minimum of three specific incidents detailing the pet's body language before, during, and after the behavior, as well as the human response, is necessary. The medical record should document previous treatments including training, medical intervention, and drug therapy. Changes in the household or management should be questioned. Inducing the behavioral response or observing the behavior on a video recorder may be necessary. However, caution should be used in regard to observing the behavior. Often the behavioral history provides sufficient information for a diagnosis. If the description of the behavior does not provide sufficient information, then observation of the patient's *first* response to a controlled exposure to the stimulus may be required. Safety factors should be in place to prevent injury to the patient or others. This should only be used as a last resort as it allows the patient to practice the undesirable behavior and carries risk. (For an example of behavior history forms, see Appendix 1)

The veterinarian and veterinary staff are instrumental in recognizing behavior issues when a pet is presented for an underlying medical problem. All medical diseases result in behavior changes and most behavioral disorders have medical differentials. A behavior disorder may lead to the clinical presentation of a surgical or medical disease. Surgical repair of wounds inflicted by a dog bite may prompt the veterinarian to recommend behavior treatment for inter-dog aggression. A cat or dog presenting with self-inflicted wounds may indicate a panic disorder or compulsive behavior (Figure 1.2). Dental disease including fractured teeth may prompt the veterinarian to inquire about anxiety-related conditions such as separation anxiety. Frequent enterotomies may indicate pica or some other anxiety-related condition. The astute veterinarian must use a multimodal approach with the integration of behavioral questionnaires and medical testing to determine specific and nonspecific links to behavioral disorders. Medical disease may cause the development of a behavior disorder. Feline lower urinary tract disease may lead to the continuation of inappropriate elimination even after the inciting cause has been treated. Many behavior disorders require and benefit from concurrent medical and pharmacological treatment.

> • All medical diseases result in behavior changes and most behavioral disorders have medical differentials.

- The astute veterinarian must use a multimodal approach with the integration of behavioral questionnaires and medical testing to determine specific and nonspecific links to behavioral disorders.

Medical differentials to behavior disorders

When faced with a behavior problem, the veterinarian must determine if the cause is medical and/or behavioral. The rationale that the problem is only either medical or behavioral is a flawed approach. Neurophysiologically, any medical condition that affects the normal function of the central nervous system can alter behavior. The nonspecific complaint of lethargy or depression may be caused by a multitude of factors including pyrexia, pain, anemia, hypoglycemia, a congenital abnormality such as lissencephaly or hydrocephalus, a central nervous system disorder involving neoplasia, infection, trauma, or lead toxicity, endocrine disorders such as hypothyroidism or hyperadrenocorticism, metabolic disorders such as hepatic or uremic encephalopathy, and cognitive dysfunction or sensory deficits. Behavioral signs are the first presenting signs of any illness.

As a general rule, veterinarians should do a physical and neurological examination and basic blood analysis for all pets presenting for behavioral changes. The practitioner may decide to perform more specific diagnostic tests based on exam findings. Additional diagnostics will vary on a case-by-case basis.

The existence of a medical condition can be determined only after a thorough physical and neurological examination. Completing a neurological examination is difficult in aggressive patients. The neurological examination may be basic and limited to the cranial nerves, muscle symmetry and tone, central propioception, ambulation, and anal tone. Other minimum diagnostic testing should include a complete laboratory analysis (complete blood count, serum chemistry profile, and urinalysis) and fecal screening. A further look into sensory perception may include an electroretinogram (ERG) or brainstem auditory evoked response (BAER). Thyroid testing (total thyroxine, free thyroxine, triiodothyronine, thyrotropin, and/or antithyroid antibodies) may be indicated based on clinical signs, suspicion, and the class of medication considered for behavioral treatment. Imaging techniques, such as radiographs, ultrasound, magnetic resonance imaging (MRI) or computed axial tomography (CT) may provide invaluable information. The workup for medical conditions and behavioral conditions is not mutually exclusive. However, exhausting every medical rule out may pose financial limitations for the client. After all, diagnosis is inferential behaviorally and medically and the purpose of establishing a diagnosis is not to categorize, but to prescribe treatment.

Behavioral dermatology

A relationship between dermatologic conditions and anxiety-related conditions exists in humans and pets. Environmental and social stress has been shown to increase epidermal permeability and increase the susceptibility to allergens (Garg *et al.*, 2001). A dermatological lesion can be caused behaviorally by a compulsive disorder, a conditioned behavior, separation anxiety, or any conflict behavior. Behavioral dermatologic signs in companion animals may include alopecia, feet or limb biting, licking or chewing, tail chasing, flank sucking, hind end checking, anal licking, nonspecific scratching, hyperaesthesia, and self-directed aggression. Medical reasons for tail chasing may include lumbrosacral stenosis or cauda equina syndrome, a tail dock neuroma or a paraesthesia. Anal licking may be associated with anal sac disease, parasites, or food hypersensitivity. Dermatological conditions may be related to staphlococcal infection, mange, dermatophytosis, allergies, hypothyroidism, trauma, foreign body, neoplasia, osteoarthritis, or neuropathic pain. Diagnostic testing may include screening for ectoparasites, skin scraping, epidermal cytology, dermatophyte test medium (DTM), woods lamp, an insecticide application every 3 weeks, a food allergy elimination diet (FAED), skin biopsy, intradermal skin testing or enzyme linked immunosorbent assay (ELISA), and a corticosteroid trial. It is important to realize that corticosteroids have psychotropic effects in addition to antipruritic properties. A favorable response to steroids does not rule out behavioral factors.

Conversely, behavioral disorders may be maintained even after the dermatological condition has resolved. Dermatological lesions may be linked to behavioral disorders and lesions can facilitate and intensify other behavior problems including aggression. Dogs with dermatological lesions are not necessarily more likely to be aggressive, but dogs with aggression disorders may be more irritable when they have concurrent dermatological lesions.

Aggression

The relationship between the viral disease of rabies and aggression is very clear. All cases of aggression should be verified for current rabies vaccination from a liability standpoint. Iatrogenic aggression in canine and feline patients has been induced by the administration of certain drugs such as benzodiazepines, acepromazine, and ketamine.

> • All cases of aggression should be verified for current rabies vaccination from a liability standpoint.

The relationship between hyperthyroidism in cats and irritable aggression is very likely present, although not definitively established. The relationship between hypothyroidism and aggression in dogs is inconclusive. Numerous case reports suggesting a link between aggression in dogs and thyroid deficiency have been published in the veterinary literature. The effect of thyroid supplementation on behavior without the benefit of a control group in these case studies offers limited evidence of a causative relationship. In a controlled study of nonaggressive and aggressive dogs, no significant differences in thyroid levels were found (Radosta-Huntley *et al.*, 2006). Thyroid hormone supplementation in rats results in elevation of serotonin in the frontal cortex (Gur *et al.*, 1999). Serotonin is a neurotransmitter associated with mood stabilization (see Chapter 9). The possible elevation of serotonin due to thyroid supplementation may result in beneficial behavioral changes in aggressive dogs. Spontaneous resolution of aggression with thyroid supplementation is probably overstated and hypothyroidism is unlikely the cause of aggression. While malaise can lead to irritability, many dogs that have hypothyroidism do not show aggression.

The presence of sensory deficits may contribute to aggressive behavior and anxiety. This is particularly important when assessing the behavior of senior patients with concurrent medical disorders. Age-related behavioral changes in the brain can lead to the presentation of clinical signs consistent with cognitive dysfunction syndrome. These signs may include disorientation, interaction changes with the owner, changes in the sleep–wake cycle, and house soiling. Activity level may be decreased or increased.

Elimination disorders

Elimination problems in dogs may be related to urinary tract infection, urolithiasis, polyuria/polydypsia,

incontinence, prostatic disease, renal disease, diarrhea, or neoplasia. Elimination problems in cats may be related to idiopathic cystitis, urolithiasis, infection, neoplasia, polyuria/polydypsia, constipation/diarrhea, or associated with long hair. Urological diagnostics may include a complete blood count (CBC), chemistry, urinalysis, urine culture, adrenocorticotropic hormone (ACTH) stimulation, water deprivation tests, imaging, cystoscopy, or a urethral pressure profile.

When one is uncertain whether it is a behavioral or medical problem, one must do some reasonable fact finding and treat the entire patient, physically and psychologically. When necessary, infer the most likely diagnosis and treat all contributing factors. Medical and psychological factors must be treated concurrently. A treatment plan that includes conventional medical treatment and behavioral intervention is necessary for successful resolution of the inciting problem.

> • When one is uncertain whether it is a behavioral or medical problem, one must do some reasonable fact finding and treat the entire patient, physically and psychologically.

Behavior disorder versus training problem

Behavioral disorders of animals are emotional disorders that are unrelated to training. Training problems relate to pets that are unruly or do not know or respond to cues or commands. These problems are common in young puppies and adolescent dogs without obedience training. These dogs lack manners. Training involves the learning of "human-taught" appropriate behaviors that are unrelated to the emotional or mental well-being of the patient. There are many different approaches to training. Some are purely positive reinforcement based and others rely primarily on the use of aversive methodology (positive punishment and negative reinforcement). Trainers may also be somewhere in the middle regarding methodology, using a combination of pleasant and unpleasant consequences. Depending on the methodology used, positive and negative associations can be made by the dog. Positive methods are less damaging and can strengthen the human–animal bond. Behaviors taught in a positive learning environment are retained longer and performed more reliably. Aversive methods risk creating a negative emotional state and may contribute to the development of a behavioral

CHAPTER 1

Figure 1.3 Therapy dog who suffers from thunderstorm phobia.

disorder. Dogs that are behaviorally normal and emotionally stable, yet lack basic obedience skills related to heeling on leash, coming when called, sitting, lying down and staying, fit into the category of a training problem. Yes, some emotionally unstable dogs may, in addition, have training problems, but training problems and behavior disorders are treated independently as separate entities. Dogs with fear or anxiety conditions can benefit from positive reinforcement-based training in much the same way as shy children benefit from team sports or other confidence-building activities. Dogs previously trained using aversive methodology often need to be retrained using positive methods for performing behavioral modification techniques as a result of the negative emotional response caused by the previous aversive training. Many well-trained dogs have behavioral disorders (Figure 1.3). Examples include separation anxiety or human-directed aggression. These disorders occur in spite of the fact that the dog may be very well trained and responsive to the handler. Dog training does not directly treat behavioral disorders and is not considered practicing veterinary behavioral medicine.

> • Behavioral disorders of animals are emotional disorders that are unrelated to training.

> • Training involves the learning of "human-taught" appropriate behaviors that are unrelated to the emotional or mental well-being of the patient.

> • Some emotionally unstable dogs may, in addition, have training problems, but training problems and behavior disorders are treated independently as separate entities.

It should be noted that there are many benefits to having a trainer associated or working within the veterinary practice. Pet owners have been shown to search the internet for information and call their veterinary hospital for their pet's behavioral and training needs. (Shore *et al.* 2008)

Qualified professionals to treat animal behavior disorders

When the pet's behavior is considered abnormal, with an underlying medical or behavioral component, comprising fear, anxiety, or aggression, owners should seek guidance from a trained professional. The veterinarian is the first person who should be contacted when a pet exhibits a problem behavior or the pet's behavior changes. Changes in behavior or behavior problems can reflect underlying medical conditions, which must be evaluated by a veterinarian. Many underlying medical problems, including pain, can alter the pet's behavior in ways that are difficult for pet owners to identify. Once medical conditions have been ruled out, behavioral advice should be sought. It is important to understand the qualifications of people who use titles that indicate they are behavior professionals. This is difficult because, unlike the titles veterinarian, psychologist, and psychiatrist, which are state licensed, the title "animal behaviorist" or similar titles can be used by anyone, regardless of their background (modified from www.certifiedanimalbehaviorist.com). Qualified animal behavior professionals include a veterinarian with special interest and training in animal behavior, a Diplomate of the American College of Veterinary Behaviorists (DACVB) or a Certified Applied Animal Behaviorist (CAAB).

> • The veterinarian is the first person who should be contacted when a pet exhibits a problem behavior or the pet's behavior changes. Changes in behavior or behavior problems can reflect underlying medical conditions, which must be evaluated by a veterinarian.

- Qualified animal behavior professionals include a veterinarian with special interest and training in animal behavior, a DACVB or a CAAB.

The American Veterinary Society of Animal Behavior (AVSAB) is a group of veterinarians and research professionals who share an interest in understanding the behavior of animals. AVSAB emphasizes that the use of scientifically sound learning principles that apply to all species is the accepted means of training and modifying behavior in pets and is the key to our understanding of how pets learn and how to communicate with our pets. AVSAB (www.avsabonline.org) is thereby committed to improving the quality of life of all animals and strengthening the human–animal bond. AVSAB membership provides quarterly electronic newsletters containing animal behavior case reports, listings of behavior continuing education, behavior book reviews, advertisements for positions in behavioral medicine; listserv access for networking and exchanging information with veterinarians, veterinary students, veterinary behaviorists, and applied animal behaviorists; and reduced cost of registration and proceedings for the annual AVSAB Scientific Meeting. AVSAB does not certify its members or guarantee its members meet a specific standard of competence or possess specific behavioral knowledge.

The American College of Veterinary Behaviorists or ACVB (www.veterinarybehaviorists.org) is a professional organization of veterinarians who are board-certified in the specialty of Veterinary Behavior. This veterinary specialty is recognized by the American Board of Veterinary Specialization. Board-certified specialists are known as *diplomates*. Veterinarians who have the honor of calling themselves diplomates may use the designation "DACVB" after their names. The requirements for veterinarians include completing the equivalency of a 1-year veterinary internship, completing a conforming approved residency program or a nonconforming training program mentored and approved by ACVB, authoring a scientific paper on behavior research and publishing it in a peer-reviewed journal, writing three peer-reviewed case reports, and successfully completing a comprehensive 2-day examination.

The Animal Behavior Society (ABS) is a professional organization in North America for the study of animal behavior. Certification by the ABS (www.animalbehavior.org) recognizes that, to the best of its knowledge, the certificant meets the educational, experimental, and ethical standards required by the society for professional applied animal behaviorists. Certification does not constitute a guarantee that the applicant meets a specific standard of competence or possesses specific knowledge. Members who meet the specific criteria may use the designation, "CAAB," after their names. CAABs (www.certifiedanimalbehaviorist.com) come from different educational backgrounds and may include a PhD in Animal Behavior or Doctor of Veterinary Medicine. CAABs, who are not veterinarians, usually work through veterinary referral to provide behavioral care.

Trainer's roles and responsibilities

The role of the dog trainer in behavior is coaching and teaching of dogs and dog owners about basic training and manners. Trainers are teachers. Some trainers function as coaches for competitive dog sports such as obedience, tracking, agility, rally, or protection. Those who work with veterinarians provide an instrumental role in implementing behavior modification as prescribed in a treatment plan.

Comparatively, as it would be inappropriate for a school teacher to diagnose or prescribe treatment for a child with a behavioral disorder, dog trainers may not diagnose or prescribe treatment for veterinary behavioral disorders (Luescher et al., 2007). Although the treatment of animal behavior disorders is considered the practice of veterinary medicine, many states have been unwilling to prosecute when treatment is done in the name of dog training.

Dog training is a largely unlicensed and unregulated profession in the United States. Currently, anyone who wishes to call himself/herself a dog trainer or animal behaviorist may do so, without any formal education or true understanding of learning theory. The trainer's reasoning for the behavior may vary greatly from the actual motivation and the training methodology may be inhumane, outdated, or inappropriate. For example, some trainers base all dog behavior and training on dominance theory. The assumption that dogs misbehave because they are striving for higher rank often leads trainers to use force or correction to modify undesirable behaviors. This negatively affects the human–animal bond and is a flawed approach (Luescher and Reisner, 2008 ;Landsberg et al., 2008).

When the pet's behavior is considered normal, without an underlying medical or mental disorder, owners may seek guidance from a trained professional. That person may be a Karen Pryor Academy Certified Training Partner (KPA CTP) (www.karenpryoracademy.com, www.greatdogtrainers.com), a Certified Professional Dog Trainer, or a Veterinary Technician Specialist (Behavior) (VTS-Behavior).

Choosing a dog trainer can be a difficult decision for the veterinarian, the veterinary staff, and the client. A dog trainer should have all the desirable attributes of a good teacher. He/she should keep up with current training tools and methods by attending workshops and continuing education conferences; should be calm, patient, open-minded, understand how dogs learn, and be able to convey this knowledge to the pet owner in a positive and motivational manner; should describe the behavior being trained, explain why it is important, and be able to demonstrate it. In a group setting, ample time should be allotted to individually assist students and allow time for practice. The AVSAB Position Statement on Punishment states: Trainers who use or advocate physical force (e.g., hitting, alpha rolling, pushing a dog into position, choke chain, or pinch collar correction) or methods/devices that have the potential to harm, as an acceptable way to train should be avoided (Eskeland, 2007). Trainers must adapt humane training methods to the individual dog or problem situation. The most outstanding trainers are motivational and positive reinforcement-based in their techniques. Trainers who do not use rewards should be avoided. Motivational trainers use rewards (e.g., food, toys, play, affection) rather than teaching the dog using fear, pain, or punishment. In this situation, the dog works for the possibility of a reward, rather than to avoid physical or psychological punishment. Punishment is rarely necessary, does not teach an appropriate desirable behavior, and should only be used as a last resort by a trainer who can fully explain the possible adverse effects. Before referring to a trainer, veterinarians should interview the trainer about vaccination requirements for attending training classes. In addition, the veterinarian or veterinary technician should observe the trainer instructing a class (Box 1.1). Are rewards used liberally? Are the handlers smiling and using upbeat voices? Are the dogs having fun? Do you hear any yelling or scolding? See any harsh physical correction? And if so, how does the instructor handle the situation? See Appendix 10 for a Trainer Assessment Form.

BOX 1.1: ASSESSING A DOG TRAINER'S COMPETENCE AND ETHICS.

- Welcomes potential clients to observe a class prior to making a decision to enroll
- Explains a skill and gives examples of how the skill is useful in everyday life
- Demonstrates the skill
- Utilizes handouts and other instructional guides
- Circulates through the students giving assistance and guidance when needed
- Remains conscious of the emotional state of all animals in the classroom setting and acts appropriately
- Arranges the classroom to optimize the success of each handler and animal
- Does not become focused on one student
- Keeps the class moving at an appropriate pace
- Can adjust the teaching plan as needed for individual student's needs
- Is professional and respectful at all times to owners/handlers
- Is appropriate and liberal with positive reinforcement to both the owners and animals
- Is familiar with TAG Teach (www.tagteach.com) and utilizes it frequently and appropriately to instruct clients (see Chapter 5)
- Uses appropriate management tools to decrease unwanted behaviors while teaching the desired behaviors
- Utilizes only humane training methods that promote and protect the human–animal bond and are not harmful to the handler or dog in any way
- Does not recommend or utilize choke collars, pinch collars, electronic shock collars or physical punishments[a]
- Does not coach or advocate the outdated and disproved "dominance hierarchy theory" and the subsequent confrontational training and relationship that follows from it
- Understands and addresses the emotional and motivational state of the animal
- Recommends and utilizes training tools such as head collars and no pull harnesses on an individual basis or as recommended and prescribed by the veterinarian
- Understands the value of education and attends continuing education seminars regularly
- Is a certified member of a standardized and policed credentialing program
- Because of variables in dog breeding, temperament, owner commitment, and experience, a trainer cannot and should not guarantee the results of his/her training, although should ensure client satisfaction
- Builds and maintains a mutually communicative, respectful, and professional relationship with veterinary professionals
- Understands veterinarians are exclusively responsible for diagnosing behavioral disorders, for medical and behavioral differential diagnoses, and for prescribing

a treatment plan which may include pharmacological intervention
- Any trainer who utilizes punishment must be able to
1. understand the scientific principles for the application of punishment,
2. articulate the most serious adverse effects associated with punishment,
3. judge when these adverse effects are occurring over the short and/or long term, and
4. explain how they would attempt to reverse any adverse effects if or when they occur.

[a]Modified from AVSAB's Position Statement on Punishment.

Before veterinary professionals refer their client to a trainer, they should be familiar with the trainer's level of education and the methodology and tools used to achieve behavior modification. One should be wary of trainers who guarantee results and refer to themselves as a behaviorist, while lacking credentials. The ideal trainer should collaborate openly with the veterinarian when faced with possible underlying medical and behavior disorders (fear, anxiety, or aggression). In doing so, the veterinarian may diagnose and prescribe behavior modification and/or pharmacological treatment. The trainer then may instruct and assist the pet owner on implementation of the prescribed behavior modification plan. A holistic team approach should be developed between the veterinary team, trainer, and client (Table 1.1).

- Before veterinary professionals refer their client to a trainer, they should be familiar with the trainer's level of education and the methodology and tools used to achieve behavior modification.

Fortunately, the trend is toward the licensing of dog trainers who have some level of education; continuing education is also required. The AVSAB Position Statement on Dominance recommends that veterinarians do not refer clients to trainers or behavior consultants who coach and advocate dominance hierarchy theory and the subsequently confrontational training. Rather, behavior modification and training should focus on reinforcing desirable behaviors, avoiding the reinforcement of undesirable behaviors, and striving to address the underlying emotional state and motivations, including medical and genetic factors that are driving the undesirable behavior.

There are numerous dog trainer schools and organizations that offer online educational correspondence courses. These through-the-internet courses offer to "certify" the participant as a "professional" in the field of dog training and behavior. Many courses are offered by self-proclaimed animal behaviorists and dog trainers to those willing to become "certified" professional dog trainers or a certified "canine behavior therapists." The person's or place's reputation, credentials, and qualifications should be determined before accepting any title or degree. Some organizations are "bogus", while others are well known and taught by professional, qualified staff. The best schools and educational programs for trainers offer their students a strong foundation in learning theory with hands-on workshops, seminars, and continuing education. Reputable certifying organizations "police" their members by holding them to a standardized level of ethics and care. If those ethics and care are violated, certification can be revoked.

The Karen Pryor Academy or KPA (www.karenpryor-academy.com) is an educational organization that offers online education and hands-on workshops in order to certify dog trainers. Graduates of KPA become part of a community of trainers who have achieved and demonstrated a consistent level of excellence and can represent themselves as a KPA CTP. Training partners must teach and train using force-free principles and techniques, are subject to a policed credentialing process and are expected to demonstrate the highest level of professionalism and ethics. KPA CTPs must demonstrate an ability to communicate clearly, professionally, and positively with associates, veterinary professionals, and pet owners. Veterinarians should seek out KPA CTPs in their area to develop mutually beneficial working relationships.

The Association of Pet Dog Trainers (APDT) is a professional organization of individual dog trainers who are committed to becoming better trainers through education. It (www.apdt.com) provides membership networking and sharing of ideas through educational conferences, newsletters, and seminars. Membership is open to any member of the public who is interested in dog training. APDT does not offer trainer certification directly. It encourages its members to make use of "dog-friendly" training methods that use reinforcement and rewards, not punishment, to achieve the desired behavior. There is no policing of training methodology or education requirements to be an APDT member.

The Certification Council for Professional Dog Trainers (CCPDT) was originally created by the APDT in 2001.

Table 1.1 The roles and responsibilities of the veterinary behavior team.

Roles and responsibilities	Veterinarian	Veterinary technician	Dog trainer
Initial client communication	X	X	X
Client education and awareness	X	X	X
Obtaining clinical history	X	X	–
Setting hospital policies & fee structure	X	–	–
Medical differentials	X	–	–
Behavioral diagnosis	X	–	–
Prognosis	X	–	–
Develops and modifies treatment plans	X	–	–
Prescribes medications	X	–	–
Implementing prescribed treatment plan	–	X	X
Follow-up communication with client	X	X	X
Follow-up communication with veterinarian	–	X	X
Follow-up behavior consultation	X	–	–
Demonstrate training methods	–	X	X
Demonstrate training tools	–	X	X
Assess pet's trainability	–	X	X
Identifying normal versus abnormal behavior	X	X	X
Problem prevention	X	X	X
Teaching puppy and kitten classes	–	X	X
Teaching manners and obedience classes	–	X	X

The CCPDT (www.ccpdt.org) was the first national certification program for professional pet dog trainers and offers an international testing program. All certified trainers must earn continuing education credits to maintain their designations. They must also agree to adhere to a code of ethics. Candidates who meet the following requirements and pass the written exam earn the title Certified Professional Dog Trainer-Knowledge Assessed and may use the designation, "CPDT-KA," after their name. The certification requirements are as follows.

1. At least 300 h experience in dog training within the last 5 years. Two hundred and twenty-five hours or 75% of experience must be actual teaching hours (group class, private lessons) as a "Head Trainer" or Instructor. Seventy-five hours or 25% of experience can be in other related areas such as working with shelter animals, assisting in classes, working as a veterinarian technician or grooming (bather position not applicable).
2. A high school diploma or equivalent.
3. One reference from each of the following:
   ◦ Veterinarian
   ◦ Client
   ◦ Colleague

4. Completion and filing of an Application for the Certification Examination for Pet Dog Trainers.
5. Signing and filing the CCPDT Code of Ethics.
6. Payment of required fee.
7. Successful completion of the CPDT examination.

CCPDT has recognized the importance of evaluating the hands-on skills of trainers. In 2011, they launched a practical assessment of a trainer's skills. A trainer who is already a CPDT-KA may be evaluated and tested on hands-on skills via video submission. If the candidate passes the hands-on practical assessment, he/she earns the title of Certified Professional Dog Trainer-Knowledge and Skills Assessed (CPDT-KSA).

The Society of Veterinary Behavior Technicians (SVBT) is a professional organization open to veterinary technicians, veterinary technician students, and the general public. SVBT's mission is to enrich human–animal interactions by promoting scientifically-based techniques of training, management, and behavior modification. SVBT (www.svbt.org) provides a forum for discussion and continuing education while working with allied professional organizations to strengthen the veterinary health care team. In 2008, the National Association of Veterinary Technicians in America (NAVTA), through the AVBT (www.avbt.net), recognized the specialty for veterinary technicians in animal behavior.

Credential requirements for AVBT include the following.

1. Graduate of an AVMA-approved Veterinary Technician program and/or credentialed to practice as a veterinary technician in some state or province of the United States, Canada, or other country.
2. Member of NAVTA and SVBT.
3. Three years (a minimum of 4000 h) work experience or its equivalent in the field of animal behavior, clinical, or research based. All experience must be completed within the last 5 years before application.
4. A minimum of 40 continuing education (CE) hours related to veterinary behavior, animal behavior, or behavioral research 5 years immediately before submitting the application.
5. Completion of the Veterinary Behavior Skills Form.
6. A case record log or research log maintained for 1 year within the 3 years immediately preceding the submission of the application.
7. Clinical – a minimum of 50 cases must be recorded or Research – one year within the 3 years immediately preceeding application must consist of behavior research or research using behavioral observations as a major portion of the study.
8. Five detailed case reports.
9. Two letters of recommendations from the following three categories: a VTS-Behavior member, a supporting Veterinarian or a DACVB.

The responsibilities of a VTS-Behavior are described in Box 1.2.

BOX 1.2: THE ROLE AND RESPONSIBILITIES OF A VTS-BEHAVIOR.

- Triage behavior concerns of clients, both in the clinic and on the phone, including determining when to refer to a Veterinary Behaviorist (i.e., prevention vs. intervention).
- Observe and triage behavior of animals in shelters, rescues, zoological parks, laboratories, and similar animal-related facilities, following procedures developed and approved by the veterinarian on record for that facility.
- Give management and safety advice to clients before their appointments.
- Take a history and perform a physical examination.
- Observe or assess behaviors in the context in which they are offered.
- Obtain samples and perform diagnostic testing.
- Discuss diagnostic procedures.
- Dispense prescribed medications.
- Discuss medication effects, side effects, and contraindications.
- Demonstrate a comprehensive understanding of operant and classical conditioning.
- Demonstrate a comprehensive understanding of behavior modification techniques.
- Assist the veterinarian during behavior consultations.
- Rehabilitate animals with problem behaviors in veterinary clinics, shelters, rescues, zoological parks, laboratories, and similar animal-related facilities, implementing procedures developed and prescribed by a veterinarian or veterinary behaviorist.
- Demonstrate good communication, rapport, and teaching ability with owners.
- Demonstrate a high level of expertise and understanding of scientifically-based positive reinforcement training methods.
- Create a positive and safe learning experience for the animal and owner.
- Execute hands-on training and behavior modification with the client, animal caretaker, or the animal after the diagnosis and recommended treatment of a behavior problem.
- Assist the client at the hospital or in-home visits to understand and implement the prescribed behavior modification and management techniques.
- Educate clients on products used to manage behavior cases.
- Teach owners to properly fit and condition patients with tools such as head collars and basket muzzles.
- Create criteria for client behavior logs.
- Be proficient in medical, behavioral, training, and research record keeping.
- Perform follow-up telephone calls, e-mail contacts, and home or hospital visits with clients as directed by the veterinarian.
- Implement changes to the treatment plan based on client feedback and consultation with the veterinarian.
- Present papers in seminars and workshops on normal behavior and problem prevention strategies to the public, clients, volunteers, staff members, and other veterinary technicians.
- Write professional scientific material for the veterinary public.
- Develop animal-behavior-related handouts for clients.
- Assist in behavior research.
- Condition animals to handling and husbandry practices common within the veterinary environment to create a more cooperative patient.
- Train veterinary staff in behavior protocols for that hospital, including scheduling, interacting with animal patients, and desensitizing patients to procedures.

- Educate clients about normal behavior and how to train their animal to be more comfortable during veterinary visits.
- Perform pet selection counseling.
- Perform problem prevention counseling.
- Counsel owners on common training techniques.
- Develop and implement programs of preventive behavior medicine. This includes creating, organizing, and updating handouts and staff training.
- Review current literature and behavioral information directed toward veterinary professionals and the general public.
- Evaluate and network with area animal trainers and other pet care professionals who provide supportive services.
- Create and teach puppy and kitten classes.
- Create and teach obedience classes for adult animals.
- Assist with behavior wellness appointments.
- Perform grief counseling.
- Promote and protect the human–animal bond.

Source: 2008 Academy of Veterinary Behavior Technician's Petition to the National Association of Veterinary Technicians of America, (Luescher et al., 2007).

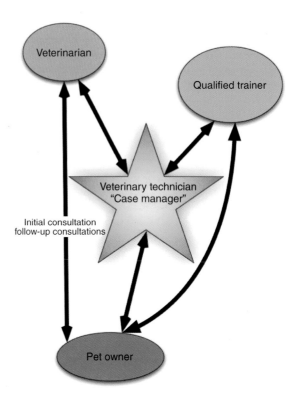

Figure 1.4 The technician's role as the "case manager" in veterinary behavior.

There are a variety of choices when looking for a dog trainer to complement veterinary behavior services. The credentials of an individual should not take the place of first-hand experience and interviewing potential training partners. When referring clientele to a trainer, clients will assume that the trainer's methodology is representative of the hospital.

- There are a variety of choices when looking for a dog trainer to complement veterinary behavior services. The credentials of an individual should not take the place of first-hand experience and interviewing potential training partners.

The role of the veterinary technician in the veterinary behavior consultation

The veterinary technician will have many roles in the veterinary behavior team. The technician will often first assess the situation and help determine the appropriate type of service needed. Not only will the behavior technician be able to triage the situation, but he/she will also assist with the clinical behavior consultation and may also act as the trainer for the hospital. Acting as the liaison for the client, trainer, and veterinarian, the veterinary behavior technician could be considered the "case manager", helping facilitate communication between all parties. Figure 1.4 shows a simple schematic of the role of the behavior technician as the "case manager."

Triaging the issues
Clients contacting the veterinary hospital are often unaware of the types of services available and necessary to address their pet's behavior. The veterinary staff or veterinary technician must triage the situation and determine whether a pet may be suffering from a possible medical/behavioral disorder, whether the situation is still in a preventative stage, or has progressed into a situation of behavior problem intervention (Figure 1.5). Medical as well as behavioral conditions may be factors that must be considered and evaluated prior to the appointment being scheduled with the appropriate personnel. Clients may contact the veterinary hospital requesting training for their pet, when in reality the pet is suffering from a behavioral disorder.

Figure 1.5 First puppy visit to the veterinary hospital. This puppy is exhibiting fear and not taking treats.

Determining whether the animal's behavior requires a veterinarian's diagnosis and attention is often a gray area that a veterinary technician must become adept at distinguishing by asking the client appropriate questions.

Generally, conditions will fall into one of two categories.

Medical and/or behavioral disorder (veterinary diagnosis required)

Medical conditions can cause or exacerbate behavioral issues and therefore must be ruled out. Any acute change in behavior should alert the veterinary technician to a primary medical disorder. Physical pain or malaise may increase irritability and contribute to anxiety, aggression, or elimination disorders. Changes in sensory perception will alter the pet's behavioral responses and social interactions. Pets with behavioral disorders in conjunction with medical disorders may present at any age. These cases must be promptly examined and evaluated by the veterinarian.

Case 1 A client calls about their cat, a 13-year old, male neutered orange tabby named Logan, who is urinating outside of the litter box. The problem could be medical, related to diabetes, kidney disease, a urinary tract infection, crystaluria or stones, and so on. The problem could be a behavioral disorder and ultimately given a diagnosis of urine marking, litter-box aversion- substrate aversion/preference or cognitive dysfunction. The patient should be seen by the veterinarian to determine the etiology and make a diagnosis.

Case 2 A client presents with their dog, a 10-month old, male intact Bull Mastiff named Rex, who has shown aggression when the owners have attempted to move him while resting. The comprehensive behavioral history limits aggression to one specific situation, moving him while resting. The dog is slow to rise and reluctant to go for walks off the property. Physical examination reveals pain and aggression with flexing and extending the coxofemoral joint. Radiographs suggest severe hip dysplasia. A veterinary diagnosis of pain-induced aggression is made. Concurrent behavioral and medical treatment is required.

Case 3 Duke is a 4-year old, male intact Boxer. The owners report they cannot trim Duke's nails and would like to be able to do so. Upon questioning the owners, the veterinary technician is told the owners have been bitten not only when trimming Duke's nails, but also when they have hugged him. Duke has growled at strangers as well.

Although the client's primary complaint is that they are unable to trim Duke's nails, his preliminary history indicates aggression with nail trimming and concurrent behavioral issues which should be addressed by the veterinarian. Because aggression has been displayed, a diagnosis by a veterinarian is required.

Case 4 Brie is a 2-year old female spayed Dalmatian. The owners would like tranquilizers for the fourth of July fireworks. The technician notices Brie is very frightened and trembling next to the owner. Upon questioning the owner, the owner reports this is Brie's usual reaction to leaving the house or toward anything "new." Brie also reportedly stares at the ceiling excessively, which could be an indication of a compulsive disorder. The technician advises that Brie's behavior and welfare could be improved through behavioral therapy with a veterinarian. A veterinary behavior consultation is recommended.

Situations in which it is unclear if the behavior is normal or abnormal, or there is a component of fear, anxiety, and/or aggression, require a veterinary diagnosis.

Prevention and training (no veterinary diagnosis required)

Some situations may not have progressed into a behavioral disorder and a veterinary technician may pre-empt the development of a behavior problem through appropriate preventive and training services. Situations may include prevention, lack of training, or conditioned unwanted behaviors.

Prevention

Prevention of behavior disorders is easier than treatment. Preventive situations most often will be with "new" puppies or kittens presenting to the veterinary hospital. Normal canine behavior and the prevention of behavioral problems should be discussed in puppy socialization classes and/or during puppy wellness visits (Figure 1.6). Kitten classes may focus on normal feline behavior and management, as well as the prevention of behavior problems.

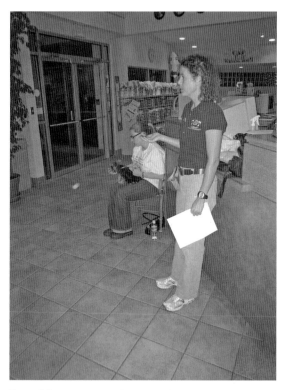

Figure 1.6 A veterinary technician conducting puppy socialization classes at the veterinary hospital.

Case 1 A client calls complaining that their 8-week old Chinese Lion Dog, better known as the *Shih Tzu*, named Mufasa, is biting the family. Is the behavior normal mouthing and biting that is commonly seen in puppies? Often owners call normal puppy mouthing "biting." The client reports that the puppy is growling and biting. His bites sometimes break the skin. Is this a fearful puppy or a lack of bite inhibition? The pet should be screened as to whether the behavior is normal puppy mouthing or abnormal behavior for a puppy. This may be accomplished through a puppy behavior wellness appointment or an in-hospital puppy socialization class. During puppy class, it can be determined if there are other areas of concern (such as guarding of resources) and a veterinary examination and diagnosis may be required.

Case 2 A 6-month old sheltie named "Cosmo" has attended puppy classes and is currently enrolled in the hospital's clicker-training classes. The owner reports Cosmo occasionally steals and chews household items (socks, paper towels, etc.). The behavior is not associated with owner departure and is not excessive. Cosmo does not show aggression in these contexts. Having Cosmo in both your puppy classes and clicker-training classes, you are familiar with him and it is obvious Cosmo is a stable and outgoing adolescent with no apparent anxiety issues. The client reports they are thrilled with Cosmo's behavior in all other aspects. Chewing is a normal behavior for adolescent dogs. The technician can recommend management, supervision, supplying a variety of appropriate chew toys, and teaching relinquishment of objects. The technician may also consider recommending a trainer to assist the client.

Lack of training or conditioned unwanted behaviors

Conditioned unwanted behaviors are behaviors that have been inadvertently reinforced by the owners and are problematic or undesirable. The behavior could be considered normal for the breed/species and not be considered excessive to the point of having a fear, aggression, anxiety, or hyperexcitability component. This is an emotionally stable pet that has not been taught cues related to good manners or presents for learned unwanted behaviors. One helpful technique is for the veterinary technician to ask the client to describe the pet's personality. This may prompt the client to express a fear or anxiety-related component. Even after elaborate questioning, one may still be unsure of the true etiology of the condition. Many dogs present during adolescence for training problems. A consistent protocol or informational handout should be followed for dealing with the specific problem. These pets may benefit from private, semiprivate, or group training lessons.

Case 1 A client informs you that their dog, a 9-month old, intact male Siberian Husky, named Bolt, needs training. Specifically, he runs away and does not come when called. You may be tempted to assume that based on the breed's genetic basis to run, that this is purely a training problem. But you do not have enough information. One must first determine the situation when Bolt runs away. Is he digging out of the yard or jumping the fence? The client reports when she opens the front door, Bolt dashes out running. Next, one must determine Bolt's motivation. Is he roaming because the neighbor's dog is in estrus? Does he want to chase things, such as small animals or children running? Does Bolt have any aggression issues (such as growling or excessive barking) with people at the door or passing the property? The client reports that Bolt is not chasing anything or anyone and has never met a person or dog he has not liked. He is very friendly. Finally, one must determine, what the client does when Bolt runs away. The client reports they chase him. His favorite game is "keep away" – he loves to be chased with a toy in his mouth. Now, after gathering a variety of information, one may assume Bolt's behavior is likely a training problem typical for the breed and related to previous learning experiences. Bolt has likely not been taught to wait at the door. Not coming when called and running away has been inadvertently conditioned by routinely being chased and playing "keep away." Private or group training sessions may be recommended to work on the training problem.

Case 2 Fang is a 6-month old, male, neutered, medium-sized mixed breed dog. The owner reports they cannot trim Fang's nails. The veterinary technician asks what Fang does when they attempt to trim his nails and the owner reports he tries to run away. The veterinary technician asks if he growls or attempts to bite the owner in these situations and the owner reports he does not; he "just wiggles." The veterinary technician asks if there are other situations such as brushing, touching body parts, or medicating

Fang that are also problematic. The owner reports, "We can do anything, but trim Fang's nails." The veterinary staff has not had difficulty handling Fang for medical treatments.

Because there is no aggression and the fear is mild and considered normal given the context and situation, the veterinary technician does not need a diagnosis from the veterinarian. Most dogs do not enjoy having their nails trimmed and mild fear/anxiety in this context is normal. The technician can instruct and demonstrate to the owner basic behavior modification techniques for desensitization to trimming nails. (see Chapters 7 and 8)

If the dog panicked to the point of losing bladder or bowel control or remains in a heightened state of arousal after being removed from the situation, then the fear and anxiety would be considered excessive and a veterinary behavior consultation should be recommended.

Table 1.2 summarizes how to determine whether the behavioral issue is associated with lack of training, preventative in nature, or intervention, and requires a veterinary diagnosis.

Box 1.3 provides a quick reference to common terminology and definitions.

BOX 1.3: COMMON DEFINITIONS.

Behavior problem: The animal's behavior is a problem for the owner. The issue could be lack of training, a conditioned unwanted behavior, a behavior disorder, or a combination of issues.

Behavior disorder: Psychological or behavioral patterns outside the behavioral norms for the species. Often there is an affective (emotional) component.

Behavioral assessment: An informal impression or evaluation of a situation; the first step in triaging a behavior problem or disorder.

Preventive care: Refers to measures taken to prevent the development of behavior problems or disorders, rather than treating the symptoms of an existing problem or disorder. Preventive care is a primary role for veterinary technicians.

Intervention care: Refers to measure taken to improve or alter an existing behavior disorder. Intervention requires a veterinary diagnosis and treatment plan.

Qualified trainer: An animal trainer who is certified from a standardized, positive-based curriculum and is policed by an organization in which certification can be revoked if the trainer acts unprofessionally or outside the organization's code of ethics.

Table 1.2 Triage.

Scenario	Comments	Veterinarian's DX?
The issue is still in "preventive" stages	See preventive definition	No diagnosis required
The behavioral issue is likely a lack of training issue or a conditioned unwanted behavior	Send to a qualified trainer (see definition)	No diagnosis required
The issue is very specific (handling feet) and the only issue. There has been no history of aggression or extreme fear. A mild fear response or avoidance is evident	Rare	No diagnosis required, but with more in-depth assessment, the handling issue may be a symptom of larger problem – then diagnosis required
There are multiple behavioral issues	Likely a complex situation and issues will need to be prioritized. Issues may be due to a general angst-based temperament	Diagnosis likely required
Multiple triggers or unknown triggers	Difficult to/impossible to manage	Diagnosis required
Issue is anxiety or fear based	Anxiolytic medication may be needed	Diagnosis required
Any history of aggression (growling, snapping, or biting not in the context of play)	Lack of bite inhibition increases risk	Diagnosis required
Any acute change in behavior	Rule out health issues	Diagnosis required
Geriatric patient with behavior changes	Rule out health issues, including cognitive dysfunction	Diagnosis required
Puppy 8 weeks of age showing aggression toward people (growling, snapping, biting not associated with normal puppy play mouthing)	Rule out health issues including neurological conditions, if behavioral usually genetic	Diagnosis required and counseling regarding the severity of the problem.
Behavior is uncharacteristically intense or out of context	Rule out health issues, possible abnormal brain chemistry or arousal issues	Diagnosis required

Prior to the consultation

The veterinary technician's responsibilities prior to the behavior consultation involve client communication tasks, office tasks including record keeping, and inventory management. Preappointment client communications may be the responsibility of the veterinary behavior technician or a trained receptionist. Providing awareness that there are viable treatment options for behavior disorders and educating clients about the difference between a training problem and a behavior disorder may be the first step in client communication. Preliminary information obtained should include the signalment (species, breed, color, sex, and age), medical problems, and behavioral issues. It is necessary to determine what prompted the call and what behavioral services are warranted (see sections titled **Triaging the issues** and **Qualified professionals to treat animal behavior disorders**). The expectations of the client should also be assessed. If the client makes an ultimatum, "If Fido growls at me one more time, he is out of here," attempting to educate the client briefly on normal canine communication and setting realistic goals for behavior intervention are important for the

client's overall satisfaction. A thorough description of the services available and what is involved, as well as the cost of the services should be understood by the client. If the pet owner is expecting the behavior issues to be "cured" in a 2-h consultation, he/she will be dissatisfied with the service and may be less likely to implement the treatment plan. When the client understands that the assessment will give the appropriate knowledge and tools to address the pet's behavior issues, he/she will be more accepting of the information and treatment plan. Informing the client that treatment options are available for their pet's behavioral issues, provides the client with some immediate relief. The client should be informed of any cancellation policies. Scheduling of the appointment may be done by the veterinary technician or a receptionist.

When any form of aggression is described by the client, the veterinary technician should advise the client to avoid triggers of aggression until the behavior disorder can be addressed through a behavior consultation. The client should also be advised to avoid punishment and manage the environment to avoid further learning of the undesired behaviors. This may include separating two dogs in the house that are fighting, avoid leaving the separation-anxiety dog alone, or blocking access to soiled areas for feline elimination disorders. The initial contact is usually a 10-15-min phone conversation. If an appointment is scheduled, requesting video footage of the pet and the problem behaviors, without eliciting aggression or endangering the pet or people, may be suggested to enhance the behavior consultation.

A detailed preliminary history should be obtained a few days prior to the appointment. The preliminary history phone conversation generally takes 15–20 min. The appointment date, time, and home address should be verified. The preliminary history should include questions regarding general management, current medications (including heartworm and flea preventives), the pet's disposition, and historical information such as the age the pet was obtained and source from which the pet was obtained. The primary undesirable behaviors should be identified and ranked in order of importance to the owner. A brief general description of the behavior should include the antecedent, the behavior, and the consequence or outcome of the behavior. The context of the behavior, including the individuals present, the location, the owner's reaction, and the pet's reaction, should be obtained.

The history form may be emailed, faxed, or mailed to the client and returned prior to the appointment. Allowing the client to complete the form decreases staff time and may facilitate multiple family members' input. While obtaining the preliminary history over the phone is more time consuming, a trained behavior technician may detect subtle indicators of other underlying behavior disorders prompting further questioning or family dysfunctions that may influence the diagnosis and treatment. For example, if the client says, "Fifi doesn't like my husband," the behavior technician would investigate this statement further. The veterinary technician may ask, "What does Fifi do that makes you say that?"

Informing the client of safety precautions for the appointment and client preparation prior to the appointment (video footage, training tools, treats, etc.) are communication tasks performed by the veterinary technician. For home behavior consultations when aggression toward strangers entering the home is identified, the client should be instructed to place the pet in a safe contained area to prevent injury to veterinary staff entering the home. If other pets live in the home, inquire about their reactivity to strangers. This helps to protect the veterinary staff. Similarly, with clinic consultations, if reactivity to other animals or people is an issue, the pet should be managed upon arrival

to the veterinary hospital to prevent an incident. This may include managing the pet outside the building or in the car until the pet can be safely escorted into the consultation room.

The pet should be hungry for the consultation. Advise the client to withhold food for 6–12 h prior to the appointment. The client should bring video footage, training collars or training devices used, the pet's favorite treats and toy, and routine medications to the consultation.

With clinic consultations the veterinarian will not be able to observe the pet in its natural environment; video footage allows evaluation of interactions with household members and other pets (Figure 1.7). Once the appointment has been scheduled, the veterinary technician should impress upon the client the importance of video footage. Resting, feeding, drinking, and exercising areas should be included in the video.

The veterinary technician is responsible for making sure the patient file and pertinent forms are prepared prior to the appointment. This provides for a smooth and efficient consultation. If the consultation is taking place within the veterinary hospital, training tools, treats, and toys should be readily accessible to the staff but out of reach of the pet. Stocking the room prevents unnecessary interruptions during the behavior appointment. Examples of such items, depending on the case, would be a variety of clickers, toys and treats, appropriate-size head halters, harnesses and basket muzzles, sound desensitization compact discs, leashes, and training books.

Any interruption may be upsetting to the patient and distracting to the client. Staff members should be

Figure 1.7 Dog interacting with feline companion in the home environment. When not providing in-home consultations, video footage is helpful in assessing the dynamics of the household.

settled in the examination room before the patient enters. Phones and pagers should be turned off prior to entering the consultation room. A sign should be placed on the outside of the consultation door notifying staff that a behavior consultation is in progress, to prevent accidental interruption. The ideal architectural design for a behavior consultation room would allow the client and pet to enter directly into the room from outside of the building. A large room with couches and no visual obstruction between the veterinarian and the clients is ideal. The staff would have a separate interior entrance to the room. Safety precautions, such as a stable tether system, should also be implemented in the behavior consultation room.

When providing home behavior consultations, the vehicle should be stocked appropriately. Similarly, a laptop computer, power charger, charged cell phone, printer, ink and paper, directions to the home, the patient file and preliminary history should all be packed into the vehicle. Inventory of behavior training tools should be assessed at least weekly, especially on items that are commonly recommended or size specific (basket muzzles, head halters).

During the consultation

The veterinary technician's responsibilities during the consultation involve working directly with the patient whenever possible, as well as assisting the client with the implementation of the treatment plan as outlined by the veterinarian. During the behavior consultation, ideally the veterinary technician should

1. offer nonthreatening body language and treats while waiting for the pet to approach and become comfortable with veterinary technician interaction,
2. assess the pet's trainability and interest in a variety of rewards (assorted treats and toys),
3. assess the pet's current level of reliability with cued behaviors required for implementation of the treatment plan (sit, stay, come, go to mat, loose leash walking),
4. introduce the pet to training tools needed to implement the treatment plan (Figure 1.8),
5. convey to the veterinarian the pet's responsiveness and reaction to training and the training tools,
6. demonstrate and explain training methods and training tools required for implementing the treatment plan,
7. encourage and give positive feedback to clients regarding their skills while utilizing the training tools (i.e., clicker, head halter) and performing the behavior modification exercises,

Figure 1.8 Desensitization and classical counter conditioning to a basket muzzle, using canned cheese.

8. clarify and problem-solve with the client to integrate the treatment plan into their lifestyle,
9. answer any questions the client may have regarding the diagnosis, prognosis, or treatment plan and refer questions to the veterinarian as needed, and
10. provide the client with resources for recommended training supplies or tools, when applicable.

The veterinarian will complete the history and temperament evaluation, make a diagnosis and prognosis, and outline a treatment plan. While the veterinarian is interviewing the client, the veterinary technician should interact with the pet in a nonthreatening manner. This includes letting the pet approach on its own, avoiding prolonged eye contact, facing sideways to the pet, and avoid reaching toward the pet. The client and other members involved in the consultation should ignore the pet. This will make the veterinary technician the only person that "pays off". The veterinary technician may toss a variety of small tasty treats in an underhand manner toward the pet.

> • While the veterinarian is interviewing the client, the veterinary technician should interact with the pet in a nonthreatening manner. This includes letting the pet approach on its own, avoiding prolonged eye contact, facing sideways to the pet, and avoid reaching toward the pet.

Once the pet is comfortably interacting with the veterinary technician, the veterinary technician may begin to assess the trainability of the pet. Some pets will warm up immediately and others may never feel comfortable enough to eat a treat throughout the entire consultation. It is important for the veterinary technician to wait until the pet is relaxed with the interactions before prompting or asking the pet to perform a behavior such as sit. Otherwise, the veterinary technician risks making the pet wary. For example, imagine meeting an unfamiliar person for the first time. As long as that person does not immediately ask something of us and is nonthreatening, we are more likely to be comfortable with the interaction.

The pet's comfort level with handling and tendency toward guarding objects and/or food will be assessed in the temperament evaluation. This is important when considering placing a head collar and utilizing treats and toys. Although the pet's body language determines how the veterinary technician will proceed, it is good to know beforehand if the pet has any known triggers, such as a sensitive area, or shows a tendency to guard food or toys. For example, a Golden Retriever presents for destructive behavior when left at home alone. The temperament evaluation reveals previous aggression when touched around the ears. This invaluable information may not be immediately offered by the client because it is not a presenting complaint. The veterinary technician should wait until the temperament evaluation is completed by the veterinarian prior to desensitizing to a head halter, harness, muzzle or introducing toys. This increases safety with handling of the patient. Toys should be on a rope or tether when introduced to the pet. This provides a non-confrontational way for the veterinary technician to retrieve the toy.

> - Although the pet's body language determines how the veterinary technician will proceed, it is good to know beforehand if the pet has any known triggers, such as a sensitive area, or shows a tendency to guard food or toys.

The veterinary technician may introduce training tools (e.g., clicker, head collar, muzzle) (see Chapter 8) and training cues needed for behavior modification exercises (e.g., sit, stay, go to a mat, loose leash walking) to the pet while the veterinarian describes the diagnosis and treatment plan. Whenever possible, the veterinary technician should take the canine patient for a walk to assess reactivity to environmental factors and temperament away from the owner. This will determine whether the owner will be capable of walking the dog and if undesirable behaviors have been inadvertently conditioned by the owner. For example, some dogs are

only reactive to other dogs while with their owner. The technician may also observe defensive or fearful behaviors that can be reported to the veterinarian. The technician may notice the dog stop taking treats, which is likely a sign of anxiety. The walk also allows the veterinary technician to assess the dog's reaction to a head collar, if applicable. The veterinary technician's insight should be conveyed to the veterinarian during the consultation.

While the veterinarian prepares the written behavior assessment summary and treatment plan, the veterinary technician should explain and demonstrate any training tools or skills required in implementing the treatment plan. This should include how to teach the pet appropriate behavior responses and their importance with regard to the treatment of the behavioral disorder. The client is more likely to comply with the treatment plan when he/she understands the significance of the exercises. Specific behavior modification exercises and desensitization to training tools should be demonstrated. The client should be provided an opportunity to practice some of the exercises with assistance and positive feedback from the veterinary technician (Figure 1.9). While observing the client's training skills, the veterinary technician may foresee potential training problems and provide insight to remediate those problems. During this time the veterinary technician should also accompany the client and dog on a walk. Not only will the veterinary technician be able to observe the dog's behavior with the client, but the veterinary technician may also assess the client's leash and handling skills. Behavior modification techniques used on walks should be demonstrated by the behavior technician. Client questions regarding the diagnosis, prognosis, and treatment plan may be

Figure 1.9 Technician coaching client on behavior modification exercises with a reactive dog.

answered by the veterinary technician or referred back to the veterinarian for clarification.

> • The client is more likely to comply with the treatment plan when he/she understands the significance of the exercises.

The veterinary behavior technician will need to develop communication skills to assist the client without putting the client on the defensive (see Chapter 5). For example, the veterinary technician observes a dog that reluctantly returns to the client when called. If the veterinary technician says, "Fido doesn't look happy when he comes to you, because he thinks you are going to punish him," the client is likely to take the comment personally and feel less competent as a trainer. Instead, the veterinary technician might say, "That is great, that Fido came when you called him. The next step in his training will be . . . ." The veterinary technician would suggest a few things to make Fido's recall enjoyable and provide the handler with tips regarding nonthreatening body language. This acknowledges the success of the client's previous training with the dog; the dog did come when called. The client is now in an open frame of mind for the "next step" to teaching the recall.

When the patient is a cat, bird, or an extremely fearful and/or aggressive dog, the veterinary technician may be more limited in the amount of interactions with the patient. Birds may be wary of new people and are less likely to be amendable to interacting with a stranger. Similarly, some cats will avoid interactions with new people or will lose interest in treats and toys quickly. Some dogs will not be comfortable enough to interact with the veterinary technician even after a sustained period of time. There will also be some canine patients that are too aggressive for the veterinary technician to handle directly. The veterinary technician will need to rely on his/her ability to explain and demonstrate implementation of the treatment plan without the pet. Coaching the client regarding problem solving and training is an important role of the veterinary technician in these cases.

> • When the patient is a cat, bird, or an extremely fearful and/or aggressive dog, the veterinary technician may be more limited in the amount of interactions with the patient.

The flow of the behavior consultation is shown in Box 1.4.

BOX 1.4: BEHAVIOR CONSULTATION FLOW CHART (DURING THE CONSULTATION).

- Appropriate safety measures in place prior to appointment or on presentation to the veterinary hospital.
- Introductions and assessment of environment (video or directly).
  - Technician may be offering the pet treats.
- History and temperament evaluation:
  - Veterinarian: summarizes the presenting complaints and obtains the temperament evaluation and completes the history.
  - Technician: offers nonthreatening body language and treats while waiting for the pet to approach and become comfortable with interaction.
- Diagnosis, prognosis, and treatment plan
  - Veterinarian: explains the diagnosis (diagnoses), prognosis, and treatment plan.
  - Technician
    - assesses the pet's trainability and interest in a variety of rewards (assorted treats and toys),
    - assesses the pet's current level of reliability with behaviors required for implementation of the treatment plan (sit, stay, come, go to mat, loose leash walking),
    - introduces the pet to training tools needed to facilitate the treatment plan,
    - takes the dog for a walk,
    - conveys to the veterinarian the pet's response and reaction to training and the training tools.
- Training plan demonstration and implementation
  - Veterinarian: prepares the written behavior assessment summary and treatment plan.
  - Technician
    - demonstrates and explains training methods and training tools required for implementing the treatment plan,
    - encourages the client and offers positive feedback while the client practices using the training tools (e.g., clicker, head halter) and during behavior modification exercises,
    - clarifies and problem-solves implementation of the treatment plan with the client,
    - answers any questions the client may have regarding the diagnosis, prognosis, or treatment plan or refers to the veterinarian, and
    - provides the client with resources for recommended training supplies or tools, if applicable.

- Conclusion of appointment:
  - Veterinarian
    - reads through written behavior assessment summary and treatment plan and obtains signature for medical record,
    - prescribes medication (when applicable) and explains possible side effects,
    - explains follow-up recommendations (written into the behavior summary), and
    - answers client's questions.
  - Technician
    - conveys any pertinent information revealed during the training exercises that may affect the treatment plan,
    - asks veterinarian's opinion on questions presented by client during training, if applicable,
    - relays to the veterinarian a summary of the training and behavior modification exercises performed.

After the consultation: follow-up care

The role of the veterinary technician regarding follow-up care is to provide continued support for the client and promote fluent communication. Clarification of the treatment plan and evaluation of the human–animal bond should be determined at each contact. The veterinary technician can evaluate through home visits, phone contacts, emails, or video tapes, the implementation of training and behavior modification exercises. Answering questions regarding the treatment plan, prescribed medications, training, and behavior modification may also be addressed by the veterinary technician.

- The role of the veterinary technician regarding follow-up care is to provide continued support for the client and promote fluent communication.

When the pet shows no signs of improvement, worsening of the behavior, or a new undesirable behavior, the veterinarian should be informed and assess whether changes in the treatment plan are necessary. With the veterinary technician's insight, the veterinarian may make changes to the treatment plan. Only a veterinarian can change the treatment plan, including changing prescribed medications or medication dosages. When improper implementation of the behavior modification

is suspected, a behavior modification appointment with the veterinary technician may be suggested. The veterinarian may determine that a follow-up behavior consultation is required to reevaluate the pet.

- Only a veterinarian can change the treatment plan, including changing prescribed medications or medication dosages.

If new problem behaviors, which were not addressed in the consultation, arise, then another behavior consultation with the veterinarian would be necessary. For example, Herman, a 5-year old, neutered male Himalayan, was seen for urinating and defecating daily on the floor next to the litter box. The veterinarian diagnosed feline inappropriate elimination with a litter-box aversion. Litter-box factors were changed and environmental and behavior modifications were implemented. Herman's behavior was significantly improved and he was found to only eliminates inappropriately when the owner is negligent about cleaning the litter boxes. After several months, the client reports that Herman is having a relapse. Further questioning reveals that Herman is now urinating on the owner's bed, bathroom rug, and the new kitten's bed. It is only urine, never stool. Not only should this warrant a thorough medical workup to evaluate Herman's urinary tract health, but it should also be recognized that this is an entirely different behavior disorder. This warrants another behavior consultation with the veterinarian because the behavior is likely anxiety-related urine marking. Although the initial complaint is the same, the cat is not always using the litter box; the description of the behavior is different.

A set protocol for follow-up care should be determined by the veterinarian and documented in the treatment plan. Follow-ups may be performed by the veterinary behavior technician. The suggested minimum follow-up care should occur 1 and 3 weeks post the initial behavior consultation. Follow-up may be either by telephone/email or in clinic with or without the pet. The 1-week follow-up centers around answering questions regarding the treatment plan. If medication was prescribed, the veterinary technician should ask the client if the pet has been started on the medication. It should not be assumed that the prescribed medication is being administered or given appropriately. Confirm the dosage and frequency of the medication. The client should be questioned regarding side effects of the medication. During the 1-week follow-up, determine which parts of the treatment plan the client has begun to implement. The 3-week follow-up includes verifying implementation of the treatment plan; discussing medication, if applicable; assessing the frequency and intensity of the behavior disorders; and determining the client's satisfaction level with the pet's behavior. Updates should be provided to the veterinarian and the treatment plan modified as directed. When providing in-clinic follow-up, avoid mistaking the follow-up assessment with a behavior modification appointment. If the client requires further assistance with training or behavior modification, an appointment should be scheduled with appropriate personnel. Ideally, this person may be a veterinary behavior technician or a dog trainer who is knowledgeable about implementation of behavior modification techniques.

• It should not be assumed that the prescribed medication is being administered or given appropriately.

After 3 weeks, continued follow-up care should be tailored to the case. Any changes to the treatment plan should be reevaluated 2–3 weeks post implementation. If no changes to the treatment plan are made and the client is satisfied with the pet's progress, reassessment should be rendered in an additional 1 month (approximately 2 months following the initial consultation). The 3-month follow-up may be either a phone- or in-clinic assessment. In-person follow-up appointments should be required every 6 months to yearly in order to continue providing behavioral assistance. The majority of veterinary computer software programs support phone and appointment reminder systems. This makes follow-up care easier to implement. Routine follow-up care initiated by the veterinary staff provides for continued guidance and support from the veterinary team, thereby facilitating and enhancing the human–animal bond.

The veterinary technician's roles encompass client communication, including education, awareness and prevention before, during, and after the consultation, as well as assisting the veterinarian with the clinical behavior consultation. Utilization of the veterinary technician provides for a more comprehensive and successful behavior service for the hospital and the client/patient.

• The veterinary technician's roles encompass client communication, including education, awareness and prevention before, during, and after the consultation, as well as assisting the veterinarian with the clinical behavior consultation.

Summary of the roles of the veterinarian, veterinary technician, and dog trainer in veterinary behavior

Table 1.1 summarizes the roles of the veterinarian, veterinary technician, and dog trainer in the veterinary behavior team. Although many of the tasks may overlap, there are clearly defined roles that are exclusive to the veterinarian because they involve the practice of veterinary medicine.

Home versus clinic behavior consultations

Offering in-home or in-clinic veterinary behavior consultations to clients can be a service added to a general practice or the sole focus of a veterinary practice. Behavior consultations in the home can provide additional insight that may affect the diagnosis and treatment plan. Perhaps a combination of in-clinic and in-home behavioral services could be offered in order to balance the advantages and disadvantages of each service.

Pros and cons of the home behavior consultation versus the clinic behavior consultation

Providing home veterinary behavior consultations have some distinct advantages and disadvantages compared to clinic behavior consultations. With the home consultation, the pet and client are in their natural environment. This increases the likelihood that the pet will exhibit typical characteristic behaviors. It is easier for the entire household to attend the in-home consultation. This may lead to better compliance and will definitely allow for better insight. By observing the home environment, management problems and environmental stressors may be more easily identified. Home consultations also allow the veterinarian and veterinary technician to observe the human social relationships and dynamics within the household. Another distinct advantage to the home consultation is direct application of behavior and environmental modification to the home setting. Home visits increase the perceived value of the service to the client. It adds a personal touch because the veterinarian and veterinary technician have spent time in the home with the client and the pet. During home consultations, the veterinarian is less likely to be interrupted by ancillary hospital staff, yet the client may have personal distractions. Home visits may be less stressful for the client and the pet. If the veterinary service is dedicated solely to treating behavior problems, providing in-home consultations eliminates operating costs associated with a building and additional personnel (Figure 1.10).

The main disadvantage of home behavior consultations is the risk of injury to staff members. It is an unknown environment and therefore safety is a major concern. Often the patient is more offensive, more protective, and has a lengthy learning history in the home environment, making aggression more prone to occur. The veterinary technician will be expected to take dogs for brief walks during the consultation. Unfamiliarity with the neighborhood, neighborhood pets, and the dog can be potential safety issues. There is risk of injury to the dog and veterinary technician due to stray dogs. Attempting to implement as many safety precautions and protocols as possible will help prevent dangerous situations. The clinic behavior consultation allows for existing safety measures and familiarity with the setting (Figures 1.11 and 1.12).

Home visits require travel time and may take longer than in-clinic consultations. This may be due to the social nature of the home appointment setting. See Tables 1.3 and 1.4 for average time commitments related to the home versus clinic behavior consultation.

Home behavior consultations typically require follow-up to be facilitated by phone or email. Ideally, an in-person follow-up would be performed 3–4 weeks following the initial consultation. This may not be financially feasible due to travel time. Private behavior modification appointments may be recommended for continued follow-up. In-clinic follow-up, training, and behavior modification appointments may be more cost- and time effective for the veterinary staff. A general

Figure 1.10 Patient evaluated in the home setting for aggression toward family members and strangers entering the home.

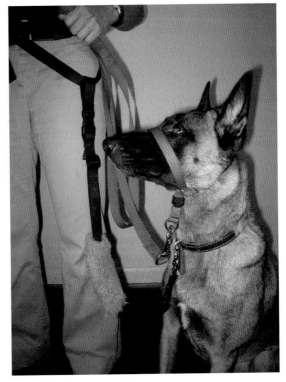

Figure 1.11 Dual leash method, with one leash attached to the head collar and waist leash attached to flat buckle collar. This adds safety and security with reactive dogs.

Figure 1.12 Coupler attaching head collar to flat buckle collar. This adds security should one device fail with reactivity.

Table 1.3 Home behavior consultations.

Initial contact phone call	10–15 min
Preliminary history	15–20 min
Appointment preparation	10 min
Travel time (varies)	30–60 min
Consultation	2–2.5 h
Fax/Call RDVM[a] (if applicable)	5–10 min
Follow-up contact	30–60 min
Total time	4–6.5 h

[a] Referring DVM.

Table 1.4 Clinic behavior consultations.

Initial call	10–15 min
Preliminary history	15–20 min
Appointment preparation	5 min
Appointment	1.75–2.25 h
Fax/Call RDVM[a] (if applicable)	5–10 min
Follow-up contact	30–60 min
Total time	2.8–4 h

[a] Referring DVM.

practice that is offering home behavior consultations may have the capability to perform follow-up appointments and behavior modification appointments in the clinic.

Veterinary-technician-driven behavior services

Besides assisting with behavior consultation, the behavior technician may also provide a variety

of other behavior services. Potential veterinary technician-instigated behavior services include behavior modification appointments, puppy socialization classes, kitten classes, pet selection counseling, new puppy/kitten appointments, basic manners/training classes, head collar fitting, behavior wellness visits, avian classes, and staff and client seminars. Many of these services will be covered in more detail in Chapter 7.

> - Besides assisting with behavior consultation, the behavior technician may also provide a variety of other behavior services.

Behavior modification appointments

Behavior modification appointments assist clients with the implementation of the veterinarian-prescribed treatment plan. Behavior modification appointments should last less than 1 h. The pet will require scheduled training breaks throughout the appointment; these breaks allow for discussion with the client. Appointments may occur in the hospital setting or at the pet's home. Behavior modification appointments performed in the home allow for further insight and implementation of the treatment plan in the pet's natural environment. This may be beneficial, especially if the initial consultation was performed in the hospital. In contrast, when applying behavior modification for fear at the veterinary hospital, the hospital is the preferred choice unless a nonstressful starting point in the hospital setting is not identified (see Desensitization, Chapter 8).

The same safety and preappointment measures implemented during the consultation should be applied to behavior modification appointments. Review the temperament evaluation prior to the appointment to determine if the pet has a history of guarding objects or food from people.

> - The same safety and preappointment measures implemented during the consultation should be applied to behavior modification appointments.

The first part of the appointment is discussion with the client regarding the status of the pet's progress. What parts of the treatment plan have they implemented? What problems have they encountered? The client should demonstrate the behavior modification exercises with the pet. While the pet is given something enjoyable to do, the veterinary technician can give feedback to the client. Always offer verbal encouragement regarding two or three things the client did well, then discuss alternatives for problem areas. Make it a joint effort, demonstrate for the client, and then allow the client to practice. The conclusion of the appointment should review the major topics covered, present realistic expectations for progression, and set a date for follow-up communication. Detailed notes should be recorded in the patient's file regarding the behavior modification appointment. The veterinarian should be provided with a status update, allowing for any necessary adjustments to the treatment plan.

Semiprivate behavior modification classes are another option. Dogs that are reactive with other dogs may benefit from "reactive" group dog classes. Careful management and safety are imperative with these classes. Dogs may be required to wear a basket muzzle throughout the class in order to minimize risk associated with handler error. Classes may be formatted in a variety of different ways. One option is to allow only one dog each week to attend the session. All the owners benefit from observing the behavior modification in practice. A volunteer decoy dog or stuffed animal may be used, depending on the dog's reactivity and the client's ability to safely handle their dog. Pets that demonstrate other behavioral disorders, such as fear and aggression at the veterinary hospital, may also benefit from semiprivate classes at the veterinary hospital focusing on behavior modification techniques. Semiprivate classes may be more cost effective than private lessons. Clients learn by observing implementation of behavior modification with other dogs. Similarly, the client is also provided with a network of people with pets presented for similar behavior disorders.

Because behavior modification appointments require specialized training and knowledge, appropriate charges should apply. An additional fee should be assessed when traveling to the client's home. Travel fees may be a variable or fixed rate, based on mileage or travel time. The travel radius should be predetermined.

- Because behavior modification appointments require specialized training and knowledge, appropriate charges should apply.

Puppy socialization classes

Poor socialization or deprivation of environmental exposure often leads to lifelong deficits and dysfunctional behaviors. Lack of positive exposure is as detrimental as a bad experience. The socialization period is a finite period of development in which the dog is genetically programmed to be more accepting of novelty. Puppy socialization classes help to provide immunity against behavior disorders (Figure 1.13).

The benefits to offering puppy socialization classes in the veterinary hospital include bonding the client to the puppy and veterinary hospital, educating the client on normal canine behavior, addressing common puppy-training issues, and providing a controlled and safe environment for play. Puppy socialization classes also help prevent behavior disorders such as inter-dog aggression, separation anxiety, and fear disorders related to lack of socialization. Teaching puppies to enjoy restraint and handling will make the veterinary staff's job easier. Puppy classes also help identify problem puppies or high-risk puppies for the development of future behavior disorders. They are intended for behaviorally normal puppies and are not designed to address abnormal behaviors. The focus of puppy class is on education and prevention. Puppy socialization classes are the number one preventive behavior service a veterinary hospital can offer its clients. Puppy classes can be started with minimal work and capital investment. Instructing and assisting puppy socialization classes can be extremely enjoyable and rewarding for the veterinary technician. Puppy socialization classes are discussed in more detail in Chapter 7.

Figure 1.13 Exploration and desensitization to the veterinary hospital and staff using treats.

- Puppy socialization classes are the number one preventive behavior service a veterinary hospital can offer its clients.

- Pet selection counseling is the first defense in the prevention of behavior disorders.

Kitten classes

Kitten classes are similar to puppy socialization classes, but because most kittens are out of their socialization period (feline socialization period is 2–7 weeks of age) by the time they are obtained, there are some distinct differences. Rather than focusing on socialization, kitten classes focus on normal feline behavior and the prevention of behavior disorders. They allow for positive exposure to the veterinary hospital, desensitization to handling, and controlled exploration, thereby bonding the client to the kitten and veterinary hospital. Understanding why cats perform certain behaviors fosters client empathy for the cat. Kitten classes provide the client with the knowledge necessary to modify unwanted behaviors. Responsible cat ownership with regard to allowing the cat outdoor versus indoor, environmental enrichment, and minimizing stress in multicat households should be addressed. Kitten classes identify and prevent behavior disorders, teach appropriate owner play, address litter-box factors, bite and claw inhibition, handling, and carrier/kennel training. Often, basic cue training such as sit, come, touch, and place are taught, using positive reinforcement training.

Pet selection counseling

Pet selection counseling is the first defense in the prevention of behavior disorders. The goals of pet selection counseling are to educate the client about normal canine behavior and breed selection, prepare the client for the new arrival, promote positive reinforcement training, and promote hospital services. If the pet does not meet the client's expectations or is a mismatch to the client's personality or lifestyle, it is unlikely to be retained. Offering prepurchasing counseling is a way to educate clients prior to their pet's first veterinary visit. This service should be promoted through client mailings, newsletters, email, telephone correspondence, and the hospital bulletin board. Because pet selection counseling is time consuming, hospitals should charge appropriately for technician/staff time. Pet selection counseling appointments can be a valuable service, enhancing the human–animal bond, as well as the client–veterinary–hospital bond.

New puppy/kitten appointments

The first veterinary hospital visit for puppies and kittens sets the trend for future visits. This can be problematic when the first visit is not enjoyable for the pet. A bad experience potentiates fear or aggression with future visits to the veterinary hospital. Ideally, for all wellness visits, clients should be encouraged to bring a hungry pet and a variety of high-value treats such as string cheese, canned cheese, peanut butter, and small pieces of hotdog. The client should be informed to offer the pet a treat in the parking lot, upon entering the hospital, in the waiting room, and in the exam room. If the puppy/kitten fails to acclimate during the first visit, reschedule the appointment and delay vaccination until the pet is comfortable and taking treats. The goal is for the pet to associate the veterinary hospital with good things (food). Consequently, regardless of the pet's actions, the pet should be offered treats. Scheduling of all new puppy/kitten visits as an extended appointment allows the pet to become acclimatized to the hospital/staff and allows for time to cover specific behavioral topics.

- The first veterinary hospital visit for puppies and kittens sets the trend for future visits.

Veterinary technicians play a critical role in educating clients and staff members about the prevention of behavioral disorders and training problems. Prevention is the most important step in the treatment of behavior. Preventative measures include educating clients about what is normal behavior for the particular breed or species. With each additional wellness visit, specific behavior topics should be covered. Behavioral topics for puppy visits should include socialization, body language, house training, teaching bite inhibition, and methodology for basic training and problem solving. Behavioral topics for kitten visits should include teaching bite and claw inhibition, litter-box training and management, handling, and carrier training. The importance of veterinary behavioral services such as puppy socialization classes and kitten classes should be stressed to the client. These topics or services may be additionally covered in instructional handouts. Receptionists should be trained to discuss behavioral services regarding preventive medicine over the telephone when scheduling appointments.

> • Veterinary technicians play a critical role in educating clients and staff members about the prevention of behavioral disorders and training problems.

Basic manners/training classes

Basic manners/training classes should focus on foundation behaviors for all young dogs and puppies. Foundation behaviors may include targeting, attention, position changes (sit, down), settle or go to a place, coming when called, and loose leash walking. Ideally, this class should follow the completion of a puppy socialization class. Classes may be group, semiprivate, or private, depending on the facility. Training should utilize positive reinforcement. Offering more advanced classes may also be incorporated. For more information on curriculum development and class formats, see Chapter 7.

Head collar fitting

Many clients and dogs presenting to the veterinary hospital will benefit from the proper fit and usage of head collars. When head collars are fitted improperly, they are likely to be rejected by the dog and may cause physical abrasion. Head collars offer clients control of their dog and facilitate humane leash walking. This increases the likelihood that clients will exercise their pet, benefiting the pet mentally and physically. Head collars are often a necessity for reactive dogs. The behavior veterinary technician should be utilized when offering this service. A specific appointment should be scheduled for a head collar fitting. The hospital should be compensated for the veterinary technician's time and knowledge when educating about head collar use (see Chapter 7).

Behavior wellness visits

Although information regarding animal behavior should be solicited during every veterinary visit, pet behavioral wellness appointments are a specific appointment to identify and prevent potential behavioral disorders and training problems. This routine appointment should be scheduled with the veterinary behavior technician. The ideal time to identify behavior and training issues is during the juvenile and adolescent periods. The onset of behavior and training problems is typically prior to social maturity. In dogs, this is prior to 2–3 years of age.

A behavioral wellness visit should also be scheduled for senior pets. Dogs are typically considered senior by an average of 7 years of age, compared to cats between 10 and 12 years of age. Senior pets should be screened for cognitive dysfunction syndrome. The format of the appointment may be conversational and/or a questionnaire.

The longer the duration of the behavioral disorder or learning history for training problems, the more difficult it is to rectify. Behavior wellness visits focus on identifying and preventing problem behaviors and training issues. Veterinary behavioral consultation services or referral to a veterinary behaviorist may be necessary, depending on the disorders or problems identified.

> • The longer the duration of the behavioral disorder or learning history for training problems, the more difficult it is to rectify.

Avian classes

In a hospital that provides care to birds, the veterinary behavior technician may consider providing avian classes. Classes may be in a lecture format, discussing management and enrichment recommendations for parrots or hands-on, providing training directly with the birds and clients. Birds should be free of contagious diseases and recently examined by a veterinarian prior to attending classes. Setting specific guidelines for health prerequisites may be determined by the veterinarian–veterinary technician team.

Staff and client seminars

The veterinary behavior team not only has the responsibility of educating the public, but also the veterinary staff, including receptionists, veterinary assistants, kennel assistants, veterinarians, technicians, and the grooming staff. Providing staff members with behavior training through staff seminars ensures that the entire veterinary team is providing and promoting consistent behavior information. Contradictory information will confuse the client and may be detrimental to the human–animal, as well as the client–hospital bond. New team members should be provided immediate education on hospital policies regarding animal behavior. At least biannual seminars to refresh and strengthen the entire team's behavior knowledge are recommended. Information provided should be well documented and not merely based on personal experience.

- Providing staff members with behavior training through staff seminars ensures that the entire veterinary team is providing and promoting consistent behavior information.

Similarly, providing the hospital's clientele with monthly seminars on a variety of behavior topics is an added service the behavior technician may implement. Examples of topics include problem prevention, body language, normal development and behavior, safety with children and pets, and avian management and husbandry. Charging clients a fee for attendance is appropriate.

Financial benefits

Behavior services not only generate additional revenue to the hospital with the addition of behavioral services, but they also assist in maintaining and enhancing the human–animal and client–hospital bond. The direct financial benefits are realized through the income produced by behavioral services. However, indirect financial benefits are equally as profound and are associated with an increase in pet retention, client referrals, veterinary visits, and a decrease in required staff assistance and examination time.

Behavioral issues have been estimated to result in 15% of pets being relinquished, rehomed, or euthanized each year (Tremayne, 2005). Even a 5% loss of a veterinary hospital's patients has a profound impact on revenue.

For example, consider the following.
- A hospital with 2500 active patients.
- An annual loss of 5% results in 125 patients.
- The average annual veterinary expenses for a pet in 2011 was $505. (From AP poll, November 2011. http://ap-gfkpoll.com/uncategorized/ap-petside-com-poll-8-in-10-pet-owners-visited-vet-in-last-year)
- Total annual loss $63,125 (125 patients × $505).
- A 10% loss would be $126,250 (250 patients × $505).
- A 15% loss would be $189,375 (375 patients × $505).

Preventive behavior services and early intervention are likely to increase pet retention and decrease financial loss due to unresolved behavioral concerns. When the human–animal bond is weakened due to behavior issues, pet owners are less likely to seek veterinary care and follow veterinary recommendations (Lue *et al.*, 2008).

Through the implementation of compassionate care that integrates low stress interactions, handling, and restraint, veterinary patients will have a more pleasant experience at the veterinary hospital. Owners, whose pets enjoy coming to the hospital, will visit more often. Similarly, satisfied clients will recommend the hospital to friends and family, thus potentially increasing clientele through referrals.

By offering puppy socialization and kitten classes, participating dogs and cats will have repetitive positive experiences in the hospital and become acclimated to handling and restraint. Consequently, examination time and the need for extra staff assistance with restraint will be decreased.

The veterinary behavior technician can be instrumental in providing direct and indirect financial benefits to his/her hospital.

Conclusion

At a minimum, the veterinary technician and veterinary staff should be familiar with preventive behavior services and even if not directly involved with the implementation of behavior services, they need to be able to provide clients with appropriate resources that will enhance the human–animal bond.

Should the technician choose, he/she can play an instrumental role in the success of preventive behavior services. Behavior can be a specialty area in which the veterinary technician can excel. The inspired behavior technician can develop and implement a variety of preventative behavior services and in doing so, increase animal retention, save animals, and improve client satisfaction while simultaneously improving the hospital's revenue.

References

Eskeland, G. (2007) Educational methods as risk factors for problem behaviours in dogs. School of Psychology, University of Southampton. MSc in Companion Animal Behaviour Counseling: 127.

Garg, A., Chren, M.M., Sands, L.P. *et al.* (2001) Psychological stress perturbs epidermal permeability barrier homeostasis: implications for the pathogenesis of stress-associated skin disorders. *Archives of Dermatology*, **137** (1), 53–59.

Gur, E., Lerer, B., Newman, M. *et al.* (1999) Chronic clomipramine and triiodothyronine increase serotonin levels in rat frontal cortex in vivo: relationship to serotonin autoreceptor activity. *Journal of Pharmacology and Experimental Therapeutics*, **288** (1), 81–87.

Landsberg, G.M., Shaw, J., Donaldson, J. *et al.* (2008) Handling behavior problems in the practice setting. *The Veterinary Clinics of North America. Small Animal Practice*, **38** (5), 951–969 v.

Lue, T.W., Pantenburg, D.P. and Crawford, P.M. (2008) Impact of the owner–pet and client–veterinarian bond on the care that pets receive. *Journal of the American Veterinary Medical Association*, **232** (4), 531–540.

Luescher, A.U., Flannigan, G., Frank, D. *et al.* (2007) The role and limitations of trainers in behavior treatment and therapy. *Journal of Veterinary Behavior: Clinical Applications and Research*, **2** (1), 26–27.

Luescher, A.U. and Reisner, I.R. (2008) Canine aggression toward familiar people: a new look at an old problem. *The Veterinary Clinics of North America. Small Animal Practice*, **38** (5), 1107–1130 vii.

Radosta-Huntley, L. A., F. S. Shofer, I.R. Reisner, *et al.* (2006) Comparison of thyroid values in aggressive and non-aggressive dogs. American College of Veterinary Behaviorists and American Veterinary Society of Animal Behavior Annual Paper and Poster Session, Honolulu, HI.

Shore, E.R., Burdsal, C., Douglas, D.K. *et al.* (2008) Pet owners' views of pet behavior problems and willingness to consult experts for assistance. *Journal of Applied Animal Welfare Science*, **11** (1), 63–73.

Tremayne J. AAFP Pens Behavior Guidelines for DVMs, Staff, Clients. DVM Magazine April 1, 2005. Available at http://veterinarynews.dvm360.com/dvm/article/articleDetail.jsp?id=155730 (accessed 21 April 2014).

2 Canine behavior and development

Andrew U. Luescher[1,2]

[1] *Purdue University, West Lafayette, IN, USA*
[2] *Foundation Barry du Grand Saint Bernard, Martigny, Switzerland*

CHAPTER MENU

It is important for a veterinary technician to understand how dogs develop and what is considered "normal" behavior. Without such a baseline, it is impossible to understand the canine perspective and what is considered outside their norm.

Canine sensory capacities

Vision

A dog's binocular field of vision is about 40–60°. Its total field of vision is about 250°. Its vision is best close-up. Dogs have good motion detection.

Canine and Feline Behavior for Veterinary Technicians and Nurses, First Edition. Edited by Julie K. Shaw and Debbie Martin.
© 2015 John Wiley & Sons, Inc. Published 2015 by John Wiley & Sons, Inc.
Companion Website: www.wiley.com/go/shaw/behavior

Dogs have much better vision in dim light than people. This is due to a reflective layer (tapetum lucidum) located behind the retina that reflects light back to hit the retina a second time. Vision in reduced light is also improved because the canine retina contains mostly rods that are more light-sensitive than cones. In addition, many rods are connected to the same nerve fiber, which further increases light sensitivity, but decreases resolution. Dogs probably do not see an equally sharp picture as humans and have a very limited depth of visual acuity.

> • Dogs probably do not see an equally sharp picture as humans and have a very limited depth of visual acuity.

Dogs have the capability to see color, particularly in the blue–violet and the yellow–green ranges. However, their retina contains relatively few color-sensitive cones. They also have fewer color-comparing neurons than humans. It has therefore been suggested that although dogs are capable of seeing color, it may not be important to them.

Hearing

A dog's hearing range is much greater than that of a human's. It is estimated that dogs hear up to 65,000 Hz (vs. 20,000 Hz in humans). However, hearing is best at around 4000 Hz, that is, well in the audible range for humans. Dogs may therefore not hear ultrasonic dog whistles very well.

Dogs can localize the source of a noise by moving their pinnae. Like humans, they can also derive the direction from which a sound is coming from the time difference between the left and the right ear perceiving the sound.

Olfaction

Dogs have a much larger olfactory epithelium than humans ($20-200 \text{ cm}^2$ compared to $2-4 \text{ cm}^2$), and up to 50 times more olfactory receptors. While dogs cannot detect some chemicals much better than humans, they can detect others (e.g., butyric acid contained in sweat) in up to 100 million times greater dilution.

Vomeronasal organ

The vomeronasal organ is a pair of channels lined with an epithelium containing chemoreceptors that open into the mouth just behind the upper incisors. Unlike other species such as horses, dogs do not show flehmen (lip-curling behavior) when investigating a substance;

rather, they lick substances they want to test (such as urine of another dog), and "tongue" them (rub tongue against roof of mouth).

The vomeronasal organ is important for detecting pheromones and therefore for social communication. Because it is connected to the limbic system, perception via the vomeronasal organ affects emotions. This is the basis for the use of pheromones such as the "dog appeasement pheromone" for behavior modification.

> • Because it is connected to the limbic system, perception via the vomeronasal organ affects emotions.

Taste

Dogs' perception of taste appears to be similar to that of humans. They are particularly sensitive to sweets and are very fond of cheese, cream, and butter. Their sense of taste is already functional at birth.

Aside from taste, palatability is largely based on smell, temperature, and texture.

Touch

The skin has receptors to sense touch, pressure, pain, body movement and position, temperature, vibration, and chemical stimulation. Touch receptors are located at the base of every hair, and especially the vibrissae. Touch can be calming, arousing, or aversive, depending on type and circumstance.

Long, firm strokes from head to hindquarters calm, reduce heart rate, and relieve stress in both the dog and the person petting the dog.

Canine communication

Dogs communicate with visual, auditory, and olfactory cues. For humans, the visual cues are usually the most obvious, and the olfactory cues are the least salient.

Visual communication

Humans are a mostly visual species, therefore the body language of dogs is particularly important for us to interpret a dog's intentions or emotions. Different postures may indicate social status, aggression, appeasement or fear, or conflict.

Figure 2.1 The tail is held high, the dog is leaning forward with a direct stare, and the ears are pricked forward (based on conformation).

Figure 2.2 The black and tan puppy is showing appeasing body language; body weight low and shifted backward, ears and tail lowered and close to the body.

Body postures

Typically a dog carrying its body weight forward, with pricked or erect ears and an elevated tail reflects a dog that is attentive and interested in environmental stimuli. The dog's emotional state may be excitement, fear, anxiety, or threat. This alert body stance may result in a variety of outcomes, including aggression and play. It is as if the dog is assessing the situation and deciding on how to proceed (Figure 2.1).

Typically, when a dog carries its body weight low to the ground and shifted backward, with ears and tail low and close to the body, it is a reflection of fear or appeasement. Appeasement behaviors are used to signal non-threat (Figure 2.2).

A dog displaying offensive aggression stands tall with ears and tail up, lips curled, with the corner of the mouth forward and only the incisors and canine teeth exposed.

Defensively aggressive dogs lower themselves and shift their body weight backward, raise the lips with the corner of the mouth drawn backward, and expose not only incisors and canines, but also the teeth on the side of their mouth (Figure 2.3).

When a subordinate social partner greets a more dominant one, it will show appeasement behavior with the body lowered, the tail low, and wagging very quickly. This is accompanied by muzzle licking and nuzzling, as occurs during food solicitation from a puppy to an adult.

Exaggerated forms of appeasement include rolling over, exposing the belly and urinating.

Piloerection (raised hackles) indicates fear, arousal, and anxiety (Figure 2.4).

Figure 2.3 The dog on the right is showing an offensive grin, front teeth exposed, mouth pursed, nose wrinkled, forward body stance. The other dog is showing a defensive grin.

Mounting usually is not related to dominance but is a conflict behavior indicating some uncertainty related to the other dog.

A review of dominant and submissive behavior patterns in wolves is provided by Bradshaw and Nott in *The Domestic Dog: Its Evolution, Behavior and Interactions with People* (Editor James Serpell 1995) (Table 2.1). The behavior patterns seen in dogs that also occur in wolves probably convey the same message as in wolves. In that aspect, we probably can extrapolate from wolves to dogs.

The description and especially the interpretation of signs in Table 2.1 should be acknowledged with a degree of skepticism. The interpretation often depends on context, and on the entirety of signals that are

Figure 2.4 Piloerection shown over the shoulders, rump, and tail, indicating arousal and uncertainty.

Table 2.1 Typical descriptions for dominant and submissive behaviors of wolves.

Dominant	Submissive
Weight shifted forward	Weight shifted back or crouched
Ears up/forward	Ears back or to the side
Mouth closed	Commissures of the lips pulled back ("grinning")
Stiff	Avoiding eye contact, licking lips
Tail up or out	Tail tucked
Places muzzle or forelegs ("feet on")over the shoulders of the other wolf	Arched back, curved neck, head low, muzzle extended
Stands stiffly over the forequarters of the prone wolf ("stand across")	Rolls to the side and lifts a hind leg
Wolf places mouth over the muzzle of the subordinate and holds it on the ground ("muzzle pin")	Sits tucked back with chin toward the chest, averts gaze, and may paw at the dominant wolf ("submissive sit")

Serpell (1995), Mech (1970), and Jenks and Ginsburg (1987).

given. For instance, an adult dog when approached by a puppy, may very well avoid eye contact. So rather than being a sign of submission or appeasement, it may simply indicate that at this time, the adult does not want to interact with the puppy. In play, roles are often reversed, so these behaviors exhibited in play say nothing about the dogs' relative relationship status.

Furthermore, traditionally it is always the action of the dominant dog that is regarded to be the initiating behavior. This disregards the fact that a subordinate or passive animal is not usually forced to show "submissive" behaviors, but actively shows appeasement behavior to be able to engage in social contact with a minimal risk of being aggressed against. The interpretation also always implies a constant competition for a more dominant position. This is likely an anthropocentric view of dog behavior. Dogs appear least stressed when their roles in the group are clear, when they clearly communicate with assertive and appeasement behavior, and when the recipient of the signals understands them and acts accordingly. If roles are unclear or signals are not understood, individuals feel threatened by each other, and aggression may ensue. This (and not holding a lower position) is a stressful situation for the dogs involved.

Play postures
Play may include pawing with a front foot, twisting jumps, open-mouth panting, and loose, relaxed tail wagging. It may include wrestling and play-fighting. The play bow (rump in the air, front legs lowered to ground) is a play solicitation and is probably a ritualized conflict behavior. It contains elements of approach and escape and signals a nonthreatening approach (Figure 2.5).

Play is characterized by elements of behavior that are out of their normal, functional sequence, and by role reversals ("winner" and "looser", chasing vs. being chased, etc.). In play, bites are inhibited if the puppy has learned bite inhibition in interactions with social partners. If this normal developmental experience has

Figure 2.5 A puppy offering a play bow to an adult dog. The puppy is signaling nonthreat and an invitation to play but is also ready to retreat pending the adult dog's response.

not been made, the bites can be severe in spite of their playful nature.

Tail wagging

"A dog that wags its tail won't bite" is a misleading statement. If the tail is carried high and stiff, and wagged with small amplitude, it often reflects high arousal and may well precede aggression. When the tail is held low, maybe between the legs, is relatively stiff and wags rapidly with small amplitude, it indicates anxiety or fear, and appeasement. Such a dog may show defensive aggression if the threat increases. If the tail is loose and relaxed, and wagged with large amplitude (the typical Labrador tail wag where the tail hits the dog's head), this indicates friendliness and playfulness.

Facial expressions

A direct eye stare indicates an alert and potentially highly aroused dog and may precede aggression. If directed toward another dog, it may indicate assertiveness and/or interest toward the other dog. Many dogs that are well trained will look in their owners' eyes for prolonged times, waiting for a cue. This does not mean these dogs are "dominant" or challenging their owners, but it indicates that they do not feel threatened. Avoiding eye contact usually indicates some degree of fear, anxiety, or conflict and may be an appeasement behavior. Therefore, we train canine patients that are uneasy with looking into the owner's eyes, to become comfortable with prolonged eye contact by teaching them a "watch-me" cue.

Ears that are pricked up (or raised at their base in lop-eared dogs) indicate attentiveness.

Ears that are folded back and flattened indicate fear or appeasement (Figure 2.6, Table 2.2). They often are folded back in play. They are also always tucked back during a bite, even in an offensively aggressive dog.

A lip-curl that exposes incisors and canine teeth only is an indication of offensive aggression (see Figure 2.3). Exposure of all teeth with the corner of the mouth retracted indicates fear, conflict, or appeasement, and may accompany defensive aggression (see Figure 2.3). However, a fearful dog that feels only mildly threatened only pulls the corners of the mouth back very little. It is important to note that a dog that is afraid can show offensive or defensive aggression.

Licking or nuzzling the mouth of a dog or a person is an appeasement behavior, or a way to initiate social contact in a friendly, nonthreatening way. The licking or nuzzling of another dog is frequently interpreted to indicate that the dog doing the nuzzling is of lower rank than the receiver of the behavior. A more precise interpretation

Figure 2.6 The puppy is pulling her ears back in response to the adult dog. The puppy is showing appeasement/fear.

Table 2.2 Signs of fear or anxiety could be.

Ears back or to the side
Tail down or tucked
Weight shifted back
Lowered head/neck (common when guarding)
Leaning or backing away
Hiding
Trembling/shaking
Pacing, running, or escape behavior
Seeking close human contact
"Grabbing" treats or not taking treats at all
Hackles raised-piloerection
Scanning
Furrowed brow
"Whale" eye
Dry, squeaky pant
Barking
Growling
Snapping

Conflict behaviors listed in Table 2.4 are also displayed in stress or anxiety inducing situations and can also be signs of anxiety or fear.

might be that the nuzzling dog has learned from previous experience that it has reason to show appeasement behavior toward the other dog.

Auditory communication

Dogs may bark when they perceive their territory to be threatened, as a warning, as a greeting, in play,

Table 2.3 Contexts in which different auditory communication are used by domestic dogs.

Sound	Behavior	
Bark	Defense	Call for attention
	Play	Warning
	Lone call	Greeting
Grunt	Greeting	Sign of contentment
Growl	Defense warning	Play
	Threat signal	
Whimper/whine	Submission	Pain
	Defense	Attention seeking
	Greeting	

Bradshaw and Nott (1995) © Cambridge University Press 1995, reproduced with permission.

out of excitement, when separated from their social group, and to get attention. The sound of the bark varies, depending on the situation. They may growl as a defense or warning, and in play. They may whimper or whine as appeasement behavior, as a greeting, when in pain, when anxious, or to get attention. Vocalization of any kind can also be used in situations of conflict or frustration (Table 2.3).

Olfactory communication

Dogs excrete scents through skin glands that may serve individual recognition. They also deposit scents via feces, urine, and anal-sac secretions. As the composition of these excretions frequently changes, it is unclear what message if any is conveyed by these means. They may indicate confidence or fear, ownership of territory or reproductive status, and possibly much more. Raised-leg urination does not only serve the deposition of urine and smell, but is also a social display. However, urine marking is also frequently a sign of anxiety. Many dogs with separation anxiety, for example, exhibit this behavior.

Ground scratching is likely a form of scent (sweat glands on feet) and visual marking. Dogs also roll in odiferous items such as feces of other species or carrion (Figure 2.7). The function of this behavior is not understood.

Conflict behavior

Dogs often display signals that appear to be contradictory. In addition, dogs may show behaviors that are apparently out of context and appear unrelated to the signals described earlier. Such behaviors may be conflict behaviors resulting from stress, frustration, or

Figure 2.7 The Dalmatian has found an interesting scent to roll in.

motivational conflict. There are many causes of stress, but stress frequently results from an environment that is unpredictable, and does not give the dog any control over events such as pleasant or aversive stimuli. Frustration results from a dog being motivated to perform a behavior, but being thwarted from performing it. A dog is in a motivational conflict if it experiences two opposing motivations, such as the motivation to approach and the motivation to withdraw. For example, a dog that wants to socialize with a person but at the same time is afraid of how the person might react is in an approach–withdrawal conflict.

> • A dog is in a motivational conflict if it experiences two opposing motivations, such as the motivation to approach and the motivation to withdraw.

Conflict behaviors include yawning, licking lips and muzzle, looking away (Figure 2.8) or toward the ceiling, visually scanning the surroundings, squinting the eyes, licking objects, lifting a paw, scratching self, vocalizing (barking, whining, or growling), wet-dog shaking, and many more. Even aggression is often shown as a conflict behavior.

Some conflict behaviors may have become "ritualized," that is, they have become part of the normal behavior repertoire of dogs and have taken on a communication function. They are "understood" by the recipient and influence the recipient's behavior. These conflict behaviors are now used as a means of communication. Some of these ritualized conflict behaviors have been described as "calming signals." It is important to realize, though, that in order to call them ritualized conflict behaviors or calming signals, an effect

CHAPTER 2

Figure 2.8 The dog turns away, licks her lips, while refusing a treat from the child. These are signs the dog is stressed about the situation or interaction.

on the recipient's behavior has to be demonstrated. It also has to be kept in mind that in any case, they are first and foremost an expression of stress, conflict, or frustration.

> • Some conflict behaviors may have become "ritualized," that is, they have become part of the normal behavior repertoire of dogs and have taken on a communication function.

> • It also has to be kept in mind that in any case, conflict behaviors are first and foremost an expression of stress, conflict, or frustration.

Ritualized conflict behaviors include averting the gaze to avoid interaction with an approaching dog, cowering and tucking the tail, rolling over and possibly urinating to inhibit aggression, growling and the "submissive grin," and whining. These behaviors have become appeasement behaviors and are used by a fearful dog to inhibit aggression from a more confident dog or a frightening human. The play bow is likely another ritualized conflict behavior. It is a combination of moving forward and an intention to jump backward. It has become a means of signaling a nonthreatening approach.

Mounting, which is often interpreted as a sexual behavior, most commonly indicates that the dog that

Table 2.4 Common conflict behaviors could be.

Freezing
Glassy eyed stare
Turning away
Turning the head
Averting eyes
Shifting eyes/brows
Licking
Squinting
Scratching
Sneezing
Sitting down
Lying down
Yawning
Mounting
Wet dog shake
Many others …

Conflict is defined as a psychological struggle, often unconscious, resulting from the opposition or simultaneous functioning of mutually exclusive impulses, desires, or tendencies. Conflict behaviors are often shown in situations of frustration, uncertainty and/ or motivational conflict and may or may not have an effect on the receiver. A key point in preventing an aggressive situation is to interpret conflict behaviors early so your actions may be appraised and possibly changed to decrease the conflict.

does the mounting experiences a conflict related to the mounted individual (which may be a person). In most cases it is not a sign of dominance or, unless displayed by an intact male toward a female in heat, a sexual advance. Most often it indicates an approach–withdrawal conflict.

As in people, aggression can also be a conflict behavior in dogs (see Table 2.4). Just imagine yourself working on the computer, but the computer does not do what you wanted it to do, and does "its own thing" instead. An aggressive outburst is a common human reaction to the stress of having lost control and lost the ability to predict what is going to happen. Similarly, dogs that lose control, are frustrated, or are in conflict may become aggressive.

Pet owners often believe their dog became aggressive "without warning." Figure 2.9 may assist owners in noticing potentially missed communication. The schematic can be used with the analogy of being stranded in an elevator with a person who is standing too close. Ritualized appeasement behaviors are comparable to you politely asking the person in the elevator to take a step back. If the person did not take a step back, you may raise your voice and place a hand in front of yourself (i.e., conflict behavior). If the person

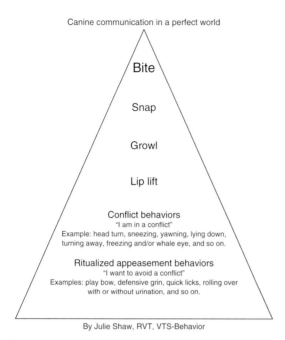

Canine communication in a perfect world

Bite

Snap

Growl

Lip lift

Conflict behaviors
"I am in a conflict"
Example: head turn, sneezing, yawning, lying down,
turning away, freezing and/or whale eye, and so on.

Ritualized appeasement behaviors
"I want to avoid a conflict"
Examples: play bow, defensive grin, quick licks, rolling over
with or without urination, and so on.

By Julie Shaw, RVT, VTS-Behavior

Figure 2.9 This is a pyramid of canine communication, outlining common behavioral signs that precede aggression.

remained too close, you may become more aggressive and threatening with the hope they will retreat (lip lift, growl, snap, etc.). Eventually you may feel the need to become violent and strike out (i.e., bite) if previous communication has not been successful. With this analogy, it becomes clear to owners their dog did not "bite without warning" but instead the communication was not interpreted clearly. In a perfect world, all dogs would precisely and routinely follow the pattern in Figure 2.9; unfortunately, that is not the case. Dogs that were punished for growling may skip directly to biting. When dogs have become confident in using aggression to resolve conflict, they may cease to show obvious conflict behaviors.

• Dogs that were punished for growling may skip
   directly to biting.

Three things are important to keep in mind. First, all these behaviors can also be shown when the dog is not in conflict, for example, because they are tired (yawning) or because they itch (scratching). Thus, context is always important when interpreting these behaviors. Second, although the ritualized conflict

behaviors have become normal social behaviors, they are still also shown when the dog is in conflict. They therefore are not an indication that the relationship of dog and owner is one of dominance and submission, nor do they allow any interpretation as to the relative social position of the dog and owner. Third, it is important to be aware of and observe conflict behaviors especially in aggressive dogs because they indicate some degree of stress, may predict imminent aggression, and point toward the reason for a behavior problem the dog may have. In training, they may indicate that the dog is confused about what is expected of him, or afraid of the training situation (punishment-based training).

During behavior modification such as systematic desensitization, conflict behaviors may indicate that the person doing the procedure has progressed a bit too quickly, or is pushing the dog too much. If a dog shows conflict behaviors when approached by a person, this indicates that the dog is uncomfortable or fearful, relative to that person. They should be noted especially when a dog interacts with children, as they may be an early warning sign for aggression. They should also be monitored throughout the treatment for behavioral issues, especially aggression, as they are a more sensitive indicator of stress or conflict than, for example, overt aggression.

Punishing conflict behaviors is obviously contraindicated. Even though punishment could be effective in suppressing particular conflict behaviors, it will not address the cause of the problem, and in many cases will increase stress and conflict which lie at the root of the problem. Punishment therefore is likely to increase the conflict behaviors, or maybe eliminate one but induce another conflict behavior. For example, a dog that was aggressive (due to a motivational conflict) to the owners and got physically punished for it, started tail chasing shortly after punishment was initiated. He was presented to the behavior clinic for persistent tail chasing for several hours a day at less than a year of age.

Canine social structure

Domestication and canine behavior
In much of the dog behavior literature, findings on behavior in wolves have been extrapolated to dogs. This section tries to show why this is not appropriate, and why wolf behavior should not be used to explain canine behavior (especially aggression) directed toward the owner (Table 2.5).

Table 2.5 Comparison of wolf and dog behavior.

Domestic dog	Wolf
Loosely structured packs generally contain between 2–5 unrelated members	Tightly structured packs generally contain between 2–20 related members
Females come into estrus twice a year. All intact females are bred	Females come into estrus once a year. Generally only high-ranking female is bred
Bitch rears puppies alone and experiences low survival rate	Pack cooperatively rears pups to ensure high survival rate
Exhibit pedomorphic behaviors throughout adult life	Pedomorphic behaviors absent in adult wolves
Generally scavengers	Highly developed predatory behavior
No real cooperative hunting	Hunt as a cohesive unit

> • Wolf behavior should not be used to explain canine behavior (especially aggression) directed toward the owner.

Dogs have been domesticated for at least 12,000 years and have been selected to remain behaviorally immature compared to wolves (Coppinger and Coppinger, 2001). This retardation of development is called *neoteny*, and the resulting retention of juvenile characteristics by adult animals is called *pedomorphosis*. Neoteny accounts for many of the pronounced behavioral differences between dogs and wolves. Dogs show many behaviors typical for wolf puppies even in adulthood: they remain playful, enjoy physical contact, are highly social, bark, paw, and nuzzle. Some breeds are more highly neotenized, and show more of the behaviors characteristic of wolf puppies than others.

Social organization in stray or feral dogs

In contrast to wild wolves, free-ranging unowned dogs do not live in well-structured family groups or packs. Instead they live in small, loosely coherent groups of 2–5 unrelated dogs. Upon the loss of members of the group, the number regenerates through the addition of abandoned or escaped pets.

The range occupied by a group of dogs is less than 0.1 sq. mile in urban areas where there are many food sources, but no high concentration of food anywhere. In these urban areas, dogs tend to be territorial, that is, they defend their territory against other dogs that might try to intrude.

In rural areas with low density of human population and therefore less abundant food sources, groups of free roaming dogs occupy home-ranges of 0.2–11 sq. miles. The larger rural home-ranges may even overlap at high resource areas (garbage dumps) but are not usually defended against other dogs.

Female dogs generally come into heat twice a year, as opposed to wolves where females come into estrus once a year. Unlike wolves, where only the pack-founding female gets bred and the pack raises the litter together in a concerted effort, in free-ranging dogs, every intact female gets bred, sometimes by multiple males. Female dogs separate from the group before giving birth and attempt to raise the puppies alone. As a result, pups born to stray dogs seldom survive to adulthood (one study showed 1 in 20 puppies born survived) and rarely account for growth or regeneration of a pack.

Predatory behavior is poorly developed in dogs compared to wolves, and depends on the degree of neotenization of a breed. Dogs are predominantly scavengers, and when they hunt, they do not hunt in a cooperative way.

All these findings suggest that the extrapolation of wolf social behavior to dogs, and especially to dogs and their relation to their human family, is inappropriate. What sense does it make, really, to claim that an infantile form (puppy) of a highly neotenized species (a species that "never grows up") tries to dominate all their social partners? This is more material for cartoons than reality.

> • All these findings suggest that the extrapolation of wolf social behavior to dogs, and especially to dogs and their relation to their human family, is inappropriate.

Social organization in dogs living in a human household

The existence of a social hierarchy in dogs is disputed. However, this belief may stem largely from a misunderstanding of what a social hierarchy is. A dominance hierarchy is a statistical construct derived from observations of dyadic interactions. Once the rank of a dog in a group is calculated, it becomes a predictor for the outcome of subsequent interactions between the two individuals in the dyad. It is not the only factor influencing the outcome. Therefore, the outcome of interactions between the same two individuals may be different in different situations (note: this does not imply that the hierarchy changes depending on the situation).

When Scott and Fuller (1965) set up pair-wise confrontations between puppies over a bone, they found that more neotenized breeds such as the Cocker Spaniel and the Beagle showed much more variation in the outcome (i.e., who gets the bone) than less neotenized breeds such as the Fox Terrier or Basenji where, with reliable frequency, the same puppy gained control of the bone. That means more neotenized breeds are more puppy-like, with a fluid social organization, while less neotenized breeds have a much more rigid social structure.

Social tensions between dogs in the same household appear to indicate that there is a dominance "hierarchy" that sometimes changes due to an animal reaching social maturity (relative to its breed), or a new addition finding its place in the social group. Genetics have a considerable influence on where in the social order an animal ends up upon reaching maturity. The concept that a dog is constantly driven to strive for a higher rank is unsubstantiated. Tensions between dogs in the household tend to coincide with unclear roles and miscommunication leading to a sense of threat and consequently aggression.

Exploratory behavior

Exploratory behavior is evident in the puppy at the latest with the beginning of locomotion. Through exploratory behavior, the dog learns details of its environment (what is food, escape pathways, location of nest, water, etc).

Exploration consumes a significant part of dogs' time and is of great importance to them. Dogs will work for the opportunity to investigate a novel stimulus: dogs have been trained to press a lever in a skinner box and as reinforcement a door would open with a different object behind it each time. This leads to the conclusion that dogs have an inherited motivation to satisfy curiosity or maintain a certain level of sensory input.

Clinically it is evident that deprivation of exploratory behavior leads to over-reactivity to stimuli and increased anxiety. Walks away from the familiar area of the home satisfy the motivation to explore and reduce reactivity and anxiety. Roaming may in part be rewarding for the same reason, in addition to providing the opportunity to scavenge, socialize, and maybe even reproduce (Figure 2.10).

Figure 2.10 Digging is a common exploratory behavior of dogs.

Ingestive behavior

Since dogs have associated with human settlements, they have been selected to be good scavengers while they have become much less proficient at hunting. They still have the potential for predatory behavior and show many of the motor patterns associated with it, especially during play. Predatory behavior has also been observed when a large group of dogs become highly excited or aroused.

The extent to which predatory behavior is developed in a dog depends on its degree of neoteny. Predatory behavior is also influenced by learning: dogs will normally not show any predatory behavior toward species with which they have been socialized at an early age. Therefore, flock-guarding dogs are socialized early with sheep. If not socialized sufficiently with humans, dogs may show predatory behavior toward people and especially children. Fighting dogs are trained to redirect predatory behavior toward their own species which is highly abnormal, and occasionally generalize to other species as well.

Dogs normally eat one large meal every few days, although they may eat small animals, carrion, fecal material, and plants in-between if available. In a caseload analysis, we found that dogs with behavior disorders that were switched from free-choice feeding to restricted feeding had a better outcome than dogs that were not switched over. Further research on the natural feeding strategies of dogs is warranted. Whether restricted or free feeding is recommended is dependent on the individual animal and environment. For example, unlimited access to food in a multiple dog household could result in competition over the food and over-indulgence. Restricting access to set meal times may provide routine and allow for more effective training when utilizing food as a reinforcer.

Anxiety reduces appetite. A dog that is trained with food rewards may refuse the rewards as the first indication of anxiety and thus inability to learn. Also, a dog that is housed at a veterinary hospital or boarding kennel may have reduced appetite. Competition over food increases consumption.

Palatability is largely based on smell, therefore appetite can be improved by moistening and warming up food. Dogs also generally prefer novel food.

Eliminative behavior

Eliminative behavior includes defecation, urination, and pre- and post-eliminative behaviors (smelling, exploring for a location, circling before elimination, and scratching the ground after elimination).

Bitches stimulate puppies to urinate and defecate by licking the perineal area and ingesting the excrement. Puppies begin to eliminate on their own at 2–3 weeks of age at which time bitches discontinue digesting the excrement. By 3 weeks of age, the pups begin to leave the nest and gradually start to defecate outside the nest.

By approximately 3 months of age, males lean forward, at 6 months they occasionally lift their leg. Leg lifting progressively increases in males until 2 years of age. Castration before puberty may delay the onset of leg lifting, but most castrated males still develop leg lifting due to the priming of their brain with testosterone while in utero.

The typical female urination posture is squatting. However, most older females lift a leg while squatting, ostensibly to mark an area with urine. This should be considered normal behavior.

Stimuli that affect elimination

It is important to know what stimuli affect elimination in order to housetrain a dog. Elimination is most common after waking up from sleep, after eating and drinking, and after exercise. The smell of previous elimination also stimulates further urination or defecation. Rectal irritation or rectal stimulation through introduction of a cotton swab also initiates defecation.

The amount of time since a dog eliminated last also affects the likelihood of defecation. While most dogs are able to refrain from eliminating all day, puppies, older dogs, and sick dogs often need to eliminate more frequently.

A rule of thumb for puppies is that they can refrain from eliminating for as many hours as they are months

old, plus one. Puppies confined for long periods and thus forced to urinate and defecate in their cage, and lie in it, may completely lose their ability to be housebroken. There may be a sensitive period when the puppy needs to be able to avoid its excrements in order to be trainable, but this has not been scientifically established.

Sexual behavior

Most males sexually mature from 9–12 months of age. While smaller breeds may mature sooner (6–9 months old), giant breeds generally mature later (12 months or older). Females are sexually mature (first estrus) at 6–9 months, although larger breeds frequently experience first estrus at a later age.

Precopulatory behavior is ritualized with great individual variation. It may include joint play-running, chasing, vocalizing, head-to-head nosing and sniffing of the female's body, particularly genitalia. The female may present to the male and solicit play. At first, the female avoids the male; then becomes more tolerant. She urinates frequently and examines the male. The bitch may mount the male, particularly if the male is inexperienced. The female becomes increasingly docile, "flagging" or moving her tail to the side.

A female is ready to be bred when she adopts a mating stance and allows the male to mount her. At this point, she shows less soliciting behavior.

Coital lock occurs after penetration. The male turns during the "tie" and the coital lock persists for 10–30 min. Separation occurs after muscular relaxation of the vagina and contraction of the bulbus glandis.

Nonestrous bitches may mount estrous bitches or vice-versa. Estrous bitches may mount males. Estrus may increase general activity, nervousness, and vocalization. Pregnancy lasts about 63 days.

Maternal behavior

Increased time licking nipples and genital area may be seen as parturition approaches. The bitch lactates (milk can be expressed) 1–7 days prepartum. Her appetite may be noticeably decreased 24–48 h before parturition. Restlessness of the bitch increases 12–24 h before parturition and body temperature drops by 2–3°F approximately 24 h before birth (most reliable indicator of imminent parturition). Nest building is seen along with a potential for aggression toward strangers. Labor signs include respiration varying from panting to slow and deep respiration, decreased activity, and agitation, particularly when not given adequate privacy.

During parturition the bitch licks her vulva and expels the puppy in the amnion. She then licks/chews through the amnion, and bites through the umbilical cord (brachiocephalic breeds are unable to do so). The puppies are licked to stimulate urination and defecation. Average time between births is 30 min but this is very variable. Long intervals may be associated with stillbirths.

Disturbances, such as strange people, can cause delays from 1–6 h. The delay can come during rest, active labor, or actual delivery with a pup in the vagina. Excitement produces adrenaline, which inhibits uterine activity.

Parent–offspring behavior
Care-giving behavior
Licking the puppy serves three functions: stimulates eating, urination, and defecation; guides the puppy to the nest by licking its head, rather than by carrying, which is seldom done by dogs;and it may also "label" the puppy with maternal pheromones.

Care-soliciting behavior
Vocalization, rooting, approach, and contact stimulate mothering.

Postpartum grooming includes the bitch licking, tearing, and ingesting the placenta and severing the umbilical cord. The length of time for placental removal varies. The bitch removes fluid from the head and mouth of the puppy and cleans herself and the bedding. Dead pups are treated the same as live pups until they are cold, then pushed aside or eaten. Nursing is initiated by the mother from 0–14 days and initiated by puppies after that until weaned (around 5–6 weeks).

Puppy activity and vocalization
Newborn puppies move only a few inches at a time and are not usually moved by the dam. Head movements are from side to side and they are attracted by heat and repelled by cold (their nose is used as a temperature probe). The puppies move against the grain of the hair and against pressure when the mother licks them. Vocalization occurs 1–4 min after birth. Whines decrease when the pups are warm or nursing; grunts can signify pleasure. The dam is insensitive to whines during whelping; if out of sight, she will not retrieve the puppy. If the dam sits on a pup, she will ignore cries unless she feels or sees it.

Play behavior

Mostly observed in young dogs, play is for learning and muscular development and coordination, as well as being inherently pleasurable. Play-fighting begins around 5–6 weeks of age.

Play is a major mechanism by which social relationships are established and maintained.

Play signals include the play bow, exaggerated approach, repeated barking, approach and withdrawal, pouncing, and leaping.

Social play is more common than solitary play in dogs.

Behavior sequences are mixed up (predatory, mating, etc.).

Role reversal occurs in play, with an adult often participating in play with a younger, weaker conspecific.

Canine behavioral development

Experiences during development have long-lasting effects on temperament and adult behavior. It is therefore important to appreciate normal and abnormal development in order to prevent, understand, and resolve behavior issues. The literature on canine development has been reviewed by Lindsay, 2000.

> • Experiences during development have long-lasting effects on temperament and adult behavior. It is therefore important to appreciate normal and abnormal development in order to prevent, understand, and resolve behavior issues.

Complexity of early environment
An animal's central nervous system develops its genetically predetermined functions only if exposed to appropriate environmental stimulation, especially early in life. A restricted environment early in life will result in an animal with abnormal sensory perception. The animal may not be able to perceive stimuli to which it was not exposed during development. An animal reared in a restrictive environment will also be emotionally unstable. In addition to emotionality, the complexity of the early environment also greatly influences learning ability. A restricted early environment may result in reduced learning ability and trainability. It is therefore important to provide an interesting and stimulating early environment. In addition, it is also important that the early environment be predictable and consistent. If

not, the animal will not only be frustrated and under stress, but it will also learn that its behavior has no impact on what is happening around it. Such animals will be in a state of learned helplessness and exceedingly hard to train later.

Effect of neonatal stress

Some degree of stress (e.g., handling, mild shock, cold temperature) in the neonatal period of dogs may accelerate growth, reduce emotionality later in life, increase social confidence, and promote resistance to some diseases. Handling sessions from the first days of a puppy's life are therefore recommended. They will not only expose the puppy to a mild stress, but also facilitate socialization when the puppy gets older. In addition to handling sessions, puppies may be removed from the nest (best while someone else walks the mother) and placed singly on a cool vinyl floor for a brief time (30 s) before being put back into the warm nest. Flashing light, noises, and motion have also been used as mild stress. The army's super-dog program used slow, refrigerated centrifuges to apply a mild stress. If done in the first few (3) days after birth when the hypothalamic–hypophyseal–adrenal (HHA) axis develops, this is expected to result in reduced behavioral and physiological reaction to chronic stress, an increased physiological reaction to acute stress, and reduced emotionality of the adult dog. Chronic stress is caused by unavoidable and long-lasting aversive conditions. As they are unavoidable, the stress reaction does not result in coping, and just drains the animal's resources. In people, such chronic stress causes stomach ulcers and other impairment of health. A strong reaction to acute stress, however, is desirable. If an animal is exposed to a sudden, intense, and potentially damaging stimulus, it may save its life if it mobilizes all its resources to escape. So both a reduced reaction to chronic stress and an increased reaction to acute stress are beneficial.

- Some degree of stress (e.g., handling, mild shock, cold temperature) in the neonatal period of dogs may accelerate growth, reduce emotionality later in life, increase social confidence, and promote resistance to some diseases.

Mild early stress also results in increased resistance to some diseases, a more stable and less emotional temperament, and increased learning ability and trainability.

- Mild early stress also results in increased resistance to some diseases, a more stable and less emotional temperament, and increased learning ability and trainability.

Sensitive periods of development

It is well documented that there are "sensitive periods" in the behavioral development of a dog. These are periods of development during which certain experiences need to be made to achieve normal development. Lack of these experiences during the critical period has lifelong irreversible effects.

For instance, between 4 and 12 weeks of age, a puppy learns how a social partner looks. During this time, the brain develops a sort of filter system in the visual cortex, which becomes sensitized to the shapes of the social partners of the puppy. In the wolf, these would be adult wolves and other pups; in the dog, they include humans and other pets. This filter system ensures that certain neurons in the visual brain are only activated when the puppy sees a social partner. After 12 weeks, this system can hardly be further modified so that the puppy will not learn (or learn only with difficulty) to accept previously unknown species as social partners.

- After 12 weeks, this system can hardly be further modified so that the puppy will not learn (or learn only with difficulty) to accept previously unknown species as social partners.

The recognition of critical periods in canine behavioral development may be one of the most important discoveries about dogs. By controlling the puppy's environment during its early life, we can influence the emotionality, temperament, sociability, confidence, and learning ability of the dog. Early and appropriate intervention can result in the dog being more adaptable, easier to train, and physically and emotionally healthier.

- Early and appropriate intervention can result in the dog being more adaptable, easier to train, and physically and emotionally healthier.

The exact time course of development varies between authors (and probably between dogs to some degree!)

Table 2.6 Developmental period of dogs.

Period	Duration
Fetal period	Up to birth
Neonatal period	0–10 days
Transition period	11–21 days
Socialization period	3–12 (–14) weeks
Fear period	8–10 (–12) weeks
Juvenile period	~3 months to puberty (~5–14 months)
Juvenile/adolescent fear period(s)?	3 weeks between 4 and 11 months?
Adolescent period	Puberty to social maturity (~2–3 years)
Adult period	Social maturity to 7+ years
Senior period	7+ years

as the sensitive periods do not start abruptly but rather phase in and out gradually. The development of dogs has been divided into the periods shown in Table 2.6.

Fetal period

The fetal period includes development of the fetus up to parturition. During the fetal period, the male brain undergoes a process that determines gender differences in behavior. Shortly before parturition, the male fetus produces a burst of testosterone. This has an organizational effect on the brain of the male fetus; it masculinizes and defeminizes the brain. Masculinization results in the organization of typical male behavior such as roaming, urine marking, inter-male aggression, and male sexual behavior. Castration is usually successful in reducing these behaviors, but does not entirely eliminate them. The effectiveness of castration in altering these behaviors is individually very variable. Defeminization results in the destruction of the mechanism that results in cyclical sexual behavior in females (intact male dogs do not have an estrus cycle and are always ready to breed), and eliminates the predisposition to show female sexual behavior. A male dog castrated after birth when given estrogen will show male and not female sexual and social behavior.

The priming of the fetal male brain is irreversible and affects all behavior that is gender-dimorphic, including various types of aggression, even in the castrated dog. Therefore, a castrated male dog is still very much male; a spayed female dog is still very much female.

Surprisingly, little appears to have been published about the effect of the nutritional status of the gestating bitch on the behavioral development of her puppies. However, it is known that poor blood supply and thus poor oxygen and nutritional supply to the fetus results in retarded or abnormal physical development. It can therefore be expected that brain development is also impaired in these cases, affecting the behavioral development and learning ability of the puppies.

Puppies can already learn in utero. If a particular flavor is fed to the pregnant bitch such as aniseed, the puppies will show a preference for that taste after birth.

Neonatal period

The neonatal period extends approximately over the first 10 days of the puppy's life (Figure 2.11). It is characterized by the puppy's complete dependence on the mother for thermoregulation, nutrition, and elimination, and by behavior that is designed to bring a puppy back into the heap of puppies and close to the mammary gland.

A puppy is born both blind and deaf, but is capable of whining to attract attention from its mother. It is born with the senses of balance, taste, smell, touch, and temperature. Until 3 weeks of age, the puppy is not able to urinate and defecate spontaneously, and is dependent on stimulation (licking) by the mother to fulfill these functions. Its nervous system is poorly developed; for the first 3 days it has "flexor dominance," that is, it curls up when picked up by the neck, and from day 4 to day 21, it has "extensor dominance," that is, it stretches when picked up. Although puppies are dependent on the mother for thermoregulation, they are born with sensitivity to temperature and will root against a warm object. Newborn puppies will also move against the grain of the hair of their mother so they will get closer to the teat, and also turn or move toward the side they are touched. From

Figure 2.11 Rye, a Border Collie puppy, at 4 days of age.

about 2–3 days of age, a puppy is able to crawl moving its head from side to side, using its nose as a touch and temperature probe. Again, all of the puppy's behaviors are designed to get it back into the heap of littermates and to the teat.

Already during this early stage, human contact and handling are important as environmental enrichment and for inducing a mild stress. As mentioned above, a mild stress can also be imposed by removing the puppy from the nest for a brief period (30 s) and placing it on a cool surface such as a vinyl floor. This may allow the animal to better cope with stress, be more trainable, and be emotionally more stable later in life.

Puppies may vocalize when hurt, when cold, or uncomfortable, or when they lose contact with their littermates or the mother. However, most bitches will not react to these vocalizations.

Learning with positive reinforcement is already possible, although the puppies' responses are very limited. Conditioned aversion has also been achieved in very young puppies.

Transition period

The transition period follows the neonatal period and reaches to about 3 weeks of age. It is characterized by fast maturation. Puppies are born in a very early stage of development. Such animals are called *altricial*. In the transitional period, a puppy catches up with those animals that are born in a much more developed state, such as foals or calves that are examples of "precocial" animals. The puppy begins to develop its senses, gains control over thermoregulation, and at the end of the transitional period, becomes able to eliminate spontaneously (and the mother stops eating its stool). From this point on, the puppies should have the possibility to leave the nest site to eliminate. Puppies that are thwarted from doing so may become almost impossible to house train.

> • The puppy begins to develop its senses, gains control over thermoregulation, and at the end of the transitional period, becomes able to eliminate spontaneously.

The puppy's nervous system is developing at a rapid pace. However, it does so only in reaction to a stimulating environment. During the transitional period, the puppy begins to develop its senses of vision and of hearing (Figure 2.12). The eyes begin to open around 12–14 days, but vision is poor. Later during this period, around

Figure 2.12 Rye, a Border Collie puppy, at 2 weeks of age.

20–21 days, the ears open. The development of vision and hearing makes the puppy more reactive to environmental stimuli. Since the puppy is also able to habituate to stimuli, and still profits from environmental complexity for normal neurological development, the provision of sensory, visual, and auditory stimuli is very important. This can be done through handling, placing the puppy for short periods in a play pen with toys, platforms, tunnels, and so on (under supervision!), and playing recordings (commercially available) of various noises. Puppies might begin to walk unsteadily as early as day 12. Puppies will also begin to play-fight, and are better able to learn, especially with positive reinforcement.

At around 3 weeks of age, the mother and father may start to regurgitate food for the puppies. Probably as an effect of domestication, not all dogs will do that. The puppies will solicit food regurgitation by pushing their noses into the corners of the parents' mouths, a behavior that later develops into an appeasement behavior. At 3 weeks of age, it is appropriate to begin feeding solid food to puppies.

Socialization period

The next sensitive period of development of a puppy is the socialization period that extends from about 3 weeks up to 12–14 weeks. The older the puppies get, the more variability there is in the timing of developmental benchmarks.

Socialization to dogs and to people has to occur during this time. If this opportunity is missed, the puppy will most likely always be fearful of dogs and/or humans. During the socialization period, the puppy should also be exposed to all situations that it is likely to encounter during its life. The best prevention of behavior problems is to take the puppy to puppy classes during that time. During the socialization period, the puppy can already learn

Figure 2.13 Rye, a Border Collie puppy, at 9 weeks of age.

some cues. It should learn bite inhibition, and begin to learn how to fit into a social group (Figure 2.13).

The socialization period has been subdivided into a period of primary socialization, normally to conspecifics (earlier on in the socialization period), and secondary socialization to other species (later in the socialization period). Forming social attachments and social play are the most prominent behavioral aspect of this period, but exploration is very important for normal development as well. During the primary socialization period, a puppy learns to interact appropriately with other puppies, learns to read canine body language, and learns about a bite inhibition and about fitting into a social group. It basically learns to be a dog. The ability to learn this is innate, and puppies will show some appropriate basic social responses when exposed to social stimuli (such as a puppy may sniff in the right places when exposed to a dog silhouette). However, if exposure to conspecific social stimuli during this period is missed (i.e., the puppy has no opportunity to practice appropriate behavior during the socialization period), a dog may show inappropriate behavior toward other dogs later in life. This would in most cases be fear, but could also be aggression or even predatory behavior. Since it is not giving appropriate signals, other dogs will also act inappropriately toward it. It would be very difficult or impossible to teach a dog later in life how to interact appropriately with other dogs, or to understand dog body language if this opportunity is missed.

A puppy taken early from the litter and raised by hand will form its paramount relationships with people. If this isolation from its own species continues until after 12 weeks, the dog may become fearful of and aggressive to other dogs. On the other hand, if the puppy is not socialized to humans during the socialization period, it

will most likely always be fearful of and possibly become aggressive to people.

- A puppy taken early from the litter and raised by hand will form its paramount relationships with people. If this isolation from its own species continues until after 12 weeks, the dog may become fearful of and aggressive to other dogs.

Although weaning may occur from 4–6 weeks of age, a puppy should never be adopted before 7–8 weeks of age, and best not before 10 weeks of age. Although this has not been studied well in dogs, clinical observations indicate that the interaction occurring within the litter at that time and the effect of the mother are too critical to a puppy's development, and early removal from the litter may result in emotional instability. In one study, puppies taken from the litter earlier (at 6 weeks) had more health and developmental problems and showed increased stress at separation from the dam. They did not socialize any better to humans than puppies taken away from the mother at a later date and provided human contact on a daily basis while with the dam.

- Although weaning may occur from 4–6 weeks of age, a puppy should never be adopted before 7–8 weeks of age, and best not before 10 weeks of age.

During secondary socialization, the puppy learns not to be afraid of (and therefore possibly be aggressive toward) other species. It can learn to predict actions of members of other species, and learns to interact with them successfully. It can learn (and it has a genetic predisposition to do so) human body language such as the meaning of pointing to an object. It also is unlikely to ever show predatory behavior toward species it regularly interacted with during the socialization period. This characteristic is utilized by breeders of flock-guarding dogs who socialize puppies very well with sheep by even letting them nurse from sheep. This also emphasizes the need for socializing puppies to children to prevent predatory behavior (designed to kill!) being directed toward children.

During the socialization period, every effort should be made to fully socialize the puppy to people of all ages, from infant to senior, and of all races. Socialization biscuits as promoted by Dr. W. Hunthausen in Kansas City,

Figure 2.15   The environment is enriched with an entire "puppy park" of novelties for this youngster to explore with human supervision.

Figure 2.14   Physically challenged child socializing with puppies in a puppy class.

are useful for this (biscuits that each are given to the puppy by a different stranger). The puppy should also be exposed to people who limp, use a cane, or are in a wheelchair, and to people wearing a variety of clothes, hats, beards, sunglasses, and so on (Figure 2.14).

In addition to socialization, the puppy should also be exposed to a wide range of different sights, sounds, and other sensory experiences, known as *localization*. Environmental complexity is still very important in assuring normal neurological and emotional development. A puppy park that contains all kinds of objects and stimuli, where the puppies spend time under supervision, is a helpful tool to provide complex sensory experience. A puppy park may contain unusual footing, objects that make noise, a water bath, objects hanging overhead, and so on (Figure 2.15). The exposure to these stimuli has to be provided with care so puppies are not frightened. If a timid puppy gets frightened by a stimulus such as a loud noise, a treat should be placed immediately into its mouth so the frightening stimulus gets associated with a pleasant experience (counter-conditioning; there is no risk of conditioning the emotion of fear by "rewarding"

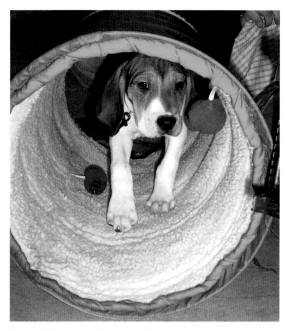

Figure 2.16   A puppy being desensitized to a tunnel at puppy class.

it with food). A puppy also needs to learn to be comfortable in a vehicle, on unstable footing, on stairs, in elevators, on an exam table, and so on (Figure 2.16).

The puppy can now learn more easily from positive experiences, and particularly from 8 weeks of age, also from negative experiences. The puppy should be trained, obviously with positive training techniques, so it learns that its behavior can operate on the environment (learning to learn). Training done at this stage is easily retained and probably enhances later trainability. Many of the exercises that are useful for problem prevention (e.g., teaching the leave it cue, food bowl safety, bite inhibition) are done most easily during this period. Even tracking is much more easily learned by an 8-week-old puppy than by a 6-month-old adolescent. Puppy classes can provide all this and more in a structured and systematic way. It is this author's belief that taking a puppy to a good puppy class during the socialization period is the best thing owners can do for their dog in its entire life. The American Veterinary Society of Animal Behavior has put out a statement available for download on their website regarding the importance of early socialization (www.avsabonline.org). In the position statement, it is stated, "In general, puppies can start puppy socialization classes as early as 7–8 weeks of age. Puppies should receive a minimum of one set of vaccines at least 7 days prior to the first class and a first deworming. They should be kept up-to-date on vaccines throughout the class." Furthermore, the statement cautions that the potential risk of under-socialization outweighs any potential health risks. See Chapter 7 for details on puppy class curriculum.

> • Taking a puppy to a good puppy class during the socialization period is the best thing owners can do for their dog in its entire life.

Fear period (8–10+ weeks)
The fear period lies within the socialization period and is included in that period by many authors. It starts at about 8 weeks of age, but the age of onset seems to vary considerably between breeds and individuals. The fear period is characterized by increased fearfulness, and likely permanent retention of the fear. Any aversive experience during that time, including shipping a puppy, is to be avoided as it may have lifelong effects on emotionality, anxiety, fear, hyperactivity and reactivity, and aggressiveness. Dogs that have been affected by adverse experiences during the fear period often cannot be rehabilitated.

If 5-week old puppies are punished, that is, with an electric shock for approaching a person, they will show fear, but approach that person again when retested later. If the puppies are between 8 and 9 weeks of age, they retain the fear of that person. Puppies older than

12 weeks are less influenced by a mild shock and may approach the person in spite of the shock, or at least can overcome their fear. Because of the increased fearfulness and the enhanced learning from bad experiences during the fear period, extra caution should be used to safeguard puppies from possibly lifelong effects of a negative experience during this time. Some dogs that are genetically predisposed to fearfulness may start to show fear during the fear period and remain fearful even in the absence of any trauma.

> • Some dogs that are genetically predisposed to fearfulness may start to show fear during the fear period and remain fearful even in the absence of any trauma.

Juvenile period
The juvenile period follows the socialization period and ends with puberty, approximately from 3 months to 5–14 months. It is characterized by rapid physical growth and increasing activity, excitability, and independence. This is a difficult stage to go through (for the owner), in particular if the puppy has not yet been trained at all. Early training pays off during this developmental stage.

Many owners of young puppies do not see the need to take their dog to puppy class. They say their puppy is so well behaved and follows them everywhere voluntarily: it is the best dog in the world without any training. Once the puppy reaches about 4 months of age, they are often greatly disappointed. Their once so voluntarily compliant puppy suddenly does not seem to care much about them anymore, and it becomes a chore to keep it under control. This is a reason why many dogs are relinquished around 5–6 months of age.

A social order may now begin to develop among the puppies, if they have remained together. Compared to wolves that have a highly structured social order, the social order among dogs of most breeds always remains one resembling that among wolf puppies. Depending on neotenization of the breed, this social order may be loose and flexible, or it may be more rigid and linear. In a few cases, social status may depend on gender, with all males being dominant over all females, such as was found to be the case in Terriers and Basenjis, two breeds that are less neotenized than most.

During the juvenile period, dogs may go through one or several more fear periods, lasting around 2–3 weeks each, during which the dog is much more easily frightened and adverse experiences can be more difficult for the dog to overcome. During these fear periods, dogs may suddenly show fear of familiar objects or situations. For example, a dog that encountered garbage cans twice a week on his daily walk, may suddenly be frightened by their sight, and not dare to go near, raise the hackles, and bark. This should not worry the owners too much. In most cases it just needs to be waited out. Counter-conditioning, response substitution, and in severe cases, systematic desensitization can be used to help the animal to get through this. Aversive training techniques, punishment, and other traumatic experiences could have a long-lasting effect on fearfulness, aggressiveness, and emotionality and should be avoided.

> • Aversive training techniques, punishment, and other traumatic experiences could have a long-lasting effect on fearfulness, aggressiveness, and emotionality and should be avoided.

The juvenile period ends with sexual maturity around 5–14 months of age, depending on individual and breed. However, attainment of sexual maturity does not imply social maturity.

Adolescent period

The adolescent period starts with puberty and ends with attainment of social maturity relative to the breed. As compared with wolves, dogs never reach social maturity. The degree of social maturity attained varies between breeds, with herd-guarding dogs remaining very puppyish, followed by retrievers and spaniels, then pointers and stalkers, with heelers and terriers becoming relatively most mature. Breeds that remain socially immature are among other things less predatory, more playful, and enjoy physical contact more; they therefore may have more desirable pet qualities than breeds that become more mature.

Dogs become increasingly more independent at this stage and cute puppy behaviors might be less tolerated by owners of the adolescent dog. Prevention and management of behaviors that are not under the owner's control will keep the dog from learning unwanted behaviors. Physical and mental exercise for the dog is essential to making this stage more enjoyable. Training problems and behavior disorders are likely to become more pronounced during this stage of development. For example, dogs might start barking at strangers entering the home or become territorial during adolescence.

Adult period

Dogs become socially mature at 2–3 years of age. Small-breed dogs will mature faster than large-breed dogs.

Play behavior might decrease as dogs reach social maturity. Social tolerances to other familiar and unfamiliar dogs can change as a dog reaches adulthood. The adolescent dog that thrived at the dog park or doggy daycare, as an adult might become less accepting of and less interested in playing with unfamiliar dogs. Play with known dogs with which they have an established relationship is often more enjoyable. Changes in the dynamics and relationships within a multidog household might change as a dog reaches social maturity. The socially mature dog might decide to challenge an older dog in the house over possession of a resource.

Senior period

Dogs become senior at 7+ years of age. Small-breed dogs live longer, and become senior at a later age (10–12 years), than large-breed dogs. As dogs age, their activity level will decrease. This might be associated with degenerative processes such as arthritis, reduced hearing, normal clouding of the cornea and/or reduced visual acuity, and muscle atrophy. Senior dogs should be screened at least annually by a veterinarian for medical disorders, as well as behavioral changes associated with aging. Some senior dogs will develop cognitive dysfunction syndrome, similar to Alzheimer's disease or dementia in humans. Early medical and behavioral treatment can greatly benefit the welfare of these dogs. Mental stimulation in the form of play and training is important for physical and behavioral wellness of all senior dogs.

Problem prevention

Complex early environment

As discussed above, providing a complex early environment is important in preventing behavior problems. Also, handling and exposing puppies to a mild stress in the first few days of life should be beneficial. Exposure to variable environments during the socialization period is important to reduce fear and aggression. Puppies should be taken on car rides and to other people's homes ideally before they are taken away from the litter, and certainly once they are with their new owner.

Socialization

Puppy classes that allow for puppy play can provide a safe way of exposing a puppy to other puppies. Under

Figure 2.17 Puppies in controlled play at puppy class.

the supervision of an expert, a puppy can learn to inter-act appropriately with other puppies with minimal risk (Figure 2.17).

Since our dogs are part of human society, socialization to humans is of paramount importance. This includes socialization to people of both genders and all races, people with physical disabilities, using crutches or being wheelchair-bound, and most of all, to children. Especially puppy owners who plan on having children should plan ahead and expose the puppy in a safe way to babies (or at least the smell and sounds thereof),

toddlers, and children of all ages, as dogs do not appear to generalize from one age group to another. Obviously, all interactions should be pleasant. In any case in which a puppy shows fear, giving it a treat immediately will tilt the balance toward a more positive experience (Figures 2.18 and 2.19).

Children also need to be educated on how to appropriately interact with a puppy, and need to be supervised around the dog at all times. They should be taught how to pet a dog and, especially, how to play with a dog. Dogs cannot be expected to put up with everything a child wants to impose on them, and many dogs will be forced to resort to aggression if a child bothers them or excites them too much. Detailed problem prevention including puppy classes is discussed in Chapter 7.

Conclusion

By getting a clear understanding of what is normal development and behavior for dogs, the veterinary technician will become astute at recognizing abnormal behavior. Through early prevention training and inter-vention before the development of serious behavior disorders, often the veterinary technician can assist in maintaining and enhancing the human–dog bond and prevent relinquishment of the dog.

Figure 2.18 Children should be included in puppy classes but in a very controlled manner. This toddler is being assisted by his mother in offering canned cheese in a syringe case. This prevents a puppy from accidently nipping the child's fingers.

CHAPTER 2

Figure 2.19 Older children can offer treats to the puppy in a flat hand while sitting in a chair or standing.

References

Bradshaw, J.W.S. and Nott, H.M.R. (1995) Social and communication behavior of companion dogs, in *The Domestic Dog: Its Evolution, Behavior and Interactions with People* (ed J. Serpell), Cambridge Univ. Press, Cambridge, p. 177.

Coppinger, R. and Coppinger, L. (2001) *Dogs: A Startling New Understanding of Canine Origin, Behavior, and Evolution*, Scribner, New York.

Jenks, S.M. and Ginsburg, B.E. (1987) Socio-sezual dynamics in a captive wolf pack, in *Man and Wolf* (ed H. Frank), Dordrecht, The Netherlands, pp. 375–399. Dr W. Junk.

Lindsay, S.R. (2000) Handbook of Applied Dog Behavior and Training: *Adaptation and Learning*, Blackwell, Ames, IA.

Mech, L.D. (1970) *The Wolf: Ecology of an Endangered Species*, Natural History Press, New York.

Scott, J.P. and Fuller, J.L. (1965) *Dog Behavior, the Genetic Basis*, The University of Chicago Press, Chicago and London.

Serpell, J. and Jagoe, J.A. (1995) Early experience and the development of behavior, in *The Domestic Dog, Its Evolution, Behavior and Interactions With People* (ed J. Serpell), Cambridge University Press, Cambridge.

Further reading

Fox, M.W. (1965) *Canine behavior*, Charles C Thomas, Springfield, IL.

Peterson, M.E. and Kutzler, M.A. (eds) (2011) *Small Animal Pediatrics*, Elsevier, St. Louis.

3 Feline behavior and development

Debbie Martin[1,2]

[1] TEAM Education in Animal Behavior, LLC, Spicewood, TX, USA
[2] Veterinary Behavior Consultations, LLC, Spicewood, TX, USA

Understanding how cats perceive the world and the social nature of cats helps us to better understand their tendencies for specific behaviors. In order to be able to recognize abnormal behavior, one must first have knowledge of normal behavior for the species. Cats have become the most popular pet in the United States (Flanigan et al., 2007). Relinquishment of cats to animal shelters is also common. About a third of cats relinquished are surrendered due to behavior problems, including Inappropriate Elimination (IE), problems between other pets in the household, aggression toward humans, and destructive behavior (Salman et al., 2000).

The veterinary behavior technician needs to be fluent in understanding felines, including their sensory capacities, communication, social behavior, and development. This knowledge will allow the technician to educate and assist cat owners.

- The veterinary behavior technician needs to be fluent in understanding felines, including their sensory capacities, communication, social behavior, and development.

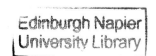

Feline sensory capacities

Cats are born with tactile, olfactory, gustatory, and vestibular abilities. Hearing, vision, and thermoregulation develop during the first weeks–months after birth (Bradshaw, 1992).

Vision

There is a wide range reported for the time period a kitten opens its eyes. It may occur anytime between 2 and 16 days (Villablanca and Olmstead, 1979). The average is 7–10 days. Although determined primarily by genetics, female kittens generally open their eyes earlier than males. Vision is not completely developed and adult-like until around 4–5 weeks of age (Bradshaw, 1992).

The cat's eyes are adapted for hunting in low light and have superior low-light vision. This is due to a combination of the large lens, pupil, and cornea, the tapetum lucidum, and a large number of rods. The tapetum lucidum, a layer of reflective cells behind the retina, reflects light back through the eye, allowing for a second chance of absorption by the rods and cones. Cats have about three times more rods (important for low-light vision) than humans and only about a sixth of the number of cones (used for color vision) (Berkley, 1976).

The visual field of cats is around 200° with binocular vision in the 90–100° range, which is similar to humans (Bradshaw, 1992). Cats are adept at noticing motion, which is advantageous when hunting field mice or preying on other small animals. Because of the blurring caused by the tapetum lucidum and decreased resolution due to the increased number of rods, the cat's visual acuity is limited (Beaver, 2003).

It has been determined that cats are able to see some color. Most likely they have dichromatic vision, with sensitivity to greenish-yellow and blue. However, their ability to see a diversity of colors is limited. The domestic cat's eye is not specialized for color vision and the importance of color is likely minimal for the species.

> • The domestic cat's eye is not specialized for color vision and the importance of color is likely minimal for the species.

The pupil of the cat can quickly constrict to a thin slit. This is to protect the light-sensitive retina. This ability is common in nocturnal animals that also spend time in full sun (Beaver, 2003) (Figure 3.1).

The physiological composition of the eyes of Siamese and Burmese cats show a difference in the ganglion cells

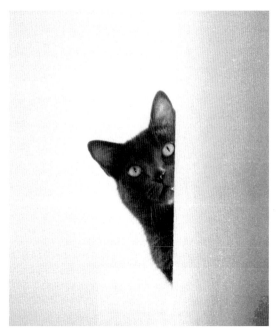

Figure 3.1 The cat is capable of quickly constricting the pupils into narrow slits to protect the retina. (*Source*: Danielle G. Theule.)

(compared to nonoriental breeds of cats)and also a lack of stereoscopic vision resulting in poor depth perception. However, they do have a normal field of vision and no difference in acuity compared to other breeds (Bradshaw, 1992).

Hearing

At birth, kittens have the neurological ability to hear. However, the ear canals are blocked by skin folds. As the kitten develops and the pinnae extend, the ability to hear increases. By 3–4 weeks of age, the hearing ability is comparable to an adult cat.

Auditory stimuli are important for the night-time hunter. The mobility of the pinnae allows the ears to rotate 180° independent of each other. This aids in the cat's ability to locate the source of sounds. The shape of the pinna also amplifies the sound (Bradshaw, 1992).

Cats hear a wider range of frequencies compared to people (humans ~20–19,000 Hz) but similar to the range of the dog (dog up to 65,000 Hz). The cat's auditory frequency ranges from approximately 20 Hz up to 85,000–100,000 Hz, with the functional or useful limit likely around 60,000 Hz (Beaver, 2003; Bradshaw, 1992). The ability to hear high frequency is conducive to detecting sounds emitted by prey such as mice.

- The ability to hear high frequency is conducive to detecting sounds emitted by prey such as mice.

Olfaction

The sense of smell is present at birth. Compared to people, a cat's sensitivity to smells is much higher. A person's olfactory epithelium is approximately $2-4\,\text{cm}^2$ whereas a cat's is approximately $20\,\text{cm}^2$ (dog's range $20-200\,\text{cm}^2$) (Bradshaw, 1992).

Cats mainly rely on visual, auditory, and tactile senses for hunting. Unlike the dog, cats do not track prey utilizing olfaction. However, olfactory cues are an important means of social communication between cats and will be discussed in more detail in the communication section of this chapter.

- Olfactory cues are an important means of social communication between cats.

Vomeronasal organ

The vomeronasal or Jacobson organ is connected to the oral and nasal cavity. When investigating a smell such as urine from another cat, the cat will open its mouth and show a "flehmen-like" response or gape; the upper lip is retracted and the mouth is held open about a quarter inch for a few seconds. This allows the scent to travel through the vomeronasal organ, which is neurologically connected to the limbic system (emotional center) of the brain. The gape response is performed on nonfood-based scents and generally only in response to odors of other cats; thus it likely is used for social information gathering (Turner and Bateson, 2000).

Taste

Cats have the ability to detect a variety of tastes. The typical adult cat responds to salty, sour, and bitter tastes. The cat's response to sugars is inconclusive, with some contradicting information in the literature. Cats, being obligate carnivores with a natural diet high in fat and protein, likely have minimal receptors dedicated to sweet tastes (Beaver, 2003; Bradshaw, 1992).

Touch

Tactile sensitivity is the first sense to develop in the cat. In fact it is functional in utero (Turner and Bateson, 2000). Although not able to regulate their body temperature at birth, kittens respond to temperature

fluctuations and as young kittens (first 1–2 weeks) will root or bury their head in warm objects (Beaver, 2003). At birth, when touched on the side of the face or abdomen, kittens will turn their head in the direction of the touch.

Perhaps adapted to aid in the feline's hunting ability and manipulation of prey, the pads, especially the front pads, have an increased sensitivity to touch and vibrations. Not only are the feet and pads densely packed with receptors, but the claws also have specialized sensory cells (Bradshaw, 1992).

The cranial and carpal vibrassae provide sensory information regarding the surroundings and may aid the cat in nocturnal hunting (Beaver, 2003). The carpal vibrassae are located on the caudal surface of the wrist. The cranial vibrassae include

mystacial – located on the upper lip and arranged in rows,
superciliary – located above each eye
genal tufts 1 and 2 – located below each ear near the mandibular angle,
mandibular – located on the chin (Figure 3.2).

Feline communication

Cats use a variety of methods for communication: visual (body language), auditory, and olfactory. The importance of each may vary depending on the context, the individual cat, and previous learning history.

Visual communication

Cats can be very subtle in their body language; a glance or look may communicate to an approaching cat to

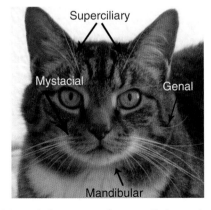

Figure 3.2 Facial vibrissae: superciliary, mandibular, genal, and mystical marked by arrows.

find an alternate route. Body language is often used to avoid or end confrontation. Many owners recognize outward signs of tension between cats such as hissing, growling, or swatting. The more subtle visual communication leading up to more intense communication may be completely overlooked. The veterinary behavior technician can help educate owners on typical feline communication and likely interpretations.

Although the individual components of body postures will be discussed, it is often necessary to look at the entire picture including the context, in order to understand the intended message. A majority of visual communication will either be referred to as *distance increasing* (go away), *neutral*, or *distance decreasing* (come closer).

> • Although the individual components of body postures will be discussed, it is often necessary to look at the entire picture including the context, in order to understand the intended message.

Body postures

The overall posture of the cat can be indicative of the general demeanor of the cat. (Table 3.1) A cat resting on its side with ears up or slightly to the side, eyes half opened, and tail dormant indicates a relaxed cat (neutral) (Figure 3.3). A cat carrying its weight forward with the hind legs slightly higher than their forelegs, tailed dropped but not tucked, ears to the side or forward, and maintaining direct eye contact is displaying an offensive threat (distance increasing) (see Figure 3.5). In comparison, a cat that turns sideways with the tail tucked or arched near the body, avoiding eye contact, and ears to the side or back is said to be displaying more defensive or fearful body language (also distance increasing). Piloerection, erecting the hair along the back and tail, may be performed by the offensive or defensive cat. However, generally with a more offensive display, the hair will only be raised along the spine and tail (see Figure 3.5) and with a defensive display, a more generalized raising of all the hair may be seen.

Rolling refers to a cat that rolls on its side and back exposing the abdomen (Figure 3.4). This posture can be seen in kittens as an invitation for play, during proestrus in females (Bradshaw, 1992), and also at times in response to a social encounter. It is generally seen in times of nonaggressive encounters (Bradshaw, 1992). However, it does not necessarily communicate a cat wants to be petted on the abdomen. Many cats will become agitated or over-stimulated if rubbed on the belly and may turn and nip or scratch the person.

Table 3.1 Body posture: a generalization of possible postures/positions and their meanings. Some cats may display a combination of body cues which seem to contradict each other, thus making it difficult to interpret.

Posture	Neutral	Distance increasing (go away)	Distance decreasing (come closer)
Resting on side, ears up or slightly to side, eyes half opened, tail dormant	√	–	–
Weight forward with hind legs slightly higher than forelegs, tail dropped but not tucked, ears to side or forward, direct eye contact	–	√ (offensive threat)	–
Turned sideways, tail tucked or arched near the body, avoiding eye contact, ears to side or back	–	√ (defensive threat)	–
Rolling or rubbing	–	–	√

Play postures

Social play is most prevalent between 4 and 16 weeks of age (Beaver, 2003). Through play, kittens often display body language associated with predatory and aggressive behavior. For example, a kitten may crouch and then spring at the other kitten (predatory) or piloerect the hair along the spine and tail and side step around the other cat (defensive aggressive displays) in mock play fighting. Perhaps other subtle signals such as facial expression and tail movement and rate, modify the meaning of the signals and signify play rather than true aggression.

Veterinary behaviorist Bonnie Beaver describes eight different play behaviors seen in kittens in her book, *Feline Behavior: A Guide for Veterinarians*. These postures include belly-up, stand-up, side-step, pounce, vertical stance or rearing, chase, horizontal leap, and face-off. Some of these same behaviors are displayed in play with objects as well.

Tail positions

The tail does not only have a functional purpose as an organ of balance in hunting and stalking prey, but is also

Figure 3.3 Relaxed state: resting on side, ears up but neutral, eyes half opened, tail still.

Figure 3.4 A cat rolling on its back as an invitation for an amicable interaction.

used to signal and communicate information regarding a cat's mood or intentions (Table 3.2).

- The tail does not only have a functional purpose as an organ of balance in hunting and stalking prey, but is also used to signal and communicate information regarding a cat's mood or intentions.

The relaxed neutral position for a cat's tail is horizontal, with slight drooping. The neutral position signifies a relaxed, confident, or slightly alert cat. A twitching tail or flicking tip of the tail can indicate agitation or high arousal and is usually a distance-increasing signal. A cat that appears to be resting calmly but with the entire tail thrashing or the tip flicking, should be approached with

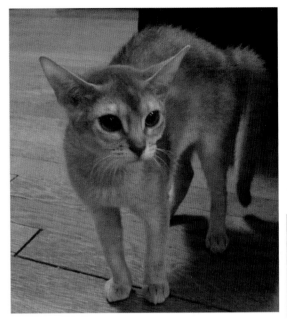

Figure 3.5 This cat displays a variety of body language. Notice the inverted L tail position, slightly raised hindlegs, piloerection along the spine and tail, direct stare, ears slightly to the side, and the whiskers forward, all indicating a more offensive threat. However, the body is turned slightly sideways and the pupils are dilated, signs indicative of defensive aggression.

caution. The tail will quiver or shake rapidly back and forth when a cat is spraying urine, as well as when it is excited, and in a friendly greeting. The tail held high winding back and forth like a flag pole is considered a friendly greeting (distance-decreasing signal). In contrast the tail held completely vertical with piloerection (known as an *upright bottle brush appearance*) indicates fear and defensive aggression – a distance-increasing signal. A tail tucked to the side or between the legs is also a sign of fear. In comparison, the tail held in an inverted L (the first inch or so is horizontal and the remainder points straight down) signifies an offensive aggression (Figure 3.5). Although a distance-increasing signal, it is also a sign of conflicting motivations. The cat is more confident and offensive than a cat displaying a tucked or bottle brush tail, but is also afraid or feeling threatened; thus the somewhat ambivalent tail position.

- A cat that appears to be resting calmly but with the entire tail thrashing or the tip flicking, should be approached with caution.

Table 3.2 Tail position and possible meanings.

Tail position	Neutral	Distance increasing (go away)	Distance decreasing (come closer)
Twitching or flicking	–	√ High arousal or agitation	–
Quivering	–	√ High arousal and when spraying	√ Excited friendly greeting usually accompanied with tail winding.
Flag pole/tail winding	–	–	√ Friendly greeting
Horizontal with slight drooping	√ Relaxed, alert	–	–
Vertical with piloerection/upright bottle brush appearance	–	√ Fear and defensive aggression	–
Tucked to side or between the legs	–	√ Fear and defensive aggression	–
Inverted L: first inch is horizontal and reminder points straight down	–	√ Fear and offensive aggression	–

Facial expressions

Table 3.3 categorizes the different facial expressions.

Head

How a cat holds its head provides insight into the intended communication, but it is difficult to decipher the meaning without looking at the face and other body parts. For example, stretching the head forward could be encouraging social interaction with another animal or person or be a greeting used to acquire more visual and possibly olfactory information about the acquaintance. When exploring a novel item in the environment, the cat will stretch its head out to gain more information about the object.

The head could be raised up high, indicating a cat that is alert, offensive, fearful, or defensive, depending on the tail and general body posture. In contrast, a cat that holds its head midline with the chin slightly down may indicate lack of interest, nonthreat, or be relaxed (neutral). Turning the head to the side and avoiding eye contact is likely used to avoid confrontation. A head tucked (held back and down) is more common in fear and aggression. Again, other visual signals such as the ear position, eyes, tail, and general posture will also enhance interpretation.

Eyes

A neutral and relaxed cat will often hold its eyes half open. Prolonged direct eye contact is a threatening signal (distance increasing) (see Figure 3.5). Ever wonder why cats in general seek out the noncat person in a room to interact with? It is usually because that person is avoiding eye contact with the cat.

Besides adjusting to light, the pupils of the eyes can give us information about the cat's mood. Dilation is seen in a variety of contexts including play, high arousal or excitement, fear, and defensive aggression. Constriction of the pupils can be seen in a content cat but also occurs during offensive aggression.

Ears

Each cat ear has 32 muscles associated with movement of the pinnae. The cat can move its ears independent of each other, rotate 180° and move them up and down. Not only are the ears utilized in locating small prey while hunting, but they are also used to communicate.

> - Each cat ear has 32 muscles associated with movement of the pinnae. The cat can move its ears independent of each other, rotate 180°, and move them up and down.

In a neutral state, the ears are forward or slightly to the side. Slightly back to flattened ears signify fear and possible aggression. An offensively aggressive cat will also carry its ears back or to the side. Perked forward can indicate interest in something. One ear might flick or orient in one direction indicating the cat is listening to something in that direction. A cat displaying one ear up and one ear flattened back is perhaps in a motivational conflict (curious but also afraid) and is displaying ambivalent body language.

Mouth/whiskers

The whiskers are to the side in a relaxed or neutral state. They will perk forward when interested or aroused by something or in an offensive threat (see Figure 3.5). In

Table 3.3 Facial expression and possible meanings: it is the combination of expressions, not just one, that will provide the key to proper interpretation.

Body part	Expression	Neutral	Distance increasing (go away)	Distance decreasing (come closer)
Head	Stretched forward	–	–	√ Could be exploration or seeking social contact
	Raised	–	√ High arousal, defensive or offensive threat	√ Alert, Excited, curious
	Midline and chin slightly down	√ Lack of interest, relaxed, nonthreat	–	–
	Turned to side and avoiding eye contact	√ Could be neutral	√ Used to avoid conflict	–
	Tucked down	–	√ Fear and defensive aggression	–
Eyes	Half open	√ Relaxed	–	–
	Prolonged direct eye contact	–	√ Offensive threat	–
	Avoiding eye contact	√ Nonthreat	√ Avoid conflict	–
	Dilated pupils	–	√ High arousal, fear, defensive aggression	√ Excited, alert, play
	Constricted pupils	√ Content, response to light	√ Offensive aggression	–
Ears	Forward or slightly to the side	√ Relaxed	–	–
	Slightly back to flattened	–	√ Fear and defensive aggression	–
	Back or to the side	–	√ Offensive aggression	–
	Perked forward	–	√ Alert, aroused	√ Curious, interested
	One ear up and one flattened	–	√ Ambivalent	√ Ambivalent
Whiskers	To the side	√ Relaxed	–	–
	Perked forward	–	√ Alert, aroused, offensive threat	√ Curious, interested
	Held back along the cheeks	–	√ Fear and defensive aggression	–
Mouth	Yawn	√ Contentment	√ Used to defuse tension	–

contrast, whiskers held back along the cheeks signify either fear or nonthreat.

The mouth is held open during a variety of vocal communications. Similar to the dog but less often, a cat may yawn to defuse tension and signal nonthreat. However, it may also signal contentment (Figure 3.6).

Auditory communication

Some cats are more vocal than others. Perhaps a cat that is primarily communicating with humans has learned people respond to auditory signals better than visual ones; thus the cat has learned to utilize a larger variety of vocalizations.

Examples of distance-decreasing sounds include the sexual mating calls, the meow, and the purr. They are generally used in amicable interactions and greetings. Kittens are capable of purring almost at birth and will purr while nursing. Purring is usually exhibited during what appears to be pleasurable circumstances. The exception is when an ill or severely injured cat purrs continuously (Beaver, 2003). Perhaps purring soothes the cat when sick or in pain.

Distance-increasing vocalizations include the hiss, growl (offensive or defensive), shriek, spit, and yowl. The yowl or howl can also be heard when a cat is in distress and communicates a call for help (Table 3.4).

Cats will also produce a variety of chirps and trills and unique vocalizations specific to each individual cat.

Figure 3.6 A cat yawning in contentment or to defuse tension. More information about the situation is necessary to determine motivation.

Table 3.4 Common auditory communication.

Meaning	Vocalization
Distance increasing (go away)	Hiss, growl, shriek, spit, yowl, or howl
Distance decreasing (come closer)	Sexual mating calls (can include a yowl), meow, purr

Olfactory communication

Olfactory communication is extremely important to the cat. Each cat has its own signature scent. When it grooms itself, it transfers scent from its saliva and from glands around the head and pads to the fur. A feline colony establishes a communal scent and it is used to recognize and identify members of the colony. Allorubbing refers to a tactile exchange between cats, whereby one cat will rub against the other, usually starting at the neck. This behavior likely is used to mix their scents and appears to be a friendly behavior. In one large farm study, females and younger cats initiated allorubbing more often than males or older cats (Bradshaw, 1992).

- Olfactory communication is extremely important to the cat. Each cat has its own signature scent.

- A feline colony establishes a communal scent and it is used to recognize and identify members of the colony.

Because scent is so important, in multiple cat households when one cat goes to the veterinarian, he may be initially rejected by the other cats upon returning home. This may in large part be due to a change in scent. Preventive measures should be taken to avoid negative encounters when reintroducing a cat (specific recommendations will be provided in Chapter 7).

Scent glands are located on the chin, corners of the lips, temples, tail base, and pads. Cats will rub their scent glands on objects within the core area of their territory to mark it with their scent. When marking with the front claws, not only is a scent from the glands deposited, but a visual mark is also left from the claws.

Cats may use urine to mark the outskirts and high traffic areas of a territory. Urine marking is considered an anxiety-related behavior. It is also associated with sexual behavior. An intact male will mark frequently in response to an estrus female. With marking, the urine is generally deposited on vertical surfaces but can also be deposited on novel items or objects with concentrated scent. The tail is held high and may quiver back and forth. Middening is the term used for marking with feces. It is relatively uncommon but if it occurs, the feces are usually deposited in high traffic locations or pathways.

Reading the entire cat

The neutral and content cat will display half-open eyes, narrow pupils, tail relaxed and still, and ears forward or mostly forward. He may purr or meow as well.

The playful cat displays partially dilated pupils, whiskers and ears forward, and tail up.

Fear and anxiety may be displayed with the pupils dilated, head tucked, ears back or to the side, body tucked or turned sideways, tail tucked or between the legs, complete piloerection, and whiskers held back. A defensive cat may growl, hiss, or spit.

Offensive aggression may be displayed with constricted pupils, direct eye contact, ears back, inverted L tail, piloerection along the spine, and head up or moving from side to side. The offensive cat may growl or yowl.

Feline domestication, social structure, and behavior

Domestication

The domestic cat is thought to be descendent from the wild cat *Felis silverstris* and specifically the African or Arabian wild cat, *Felis silverstris lybica* (Clutton-Brock, 1987). The oriental breeds may have descended from the Indian Desert Cat, *Felis silverstris ornata* (Bradshaw,

CHAPTER 3

1992). *F.s. ornata* was a leaner cat compared to the stockier *F.s.* lybica. The formal classification of the domestic cat is *Felis silverstris catus*.

Domestication was a gradual process but likely started around 4000 BC in Egypt. Around 1600 BC, cats appear to have become involved in everyday human activities as depicted in artwork during that time. Domestication of the cat resulted in less behavioral changes compared to other domesticated animals. The notable changes included a reduced brain size, a change in hormone balance (decreased adrenals), and retention of juvenile behavior characteristics into adulthood (neoteny) (Bradshaw, 1992). What is unique to the domestication of the cat is that domestication may have occurred as a result of religious beliefs rather than just utilitarian purposes. Although cats certainly were instrumental in controlling rodent populations, they were also considered sacred by the ancient Egyptians. Recognition of a cat goddess was even part of the ancient Egyptian religion (Bradshaw, 1992).

- Domestication of the cat resulted in less behavioral changes compared to other domesticated animals.

Social organization of domestic cats

Many issues arise in the human domestic environment when the innate behavior of the cat is not understood or taken into consideration. By studying the natural tendencies of the domestic cat in a less restricted environment than a human household, one is able to identify trends in behavior when given a choice. Information regarding the dynamics of intraspecies relationships of cats has mainly been obtained through the study of groups of cats living in a specific outdoor location.

Although *Felis silverstris lybica* was solitary, the domestic cat appears to vary widely in regard to sociability. The domestic cat has the ability to be either solitary or social (social flexibility) depending on early experiences and genetics. In regard to friendliness to humans, the genetics of the sire appears to have a more profound impact than early experience (Reisner et al., 1994).

- In regard to friendliness to humans, the genetics of the sire appears to have a more profound impact than early experience.

Feline groups or colonies will form, depending on the availability of resources (primarily food). A colony may consist of 30–50 cats but a majority of colonies consist of 10 or fewer. The colonies mainly consist of females and their young.

This matrilineal group will cooperatively rear litters together and will defend their home range from unknown cats (male or female). Females tend to stay their entire life with the colony in which they were born. Within a colony cats will have preferred associations.

Juvenile males will usually leave the colony by 2–3 years of age. Mature males may form loose associations with a group or multiple groups but are more solitary than females.

Regarding home range and territory, the home range will be larger than the core territory of the cat. The exception is the house cat, for which the home range and territory will often be the same. The home range of several males may overlap but the territory will be defended against other cats (Beaver, 2003).

Home ranges vary greatly in size. On average, a male cat will have a home range 3.5 times larger than females in the same area (Liberg and Sandell, 1988). In a human household, adult male cats will on average utilize 5.4 rooms and adult females 3.9 rooms (Bernstein and Strack, 1996). A cat will utilize approximately 360 sq ft (40 sq yd) of living space (Heidenberger, 1997). Cats may time-share favored resting space on a rotational basis within the household.

This tendency to be territorial, or unaccepting of new cats, is a trend seen in mature house cats as well. In a multiple cat household, providing ample resources and increasing vertical living space allows for several core territories, thus decreasing social tension. Cat trees and perches add additional square footage to the territory (Figures 3.7 and 3.8). Strong bonds can form between cats if they are together as kittens. Littermates will have a closer relationship with each other than two unrelated individuals (Bradshaw and Hall, 1999). When introducing a new cat to a household with existing cats, a systematic approach should be taken to provide for the best chance of successful integration. A detailed process of how to properly introduce cats is given in Chapter 7.

- In a multiple cat household, providing ample resources and increasing vertical living space allows for several core territories, thus decreasing social tension.

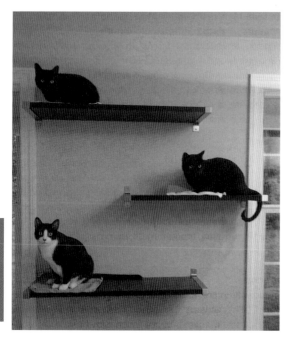

Figure 3.7 Shelves with perches for cats allow for increased vertical living space.

Sexual behavior

The female cat will reach sexual maturity on average between 3.5 and 12 months of age. Cats are seasonally polyestruous, meaning they will have several estrous cycles per season. Although some individual cats will cycle year round, most cats in the United States cycle from February to April and June to August (Beaver, 2003). Most cats are anestrous in the Fall from September through December.

Proestrus is accompanied by an increase in activity, object rubbing, and less aggression toward an approaching male. Within a 24-h period, the female will increase rolling, rubbing, and kneading. At this point, she will allow close contact from a male but not tolerate any attempts at being mounted (Bradshaw, 1992).

In estrus, rolling is discontinued and instead the female assumes a lordosis position whereby her head is close to the ground, the back is arched ventrally, the hind limbs are up and the tail is raised and to the side. She is receptive to being mounted by a male. During copulation, the male will grasp the female by the nape of the neck with his jaws. Multiple copulations are necessary to induce ovulation (Bradshaw, 1992). Cats are considered induced ovulators because of the need for copulation to trigger ovulation. The reproductive cycle of the cat is an efficient one. It is estimated that in 7 years, one female

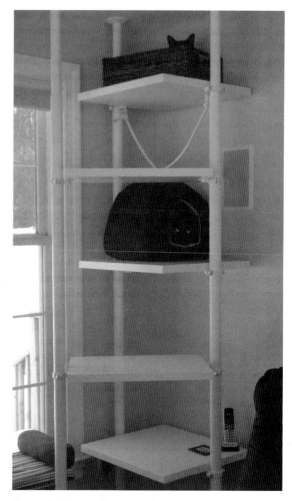

Figure 3.8 Floor-to-ceiling cat perches.

cat and her offspring could be responsible for 781,250 kittens.(Mahlow and Slater, 1996; Olson and Johnston, 1993)

Cats are polygamous and the estrus female may be bred by multiple males. In fact, several males will congregate around a receptive female. Interestingly enough, it is noted that when this occurs, there is less aggression between the males (Bradshaw, 1992). One would think that competition for an estrous female would elicit increased aggressive encounters in the toms. However, that is not the case.

Males become sexually mature around 9–12 months of age. A surge in testosterone at around 3.5 months of age can be evidenced by testosterone-induced behaviors such as mounting in play as early as 4 months of age. Although there has been at least one report of infanticide (tom cat killing kittens sired by other males in a colony), it does not appear to be common practice in domestic feral cats (Bradshaw, 1992).

Maternal behavior

Gestation lasts about 63 days. About 1 week prior to parturition, the queen will select a den site. As mentioned earlier, cat colonies consist primarily of a matrilineal group. A communal den near the food source is a successful strategy that results in a lower mortality rate when compared to individual dens further from the food source (Bradshaw, 1992). Adult female cats in the group will assist with the care of the young. Even during parturition, another female cat may assist with cleaning and drying the young immediately postpartum.

Epimeletic, care giving, behaviors exhibited by the queen include

- licking the kittens to clean them and stimulate urination and defecation during the first weeks of life,
- initiating nursing,
- retrieving kittens that have wandered from the litter, and
- responding to kitten vocalizations.

Kittens will exhibit care seeking, et-epimeletic, behaviors such as distress vocalization when cold or hungry.

The cat–human relationship is probably similar to a kitten–mother relationship whereby the people act as the care giver and the cat will display care-seeking behavior.

- The cat–human relationship is probably similar to a kitten–mother relationship whereby the people act as the care giver and the cat will display care-seeking behavior.

Ingestive and predatory behavior

The suckling reflex is present at birth. During the first 3 weeks of life, the queen initiates nursing. Teat preference is established during the first few days of life and lasts approximately 1 month (Beaver, 2003). Kittens will continue to nurse on average until 8–10 weeks of age. Weaning is a gradual process. Kittens can start to eat solid food around 1 month.

Cats are carnivores and if raised in a feral or semiferal setting, the queen must teach the kittens how to hunt. When the kittens are around a month old, the mother will bring dead prey back to the litter and later (around 2 months) injured but live prey. Chasing and catching prey is an innate behavior that needs to be practiced to be perfect. However, manipulating, killing, and ingesting

prey is learned (Beaver, 2003). Kittens will hunt what their mother hunted. If a cat was not taught to hunt as a young kitten, only about half will be able to learn to hunt as an adult and it is a much lengthier process (Beaver, 2003).

Cats prefer to eat small meals frequently. Consequently, free choice feeding is less stressful for the cat (Finco et al., 1986).

- Cats prefer to eat small meals frequently. Consequently, free choice feeding is less stressful for the cat.

Eliminative behavior

During the first 3 weeks of life, urination and defecation must be stimulated by the urogenital reflex. This is generally accomplished by the queen licking the perineal region. The queen also ingests the excrement, thus keeping the nest clean and odor free. Kittens begin to be able to eliminate on their own by 3 weeks of age. By 1 month of age, kittens will start to explore dirt and litter and dig or rake the substrate with their forepaws. Because ingestion of substrate may also occur during this early exploration, caution should be used with clumping and expanding litters with young kittens (Marder, 1997).

Cats generally prefer large, open, linerless litter boxes with an unscented fine-grained substrate. (More information on litter box training and preference can be found in Chapter 7). A typical urination includes digging a small hole in the substrate, squatting to urinate, and then covering the urine by pulling the substrate over the spot with the forepaws. Not all cats perform the digging or covering behavior. The adult cat urinates on average 2–3 times a day.

Cats may not dig as much prior to defecation (Pannaman, 1981). Within the core area, it is common for the feces to be covered following defecation. Although it has been noted that uncovered feces may be left along hunting paths and elevated surfaces and is more common in territorial males (Cooper, 1997), it is generally thought that marking with feces, middening, does not occur (Beaver, 2003) or is rare in the domestic cat. The number of defecations in a 24-h period is variable and dependent on diet and the individual. Commercially available condensed diet may limit defecation to less than once a day.

Feline inappropriate elimination (FIE) problems account for a vast number of behavioral complaints by owners. Inappropriate elimination damages the human–animal bond and often results in relinquishment. A thorough medical workup is warranted for any cat exhibiting inappropriate elimination. Medical factors may cause or exasperate an FIE issue. At the very least, they will undermine the success of treatment if not identified and addressed. Generally, FIE will fall into one of two categories.

1. House soiling: The cat has either a preference for a different substrate than what is being provided or an aversion to the existing options. An aversion or avoidance of the box can be facilitated by social or environmental stress in the household.

2. Marking: It is a sexual or an anxiety-driven inappropriate elimination issue.

Often a case will present that is a combination of house soiling and marking rather than one or the other.

- Feline inappropriate elimination (FIE) problems account for a vast number of behavioral complaints by owners.

- FIE damages the human–animal bond and often results in relinquishment.

- A thorough medical workup is warranted for any cat exhibiting inappropriate elimination.

Urine marking

Although urine marking often occurs on vertical surfaces on the outskirts of the territory, it can also be performed on horizontal surfaces within the territory. Anxiety associated with a novel item brought into the house may stimulate a cat to urinate on the object. The concentrated scent of an absent owner could produce frustration or anxiety resulting in urine marking of the person's side of the bed. Stress associated with changes in routine, other cats in or around the home, social tension between existing cats, novel items or smells could all be triggers that result in urine marking.

Urine marking occurs in males and females, as well as intact and neutered cats. However, prevalence is higher in intact males due to urine spraying associated with sexual behavior. Urine marking has a genetic component to it (Halip et al., 1992). Neutering of the male and female cat can considerably decrease marking: 90% in males and 95% in females (Hart and Cooper, 1984).

It was initially thought that urine marking was performed with only small amounts of urine. However, recent studies by veterinary behaviorist Jacqueline Neilson have indicated that the volume of a regular void and void associated with marking are similar in quantity.

Exploratory behavior and activity levels

Domestic cats generally spread their activity throughout a 24-h period with a majority of activity occurring during the day. Rather than being crepuscular (active at dusk and dawn) or nocturnal, they are likely partially diurnal (Bradshaw, 1992). Depending on the environment of the cat (house cat vs. feral cat), an individual cat's circadian rhythm may be affected by the activity level of a household or availability of food or prey. A feral cat will be forced to hunt at a time that its preferred prey is active. However, many feral cats hunt a variety of small animals that have various peak activity levels in a 24-h period.

- Domestic cats generally spread their activity throughout a 24-h period with a majority of activity occurring during the day. Rather than being crepuscular (active at dusk and dawn) or nocturnal, they are likely partially diurnal.

To provide the indoor cat with appropriate exploration and activity, cat owners will need to provide enrichment to meet the cat's needs (Figure 3.9). Specific strategies will be covered in Chapter 7, including providing a variety of interactive toys and food storage devices, scheduling set play and training times, and providing vertical living space for exploration and hiding.

Grooming behavior

Cats spend a large amount of their awake-time grooming. In fact, about 50% of awake-time or about 3.6 h of a 24-h period is spent grooming. (Eckstein and Hart, 2000; Pannaman, 1981).

During the first few weeks of life, the queen grooms the kittens until they learn to perform it on their own. Self-grooming starts around 2 weeks of age. Beaver reports that kittens that were not well groomed early in life, are more likely to be less fastidious groomers as adults (Beaver, 2003). Cleanliness is likely learned and strongly influenced by experience during the first few weeks of life.

Grooming appears to have four main functions (Beaver, 2003). The most obvious is maintenance of healthy skin and coat. Grooming will remove extra hair to prevent matting and also remove ectoparasites. Another function of grooming is to dissipate heat as it provides for evaporative cooling (Hart, 1976). The third purpose may be an affiliative behavior between cats when one cat grooms another. The final purpose of

Figure 3.9 Providing exploration and enrichment: two cats exploring ways to dislodge the balls from the hanging fabric.

grooming may be as a calming behavior for the cat or a communicative one. A cat when placed in a stressful situation may start to groom. Perhaps self-grooming is used to help soothe the cat, or decrease tension. Rather than reacting to the stimuli, the cat stops what it is doing and begins to groom. This is an example of a displacement behavior.

> - The four main functions of grooming:
>   1. Maintain healthy skin and coat
>   2. Dissipate heat
>   3. Affiliative behavior between cats
>   4. Calming or communicative

With normal self-grooming, a majority of it is performed with the tongue and teeth: oral grooming. It is usually performed from the fore body to the tail. The forepaws and hindpaws are used to reach areas that the cat is unable to reach with its mouth. The cat will lick its forepaws and then wipe its neck, ears, head, and face. Utilizing the hindpaws to scratch the neck and behind the ears is the least frequent grooming behavior performed.

The front nails will be maintained by scratching them along a surface. This behavior has a dual purpose of maintaining nail health as well as use in olfactory and visual communication.

A decrease or increase in self-grooming behavior may be a sign of a medical or behavioral condition and warrants investigation by a veterinarian.

> - A decrease or increase in self-grooming behavior may be a sign of a medical or behavioral condition and warrants investigation by a veterinarian.

Mutual grooming or allogrooming is performed by one cat to another cat. The head and neck areas are the most frequent locations groomed. Allogrooming occurs while the cats are at rest. Some cats will rest next to each other but not groom one another (Bradshaw, 1992). It appears to be a friendly behavior by the initiator; however, some recipients may not be accepting of being groomed.

Feline behavioral development

Feline behavioral development is affected by numerous factors. Genetics plays a role. In fact, friendliness toward humans is directly linked to the tom (Reisner et al., 1994). However, early experience and learning also has an effect. Behavior is a combination of genetics and experience or learning. The genetic platform may prime the individual for specific behavior, but without experience those characteristics will not reach fruition.

> - The genetic platform may prime the individual for specific behavior, but without experience those characteristics will not reach fruition.

At birth, the nervous system is still developing. Without appropriate stimuli, sensory perception may not develop normally. To optimize development, an enriched environment is necessary.

Developmental periods and life stages
The developmental periods of cats have not been as clearly defined as with dogs. The Humane Society of the

CHAPTER 3

United States and Denver Dumb Friends League identify a neonatal period (0–2 weeks), socialization period (2–7 weeks), most active play period (7–14 weeks), ranking period (3–6 months), and adolescence (6–18 months). AAFP-AAHA: Feline Life Stage Guidelines (Vogt et al., 2010) suggest a broader age classification system to help focus attention on specific physical and behavioral characteristics. They are Kitten (birth to 6 months), Junior (7 months to 2 years), Prime (3–6 years), Mature (7–10 years), Senior (11–14 years), and Geriatric (15+ years).

Classification of age ranges can help guide the veterinary professional in regard to typical life changes that may occur during a specific time. Sensitive periods of development are different than classification by life stages. Cats have some sensitive periods early in development when, if particular stimuli are not provided, normal development cannot occur. A sensitive period represents a time that is conducive to specific learning or experiences. The most sensitive period of development in cats is from birth to 3–4 months of age.

In an attempt to simplify terminology, this author will use the same terms that were used to define the canine developmental periods of life and apply these periods and life stages to cats. Obvious differences will be the demarcation of age for specific stages and developmental milestones specific to the species.

Although ages will be used to define a period, these are only guidelines. Each individual will develop at slightly different rates (Table 3.5).

Fetal

The fetal period occurs in utero and ends at birth. The nutritional, emotional, and physical status of the queen will have a profound impact on the development of the fetuses. Chronic stress and poor nutrition of the queen can affect not only the physical development but also the psychological development of the kittens.

A malnourished queen (both prenatally and during lactation) is more likely to have kittens with poor learning abilities, poor social skills with other cats, and increased emotionality, including abnormal levels of fear and aggression (Turner and Bateson, 2000).

> • A malnourished queen (both prenatally and during lactation) is more likely to have kittens with poor learning abilities, poor social skills with other cats, and increased emotionality, including abnormal levels of fear and aggression.

Neonatal

The neonatal period is from birth to about 10–14 days of age. The kittens are completely dependent on the queen for survival: nursing, thermoregulation, and elimination. Time is spent sleeping and nursing. Although cats are born with tactile, olfactory, gustatory, and vestibular abilities (ability to right themselves), they are blind and mostly deaf. Consequently they are fairly insulated from the world during this period.

Maternal nutrition and quality of milk influence the developmental rate of the kittens and deficits can produce lifelong deficiencies.

In contrast, mild stressors including gentle handling of the kittens or placing them on a cool surface for a few seconds, may have beneficial effects. A study with Siamese kittens revealed kittens that were held and stroked gently for a brief time every day during the first few weeks of life, opened their eyes earlier, left the nest sooner, and developed color points faster (Meier, 1961). Mild neonatal stress can produce beneficial effects including decreased emotionality and increased resistance to some diseases.

> • Mild stressors including gentle handling of the kittens or placing them on a cool surface for a few seconds, may have beneficial effects.

Transition

The transition or transitional period overlaps with the neonatal and socialization periods. It is defined as lasting from 10 to 21 days. The markers that signify this period include increased sensory abilities and increased mobility. The eyes open around 7–10 days (range 2–16 days).

Table 3.5 Developmental periods and life stages of cats.

Period	Duration
Fetal	Up to birth
Neonatal	Birth to 10–14 days
Transitional	~10–21 days of age
Socialization	2–7 (–10) weeks
Juvenile	~2 months to sexual maturity (~4–10 months)
Adolescent	Sexual maturity to social maturity (~2–4 years)
Adult	Social maturity to 11+ years
Senior	12+ years

The ears begin to open by 5 days with a response to loud sounds noted at that time. By 2 weeks of age, kittens will orient toward natural sounds (Olmstead and Villablanca, 1980). The teeth begin to erupt just before 2 weeks of age. At around 3 weeks, kittens begin to walk. Also at around 3 weeks of age, the kitten is better able to regulate its body temperature. Thermoregulation is fully developed by 7 weeks of age (Turner and Bateson, 2000).

Because of the developing senses and increased mobility, kittens become more aware of their surroundings and begin to interact more with stimuli (Figure 3.10).

Socialization

The socialization period lasts from 2 to 7 weeks of age and perhaps up to 10 weeks. This period is marked by decreasing reliance on the queen for survival and increased interaction with social and environmental stimuli. The socialization period is the most important sensitive period in the cat in regard to living in the human domestic household. The cat is primed to be able to bond with a variety of species through this time. Positive social experiences with other species allow the cat to become socialized and more accepting of those species throughout its lifetime. Although not impossible after this sensitive period, socialization is more difficult and less effective. Handling prior to 2 weeks of age does not have an effect on acceptance of humans. However, handling by humans after 2 weeks and before 7 weeks of age produces cats that are more responsive to people than those that were not handled (Beaver, 2003). If during the socialization period, kittens are gently handled by multiple people rather than just one person, they will be less fearful of people.

> • The socialization period is the most important sensitive period in the cat in regard to living in the human domestic household.

> • If during the socialization period, kittens are gently handled by multiple people rather than just one person, they will be less fearful of people.

Three to six weeks of age is the most influential time in regard to intraspecies (cat–cat) social development (Overall, 1992). Early weaning (before 5 weeks of age) and removal from the litter will cause inadequate

socialization with other cats. Possible behavioral consequences to early weaning include over attachment to humans, self-mutilation, lack of bite or claw inhibition, abnormal mating or maternal behavior, timidity, and fearfulness with or without aggression (Beaver, 2003). Social play with littermates is prevalent at 4 weeks of age and continues throughout the socialization period.

> • Possible behavioral consequences to early weaning include over attachment to humans, self-mutilation, lack of bite or claw inhibition, abnormal mating or maternal behavior, timidity, and fearfulness with or without aggression.

During the socialization period, kittens begin to eat solid food by 4 weeks of age and are completely weaned by 7–10 weeks. Starting around 3 weeks and cumulating at 5–6 weeks, kittens are able to voluntarily eliminate, thus no longer being dependent on the queen for stimulation. By 6–8 weeks of age, kittens will display an adult-like response to threatening social stimuli (Kolb and Nonneman, 1975). The end of this period is marked by the development of a fear response. See Figure 3.10 for a summary of developmental milestones during the first 3 months of life.

Juvenile

The juvenile stage is approximately from 2 months to sexual maturity (average 4–10 months of age). During this stage, object play becomes more prevalent and social play begins to slowly decrease by 12–14 weeks of age (West, 1974). Perhaps this is in part due to the need to develop fluent hunting skills in a feral setting. Thus the cat is perhaps genetically programmed to evolve in this manner for survival. Dexterity and motor skills are perfected during this stage.

Dr. Bonnie Beaver notes a normal period of human avoidance occurring around 7 weeks of age. Even kittens that have been socialized well with humans will show avoidance. However, the well-socialized kitten will rebound around 10 weeks of age and no longer display avoidance (Beaver, 2003).

Through the juvenile and into the adolescent stage, cats become less accepting of unfamiliar cats. Integration of a new cat into a household after a cat has reached sexual maturity can be more challenging. The bond between the cats may not be as strong if they were not introduced as young kittens. The end of this period is recognized by reaching sexual maturity.

CHAPTER 3

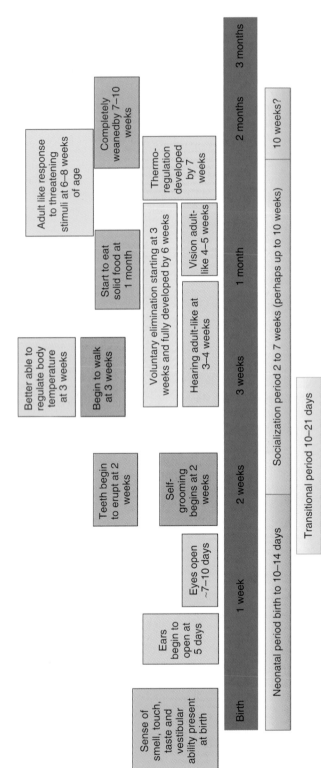

Figure 3.10 Developmental changes in the first 3 months of life.

Adolescent

The adolescent stage occurs from sexual maturity to social maturity. Social maturity is probably reached around 2–4 years of age (Overall, 1995). During adolescence, the cat continues to develop independence and males will often disperse from the colony.

Adolescent felines living in the human household will require sufficient mental and physical activity through environmental enrichment. Positive-based training not only provides enrichment but also enhances the human–animal bond (Figure 3.11a and b).

Adult

The adult stage is defined as commencing around social maturity and concluding around 11 years of age. There are no clear delineations for this stage.

Continuing to provide the indoor cat with sufficient exploration and play opportunities is important to maintain a physically and mentally healthy adult cat.

Senior

The senior or geriatric stage for cats is defined as 12+ years of age. Special care should be taken to ensure that a harmonious relationship continues between the aging cat and the owners.

Identifying and addressing medical issues that may have an impact on behavior help to maintain a strong human–animal bond. It might be necessary to educate clients that cats with mobility issues due to osteoarthritis may find a tall litter box located down a flight of stairs too difficult to navigate. Cognition issues in aging cats can lead to changes in sleep–wake cycles, excessive vocalization, pacing or restlessness, anxiety, and house soiling. Detecting early signs of cognitive dysfunction and providing early treatment may help to alleviate signs and slow the progression.

CHAPTER 3

M. Heigl

(a) (b)

Figure 3.11 (a) and (b) Examples of behaviors a young cat has been trained to perform using positive reinforcement.

Conclusion

The domestic feline is an adaptive animal that can live in groups or solitarily, depending on early experience. Cats have a complex communication system involving visual, auditory, and olfactory communication. Colonies of cats are generally comprised of females and their young. Cats are not accepting of unfamiliar cats and will protect their core territory.

As you will learn in Chapter 7, the veterinary technician can play a pivotal role in the prevention of behavior problems and disorders. Through a thorough understanding of normal development, sensory perception, social behavior, and innate behavior for a species, the veterinary behavior technician can empower others with this knowledge. Knowledge provides understanding and empathy and creates a client who is more likely to implement changes to help the cat be successful, improve the cat's welfare, and maintain the human–animal bond.

> • Knowledge provides understanding and empathy and creates a client who is more likely to implement changes to help the cat be successful, improve the cat's welfare, and maintain the human–animal bond.

References

Barry, K.J. and Crowell-Davis, S.L. (1999) Gender differences in the social behavior of the neutered indoor-only domestic cat. *Applied Animal Behaviour Science*, **64** (3), 193–211.

Beaver, B.V. (2003) Feline Behavior: A Guide for Veterinarians, *Second edition* edn, W. B. Saunders Company, Philadelphia.

Berkley, M.A. (1976) Cat visual psychophysics: neural correlates and comparisons with man. *Progress in Psychobiology and Physiological Psychology*, **6**, 63–119.

Bernstein, P.L. and Strack, M. (1996) A game of cat and house: spatial patterns and behavior of 14 cats (*Felis catus*) in the home. *Anthrozoös*, **9**, 25–39.

Bradshaw, J.W.S. (1992) *The Behaviour of the Domestic Cat*, CABI Publishing, Wallingford.

Bradshaw, J.W.S. and Hall, S.L. (1999) Affiliative behaviour of related and unrelated pairs of cats in catteries: a preliminary report. *Applied Animal Behaviour Science*, **63** (3), 251–255.

Clutton-Brock J. (1987) *A Natural History of Domesticated Mammals*. Cambridge University Press, Cambridge, and the British Museum (Natural History), London.

Cooper, L.L. (1997) Feline inappropriate elimination. *The Veterinary Clinics of North America. Small Animal Practice*, **27** (3), 569–600.

Eckstein, R.A. and Hart, B.L. (2000) The organization and control of grooming in cats. *Applied Animal Behaviour Science*, **68** (2), 131–140.

Finco, D.R., Adams, D.D., Crowell, W.A. *et al.* (1986) Food and water intake and urine composition in cats: influence of continuous versus periodic feeding. *American Journal of Veterinary Research*, **47** (7), 1638–1642.

Flanigan, J., Shepherd, A., Majchrzak, S. *et al.* (2007) *US Pet Ownership and Demographics Sourcebook*, American Veterinary Medical Association, Schaumburg, IL, pp. 1–3.

Halip, J.W., Luescher, U.A. and McKeown, D.B. (1992) Inappropriate elimination in cats, part 1. *Feline Practice*, **20** (3), 17–21.

Hart, B.L. (1976) The role of grooming activity. *Feline Practice*, **6** (4), 14, 16.

Hart, B.L. and Cooper, L. (1984) Factors relating to urine spraying and fighting in prepubertally gonadectomized cats. *Journal of the American Veterinary Medical Association*, **184** (10), 1255–1258.

Heidenberger, E. (1997) Housing conditions and behavioral problems of indoor cats as assessed by their owners. *Applied Animal Behaviour Science*, **52** (3, 4), 345–364.

Kolb, B. and Nonneman, A.J. (1975) The development of social responsiveness in kittens. *Animal Behaviour*, **23**, 368–374.

Liberg, O. and Sandell, M. (1988) Spatial organisation and reproductive tactics in the domestic cat and other felids, in *The Domestic Cat: The biology of its Behaviour* (eds D.C. Turner and P. Bateson), Cambridge University Press, Cambridge, pp. 83–98.

Mahlow, J.C. and Slater, M.R. (1996) Current issues in the control of stray and feral cats. *Journal of the American Veterinary Medical Association*, **209** (12), 2016–2020.

Marder, A. (1997) Managing behavioural problems in puppies and kittens. *Friskies PetCare Small Animal Behavior*, **15–24**.

Meier, G.W. (1961) Infantile handling and development in Siamese Kittens. *Journal of Comparative Physiology and Psychology*, **54**, 284–286.

Olmstead, C.E. and Villablanca, J.R. (1980) Development of behavioral audition in the kitten. *Physiology and Behavior*, **24**, 705–712.

Olson, P.N. and Johnston, S.D. (1993) New developments in small animal population control. *Journal of the American Veterinary Medical Association*, **202** (6), 904–909.

Overall, K.L. (1992) Preventing behavior problems: early prevention and recognition in puppies and kittens. *Purina Specialty Review*, 13–29.

Overall, K.L. (1995) Behavioral knowledge can help smooth introduction of new pet to household. *DVM Newsmagazine*, **26** (116S, 12S, 13S).

Pannaman, R. (1981) Behavior and ecology of free-ranging female farm cats (*Felis catus* L.). *Zeitschrift für Tierpsychologie*, **56**, 59–73.

Reisner, I.R., Houpt, K.A., Hollis, N.E. and Quimby, F.W. (1994) Friendliness to humans and defensive aggression in cats: the influence of handling and paternity. *Physiology and Behavior*, **55** (6), 1119–1124.

Salman, M.D., Hutchison, J., Buch-Gallie, R. *et al* (2000) Behavioral reasons for relinquishment of dogs and cats to 12 shelters. *Journal of Applied Animal Welfare Science*, **3** (2), 93–106.

The Humane Society of the United States. (2010) Cat Chat: Understanding Feline Language; February 5, 2010.

Turner, D.C. and Bateson, P. (2000) *The Domestic Cat: The Biology of its Behaviour*, 2nd edn, Cambridge University Press, Cambridge.

Villablanca, J.R. and Olmstead, C.E. (1979) Neurological development in kittens. *Developmental Psychobiology*, **12**, 101–27.

Vogt, A.H., Rodan, I., Brown, M. *et al.* (2010) AAFP-AAHA: Feline Life Stage Guidelines. *Journal of Feline Medicine and Surgery*, **12**, 43. doi: 10.1016/j.jfms.2009.12.006

West, M. (1974) Social play in the domestic cat. *American Zoologist*, **14**, 427–436.

CHAPTER 3

4

The human–animal bond – a brief look at its richness and complexities

Julie K. Shaw[1] and Sarah Lahrman[2]

[1] TEAM Education in Animal Behavior, LLC, Spicewood, TX, USA
[2] Purdue Comparative Oncology Program, Purdue University, West Lafayette, IN, USA

The celebration, protection and nurturing of the human–animal bond is veterinary medicine's North Star. It is the reason our profession exists and thrives and is trusted and admired. Veterinary practice must be a blend of science and soul. Successful veterinarians [veterinary technicians] know that the human–animal bond is the fuel that powers the emotional side of our profession. The bond allows us to thrive and not just survive in the greatest profession on earth.

Marty Becker, DVM and author, as quoted from the mission and vision statement of the Association of Human–Animal Bond Veterinarians.

The human–animal bond (HAB) was defined in a statement from the American Veterinary Medical Association in 1998 as

A mutually beneficial and dynamic relationship between people and other animals that is influenced by behaviors that are essential to the health and well-being of both. This includes but is not limited to, emotional, psychological, and physical interactions of people, other animals, and the environment.

The veterinarian's [veterinary technician's] role in the human–animal bond is to maximize the potentials of this relationship between people and other animals.

(Statement from the Committee on the Human–Animal Bond in JAVMA vol. 212, No. 11, p. 1675, June 1, 1998)

The primary aim of veterinary behavioral medicine is to strengthen and protect the HAB while allowing both the human and the animal to live a high-quality life. The strength of the HAB is directly related to the animal's behavior (Sherman and Serpell, 2008). A well-behaved animal improves people's lives by improving their general health and sense of well-being (Serpell, 1995). Animal behavioral problems place enormous stress on the HAB and are often the reason for the pet's relinquishment (Patronek *et al.*, 1996).

Veterinary technicians are in the ideal position to support pet owners in building a strong HAB by assisting them to choose the best pet for their life style during pet-selection counseling (see Chapter 7) and continuing to strengthen the bond through problem-prevention strategies, including puppy and kitten classes (Chapter 7). The primary goal of developing and strengthening the HAB must stay in the forefront of our minds, especially when very difficult situations arise, including removal of a pet from a home or euthanasia for a behavioral disorder. The veterinary technician can support the client during such times by assisting the grief process, continuing to promote, support, and protect the HAB, (see section titled **Grief counseling** in Chapter 5.) The ultimate goal of companion animal behavior is to promote, support and protect the human–animal bond. That must never be forgotten.

- The ultimate goal of companion animal behavior is to promote, support and protect the human–animal bond. That must never be forgotten.

Julie Shaw, RVT, VTS (Behavior)

The HAB past, present, and future

An animal was first distinguished as a pet when it was begun to be seen as "humanized." Three characteristics occurred to elevate an animal to the "pet" category: it was allowed in the house, given a name, and not eaten (Levi-Strauss, 1966).

The concept of a special connection between animals and people (the HAB) was met with significant resistance when it was presented by Dr. Leo K. Bustad in the 1980s. His first attempts to bring the HAB to the forefront were met with scorn, disbelief (Hines, 2003), and skepticism. Initially, the veterinary field was also disbelieving of his ideas.

The pioneers of the HAB movement campaigned and with the assistance of the media, provided research for their theories. Working with veterinary medicine,

the media, conferences, and publications, the special bond noted between a pet and its owner became widely accepted by society (Hines, 2003). Research on the health benefits of animals began in the 1960s. The majority of research focused on the effects of animals on human health, cardiac benefits, alerts of health emergencies, and the health of the elderly and children (Hering, 2008). Further studies came to similar conclusions reporting that people with some type of animal exposure typically had lower blood pressure and decreased stress levels (Pachana *et al.*, 2011; Siegel *et al.*, 2011).

Acceptance has allowed the HAB to evolve greatly over the past 50 years, and it continues to set higher standards for the care of companion animals. The role of the companion animal has changed from that of a working animal to that of a valued family member. When the animal is no longer present, the family unit must regroup to fill the void.

Future US census reports may include questions pertaining to family pets, allowing exploration of subtle positive effects of animals on the family unit (Beck and Katcher, 2003). Future data may indicate that the HAB is growing in strength because of an increase in life expectancy (Miniño, 2011), people marrying later in life (Census, 2010), choosing to not have children, or to have children later in life (Livingston, 2010). The role of veterinary medicine will likely change and increase in scope as the HAB continues to advance. The mental and emotional health of pets must become a routine component of the animal's holistic treatment. Pet insurance companies may play a more prominent role in our profession and begin to readily include behavioral health, including prevention such as puppy and kitten classes, into their insurance policies.

It is certain the HAB will continue to gain strength and depth as companion animals continue to fill the voids that we sometimes feel as humans. Veterinary medicine must be prepared to meet the expanded needs that are required to support the HAB.

- The mental and emotional health of pets must become a routine component of the animal's holistic treatment.

Special bonds
Animal-assisted therapy

The earliest animal-assisted therapy (AAT) programs dated back to 1790 in England, where companion animals were used to treat mental health patients. During World War II, soldiers with mental and emotional trauma worked on farms at the hospital as therapy (Hering, 2008). Today, animals are being integrated into hospitals, nursing homes, and schools. When animals are brought into these settings, those involved feel more at home, and some normalcy is brought into their lives (Butler, 2004).

"Pet therapy" is an outdated and inaccurate term that should no longer be used. Human service providers now use the term Animal Assisted Therapy to describe therapy involving an animal, with specific therapeutic goals for the patient and measured progress reports. For instance, during the AAT, asking a patient to throw a ball to an animal to retrieve to improve the patient's range of motion. Animal-assisted activities (AAA) are more spontaneous activities without specific patient treatment goals (Walsh, 2009).

Animals to be used in an AAA/AAT program should be qualified through programs such as Therapy Dogs International, Inc. (TDI), Therapy Dogs Incorporated (TDInc), or the Delta Society. Qualifying organizations evaluate both the handler and the animal for suitability for therapy work. AAA/AAT benefits the handler, the animal, the facility staff, and, most importantly, the patient (Figure 4.1) (Ensminger, 2010).

The use of AAA/AAT will continue to proliferate to our most innovative schools, prisons, and community programs (Walsh, 2009), and research data from such programs will continue to define the benefits of AAT.

Assistance (service) dogs

An assistance animal is any animal that performs tasks for the benefit of a person with a disability. On 15 March 2011, the Department of Justice published revised final regulations to the Americans with Disabilities Act (ADA), clarifying and refining issues that arose over the last 20 years pertaining to the use of assistance (service) animals. The term "assistance animal" is a broad term, whereas the ADA defines "service animals" as dogs that are individually trained to perform work or perform tasks for people with a disability. Examples of such work include guiding people who are blind, alerting people who are deaf, pulling a wheel chair, alerting and protecting a person who is having a seizure, reminding a person with mental illness to take prescribed medications, calming a person with post-traumatic stress disorder during an anxiety attack, or performing other duties (ADA, 2011). "Other duties" may include alerting to a diabetic crisis or assisting a child with autism. Dogs whose sole function is to provide comfort or emotional

Figure 4.1 AAA/AAT benefits the handler, the animal, the facility staff, and the patient.

support do not qualify as service animals under the current revised ADA.

The ADA includes only dogs as service animals, although a new, separate provision pertaining to miniature horses has been included. Miniature horses are most often used in guide work because of their long life expectancy. Entities covered by the ADA must modify their policies to permit miniature horses where reasonable.

When it is not obvious what service the animal provides, only two questions may be asked by the staff: is this dog a service animal required because of a disability? What work or task has the dog been trained to perform? Questions pertaining to the person's disability, requirement of medical or training documentation, or a request for demonstration of the ability of the animal to perform work are not allowed and are prohibited by law.

Figure 4.2 Dylan Shaw (aged 3 years) with his first service dog "Faith" (aged 8 weeks).

Figure 4.3 Dylan Shaw (aged 19 years) with his second service dog "Hero" (aged 10 years).

The clarification and change to the ADA pertaining to service animals are a testament to the growing value of the HAB. There is no doubt these highly trained animals benefit their challenged partners in a multitude of ways. To quote one child on the death of his service dog, "It is like losing a Mom, a best-friend and an arm all at the same time". (Quote from Dylan Shaw, who used a service dog from the age of 3–18 years (Figures 4.2 and 4.3).

Difficult to understand relationships

It would be easy and more palatable to focus only on the most common and acceptable human–animal relationships as described previously. As veterinary technicians, we should also be able to detect potential situations in which animals and/or people might be at risk. By educating ourselves in these areas we may be able to take steps toward preventing such relationships from occurring.

Motives for animal abuse

Possibly, the most difficult to understand and the largest distortion of the human–animal relationship is animal abuse or cruelty. Animal cruelty can be somewhat a subjective judgment, but in this chapter, it is defined as willful infliction of pain, injury, or harm on a nonhuman animal (Kellert and Felthous, 1985).

Kellert and Felthous determined motivations for animal cruelty among criminals and noncriminals during their childhoods. It should be noted that motives are usually multidimensional, with multiple motives occurring. The following nine motivation categories were identified in their research:

1. To control or gain compliance from the animal. Excessive use of violence or punishment to shape an animal's behavior.
2. To retaliate against the animal for a previous infraction. Taking obvious delight in excessively punishing a "wrong" behavior, such as digging in the garden.
3. To satisfy a prejudice against the animal or species. Designating groups of animals as "good" or "bad," such as all cats are evil. This type of prejudice is often culturally related.

4. To express aggression through the animal. Using cruelty or violence in an attempt to "make the animal mean" or to "toughen it up." This motivation is often seen in the dogfighting culture.
5. To enhance one's own aggression. Some subjects in the study described "practicing" their techniques on animals before attempting aggression on humans or to impress others (e.g., friends or gang members).
6. To shock for amusement, usually in an attempt to "be funny" to gain attention.
7. To retaliate against another person. This is a technique often used in spousal abuse cases to control the spouse. The abuser threatens to hurt the animal if their demands are not followed. (Faver and Strand, 2003). National and state surveys of domestic violence victims consistently find that as many as 71% of battered women report that their male partners had threatened to or had, in fact, harmed or killed their pets (Randour and Hardiman, 2007). An early study found that there was animal abuse in 88% of families who were under state supervision for the physical abuse of their children (DeViney, 1983). Animals may be used by perpetrators to coerce children into silence by threatening to harm the animal (Davidson, 1998).
8. Displacement of hostility from a person to an animal. An example of this is a person, driven by frustration or aggression toward a "feared" authority figure, hurts an animal "to get even" with the authority figure. One study stated two out of five children who were bullied and victimized at school performed some type of cruelty to an animal to let out their frustration and anger. A study by Baldry indicated that children who lived in a home in which violence against a parent, themselves, or an animal occurred were three times more likely to abuse animals. Whether the cruelty to animals occurred because of displacement or because violence was normalized is not known (Baldry, 2005).

   One of the earliest reported symptoms of childhood conduct disorder is cruelty to animals (Frick Benjamin and Paul, 1993). Conduct disorder in children refers to a group of behavioral and emotional problems, including great difficulty following rules and behaving in a socially acceptable way. Other children, adults, and social agencies unfortunately, view them as "bad" or delinquent, rather than mentally ill (AACAP, 2004). Children who are cruel to animals are also more likely to exhibit more severe conduct disorder problems than other children (Luk et al., 1999).
9. Nonspecific sadism. A desire to inflict injury, suffering, and death without provocation, with the primary goal of gaining pleasure from the act. Sadism is often used to compensate a person's feeling of weakness (Kellert and Felthous, 1985; Perez-Merz et al., 2001).

Dogfighting
The Humane Society of the United States estimates that there are at least 40,000 dogfighters in America, although that number seems to underestimate the street-fighting epidemic in urban areas (Gibson, 2005). Dogfighters are violent criminals who engage in a multitude of peripheral criminal activities, including organized crime, racketeering, drug distribution, and gang activity (Gibson, 2005; Randour and Hardiman, 2007). Dogfighting is a cunning and insidious type of underground, organized crime and is an incredible source of income for gangs and drug trafficking (Gibson, 2005).

Generally, pit bulls are gentle yet fiercely loyal toward humans. Those qualities have made them attractive to dogfighters because they can withstand neglect and significant abuse from their owners while remaining loyal and nonaggressive to the abusers (Gibson, 2005; Blazina et al., 2011).

Children – the other victims
The atrocities seen in dogfighting environments appall seasoned law enforcement officials, yet children who grow up in a dogfighting life style believe violence is normal. Over time, their exposure causes them to be calloused to suffering and desensitized to criminalization.

The routine exposure of the children to animal abuse and neglect is a major contributing factor for those children to later develop social deviance. Children between the ages of 8 and 10 years living in neighborhoods with strong gang activity can be found holding their own fights or as spectators at fights that are being held. Dogfighting is a desensitization tool for young gang members. Gene Mueller, DVM and past President of the Anti-Cruelty Society in Chicago, Illinois said, "You want to find the perfect way to desensitize a kid so he'll kill that anonymous gangbanger from three blocks over? Give him a puppy and let him raise it. Then let him kill it. I guarantee that will desensitize that kid" (Gibson, 2005). Young gang members are often required to kill their own losing dog to regain lost respect (Blazina et al., 2011).

As children become desensitized to violence, the cycle is perpetuated and passed on to another generation.

The "dogmen"
"Dogmen" are individuals who fight their pit bulls against others in "matches"(Evans and Forsynth, 1998).

A study by the Society of Animals determined five major characteristics "dogmen" use to justify dogfighting.

1. Denial that the dogs are victims. "Dogmen" believe their dogs "like" to fight and denying them the opportunity would be cruel. They rationalize the dog does not have to fight, it chooses to, therefore it cannot be a victim.
2. Denial of responsibility. Dogmen interviewed believed they were not hurting anyone and there was no harm in the "sport." They compared themselves to being a "coach" to an athlete.
3. Denial of injury. Many "dogmen" contest their dogs are well taken care of before and after the fight and what happens in the ring is pleasurable to the dog.
4. Appeal to higher loyalties. Dogfighters contend their "sport" is dated back to the eighteenth century and was attended by European aristocracy. They argue they are not criminals but "good people." They compare dogfighting laws to being "penalized for jaywalking."
5. Condemnation of the condemners. "Dogmen" believe dogfighting is a cultural tradition and they are being prevented from practicing their tradition, in turn causing "cultural genocide." They believe they are "normal folks" who are different in some ways and try to rationalize their behavior as reasonable if not conventional. They believe the animal humane organizations are extremist and are causing their dogs to suffer by not allowing them to fight (Evans and Forsynth, 1998; Evans *et al.*, 1998; Gibson, 2005).

It is rare that fighting dogs will be seen in a veterinary hospital for fear of arrest, but characteristics to be aware of are pattern of bite wounds on head, neck, and legs (Patronek, 1997).

Animal hoarders

By definition, an animal hoarder is a person who continues to obtain animals (usually one species) without providing the proper care for the animals already present, ignoring the deteriorating environment and denying there is a problem present (Patronek and Nathanson, 2009).

Animal hoarders frequently believe themselves to be rescues or "no kill" shelters and often live isolated or secretive lives. When questions or concerns are raised, they may become defensive. The National Database for Animal Cruelty has reported animal hoarding cases have increased fivefold in the past 10 years. It is estimated that there are approximately 600–2000 cases reported each year, with 60% being repeat offenders. Hoarders are most commonly female, middle aged to older, and live alone. Male hoarders often live in homes with their families (frequently multigenerational) (Arluke, 2009; Patronek and Nathanson, 2009).

Although hoarders are represented as criminals in the media, research of those affected by the disorder has found many hoarders develop symptoms of personality disorders, delusions, dementia, addiction, attachment disorder, control issues, and obsessive-compulsive disorder. Animal hoarders perceive themselves as animal caregivers, suggesting animal hoarding is largely an egosyntonic disorder (Patronek and Nathanson, 2009).

Animal hoarding can be brought on by difficult childhood experiences (i.e., absent parents, several relocations, divorce, etc.). Other traumas have included loss of a stabilizing adult relationship, a serious health crisis, or loss of a major bodily function. It has also been noted that persons with personality traits suggesting self-regulatory defects may be at a greater risk for complicated grief (pathological grief), with symptoms resembling post-traumatic stress disorder and often associated with extreme fear of abandonment. Hoarders appear to become enmeshed in a grief that incorporates animals as a method of healing (Patronek and Nathanson, 2009). Those affected with this condition see animals as the one stable factor in their lives (Vaca-Guzman and Arluke, 2005; Arluke, 2008).

State laws require pet owners to provide sufficient food and water, a sanitary environment, and the minimal necessary veterinary care. Animal hoarding cases often end in the euthanasia of multiple animals because of the lack of these requirements and the condition of the animals when the hoarders are discovered. Hoarders often do not recognize they are living in an unhealthy environment that includes excrement in the living space. Indifference to the squalor and animal suffering appears to indicate a severe lack of insight indicative of disassociation (Patronek and Nathanson, 2009).

Most counseling for animal hoarding is not patient initiated but rather court ordered and therefore has low compliance. Treatment is difficult with many complicating factors, including impairments of cognition, lack of insight, poor abstract thinking, difficulty understanding cause and effect, poor problem-solving skills, and difficulty organizing and completing a task. Exaggerated perception of threat, hyper vigilance, and distrust of authoritative figures makes developing a therapeutic relationship difficult. It is challenging for them to relate to another person when animals have been their primary relationship (Patronek and Nathanson, 2009).

Client characteristics to be aware of include clients who bring in multiple pets at different times and seem to have a large number of animals. Clients may request a medication for a pet the veterinarian has no record of seeing (i.e., ear medications or antibiotics), and animals may smell of urine and feces (Arluke, 2009). Watch for a lack of continuity of care for individual animals, office visits for trauma, and preventable contagious and parasitic diseases may be common. The client may request heroic efforts for a newly acquired pet with a poor prognosis and may visit many different veterinary hospitals.

In such cases of neglect, it is often productive to educate rather than condemn. When possible framing discussions on whether the needs of the animal are being met rather than on the "bad" behavior of the owner helps to depersonalize the discussion, allowing the veterinary professional to become an educator and animal advocate rather than passing judgment on a person (Patronek, 1997).

Puppy mill operators

The last relationship to be discussed is the relationship of puppy mill operators with their "product." This was a very difficult area to find references for, and much of the information comes from direct interviews with Tim Rickey, Senior Director of Field Investigations for the ASPCA and Linda Campbell, RVT, VTS-Behavior, Director of Behavior and Training for the Humane Society of Missouri.

Puppy mill operators consider themselves "farmers," and the seven states that have the majority of puppy mills are largely agricultural states: Missouri, Nebraska, Kansas, Iowa, Arkansas, Oklahoma, and Pennsylvania. They are unlike farming families who have a code of ethics and knowledge they pass down to generations.

The owners of puppy mills are not bonded to the animals they produce. There is a harsh, distant emotional detachment. They consider the animals as livestock or simply a commodity. The animals are objectified with little human interaction and no human emotional connection. The breeding bitch is considered the "machine" that produces the product (the puppy). The goal is minimal investment with the highest profit possible. When a "machine" stops producing, it is discarded and easily replaced at minimal cost.

The business of puppy farming is often a second career, after retirement or loss of a job. It is seen as a quick financial fix they can get "in and out of" quickly. One common denominator found in the puppy mill owner population is lack of general higher education.

A significant difference between animal hoarders and puppy mill operators is that when a hoarder's animals are removed, complete emotional devastation and destruction can occur, whereas when a puppy mill is shut down, it is seen as a destruction of their livelihood.

Defining healthy versus unhealthy bonds

The relationship we share with our pet is unlike any other relationship in our lives. It has the complexities, challenges, and rewards of a parent–child relationship, teacher–student relationship, and deep friendship.

Defining and developing a healthy HAB

Healthy relationships add to the well-being of everyone in the relationship and should be pervasively positive in their nature. Mutually healthy relationships meet both the human and the pet's psychological, emotional, and physical needs.

The foundation of a healthy human–animal relationship includes respect and trust. Respect develops through consistent clear communication and predictability. Respect of the animal's unique and specific species differences are valued. Appreciating those differences encourages pet owners to be fair in their expectations of the pet. For example, teaching an animal not to drink from the toilet is an easy task to train, but owners need to realize drinking from the toilet is "normal" or innate behavior for the animal.

Trust develops when the relationship is consistent and based on looking for the "good" in the relationship. There is no place for fear, intimidation, or coercion. Anxiety and fear develop when animals, human, or nonhuman cannot predict "what will happen next." There should be a "balance of power" in which mutual goals are met. The ability to exercise some control over the environment is empowering and a primary survival behavior. People and animals should have the ability to remove themselves from a frightening or stressful situation when possible.

Emotionally healthy animals are affectionate without being needy or overly attention seeking. They can be separated from people without undue stress. They are friendly or at least tolerant of their own species, children, family members, and strangers. They should be able to play well with others and exhibit impulse control during play. They have the confidence to be inquisitive and are not overly fearful of new objects, places, people, or events. An emotionally stable animal will "rebound" quickly from a "scary" event or stimulus. Change does not cause extreme or long-lasting anxiety and stress (McCurnin, 2010).

BOX 4.1: SIGNS OF AN EMOTIONALLY HEALTHY PET.

- □ Affectionate without being needy
- □ Not overly attention seeking
- □ Can be separated from people without undue stress
- □ Friendly or at least tolerant to conspecifics, children, family members, and strangers
- □ Plays well with others and exhibits impulse control in play
- □ Confidence to be inquisitive
- □ Not overly fearful of new objects, places, people, or events
- □ Rebounds from "scary" events or stimulus
- □ Change does not cause undue anxiety or stress

Modified from Animal Behavior Associates, Inc. Copyright 2002 All Rights Reserved. www.AnimalBehaviorAssociates.com with permission from authors, Suzanne Hetts, Ph.D. Daniel Q. Estep, Ph.D.

Ironically, emotionally healthy humans share many of the same qualities of emotionally healthy pets, including the ability to deal with stress and bounce back from adversity. They show flexibility to learn new things and adapt to changes in the environment. Emotionally healthy humans are also self-confident, independent, and not overly fearful (Helpguide.org, 2010).

Potential unhealthy pet relationships

If we accept that animals benefit humans, we must also examine potentials for adverse responses in some populations (Beck and Katcher, 2003).

Unhealthy relationships commonly bring out stress and leave a feeling of being "used up" with an overall negative outlook. Signs of an unhealthy relationship include neglecting self-care, routinely giving up activities or relationships that make you happy for the pet's emotional and psychological needs. Feelings of pressure and persistent anxiety when away from the pet may occur. Other signs may include feelings of anxiety "walking on egg shells" and uncertainty of what may happen next. Fear for yourself or others (including other pets) or having a feeling of being unsafe when around your pet is a constant stress. Fear in any relationship is a strong indicator that the relationship is not healthy and a significant sign the HAB has been seriously damaged or broken (see Table 4.1).

Table 4.1 Pet owner strain related to a pet's behavioral disorder and possible indications of an unhealthy HAB.

Life area	Manifestation of strain
Mental and emotional	□ Stress and a feeling of being "used up"
	□ Worry or anxiety
	□ Anger toward your pet
	□ Fear your pet may hurt you or a loved one
	□ "Aloneness" and alienation
	□ Feelings of "hopelessness" when it comes to your pet
	□ Feelings of "not being able to go on" if your pet were to die
Health	□ Health issues because of stress (weight loss or gain, headaches, etc.)
	□ Declined self-care
	□ Decreased energy
	□ Injury from your pet
Social	□ Embarrassment
	□ Shame or guilt
	□ Fear of stigma/social disapproval
	□ Alienation
	□ Limit or cease having house guests
	□ Guilt when socializing outside the home
	□ Neglected relationships or giving up relationships that make you happy to tend to your pet's psychological and emotional needs
	□ Fear of being away from your pet
	□ Giving up hobbies
	□ Fear of injury to strangers
Financial	□ Distraction during work day
	□ Financial liability/lawsuits
	□ Property damage and destruction
	□ Cost for treatment, medication, training, and so on
Family environment	□ Fear for safety of family members
	□ Discord with significant other
	□ Strained relationship with extended family members
	□ Alienation by extended family

Modified from Mendenhall, Mount 2011; Anonymous, 2011 Client essays.

Identifying at-risk populations for unhealthy HAB

More research needs to be performed to fully define at-risk populations, but it has been suggested that an over attachment to animals could decrease bonds to people. Research by Brown and Katcher found people with high levels of pet attachment had three times greater chance of showing clinical levels of dissociation compared to those with low levels of pet attachment. Dissociation is defined as the inability to integrate various parts of an experience, such as thoughts, feelings, or images into their stream of consciousness (Carlson *et al.*, 1993). People already with impaired ability to connect with other humans may substitute the connection with animals and therefore lose the human social support system (Brown and Katcher, 1997, 2001).

High levels of dissociation have been strongly correlated with traumatic experience, including childhood abuse or exposure to combat. It is therefore plausible that a subset of people highly attached to animals may have histories of abuse or trauma. It is speculated that some people with both high pet attachment and high dissociation may be attempting to create a reparative relationship from trauma and find animals a safe, stable, and trusting relationship substitute for a human relationship (Brown and Katcher, 1997).

Participants from animal-related professions, including veterinary technicians, had dissociation scores much higher than people from non-animal-related fields. The 113 veterinary technicians in the study had clinical dissociative experiences scale (DES) (Bernstein and Putnam, 1986) scores of 22%, which are five times higher than that in the normal population.

Previous research has found no significant personality type or trait to predict attachment to pets. It is possible that until the research by Brown and Katcher, no one had looked at the relationship to trauma and dissociation correlating the HAB. These findings are important as we interact with our clients. Although most attachments may not have an underlying dissociative connection, it is an association that should be at least passively acknowledged. Our clients may be using their attachment to their pet as a bridge to attachments with humans or to avoid human relationships.

Strengthening the HAB and preventing pet relinquishment

Pets with behavioral problems are more likely to be euthanized, abandoned, rehomed, or relinquished to animal shelters (Sherman and Serpell, 2008). Nearly 90% of owners report behavioral concerns with their pet, and "behavior problem" is the primary reason cited for relinquishment. In this case, "behavior problem" was not differentiated from a true affective behavioral disorder. Another important reason for relinquishment includes false expectations in regard to the time, effort, and cost of care for a pet.

Characteristics that increase the potential for relinquishment include mix breeds, unneutered dogs younger than 6 months, dogs not obtained as puppies, and dogs obtained from shelters at low or no cost.

The National Council on Pet Overpopulation discovered 96% of dogs relinquished to shelters had no proper training (Miller, 2001). First-time owners were less likely to give up their pet, whereas men younger than 35 years were more likely to relinquish their pet. Dogs kept for extensive amounts of time in a crate, basement, or garage were at higher risk likely because of a weak owner attachment.

Veterinary care and advice are the most important protective factors. Dogs that were taken to a veterinarian at least once a year were 23 times less likely to be relinquished than those that were not. Dogs were less likely to be surrendered if advice came from a veterinary versus a nonveterinary professional. Surprisingly, dogs given as gifts were at less risk. Those obtained at a high price also had a lower risk factor. Dogs that were allowed in the living area of the home and that received training were also more protected from relinquishment (Salman *et al.*, 1998; Scarlett *et al.*, 1999; Salman *et al.*, 2000; Luescher and Martin, 2010).

The risk factors for cat relinquishment differ somewhat from those of dogs. First-time cat owners, intact cats, mixed breed cats, and cats younger than 6 months were at a higher risk. Inappropriate expectations and lack of information on cat behavior contributed to relinquishment. Behavioral problems and disorders that increased risk included inappropriate elimination, scratching in unwanted areas, and aggression toward people. Cats that did not visit the veterinarian, were kept in a basement or garage, or had access to the outdoors were at a higher risk to lose their homes. Cats found as strays or acquired with little planning were at less risk, and cats that were declawed and visit their veterinarian were more protected from relinquishment (Salman *et al.*, 1998; Scarlett *et al.*, 1999; Salman *et al.*, 2000; Luescher and Martin, 2010).

Veterinary technicians play a key role in preventing pet relinquishment by educating clients and building a relationship of trust that will be maintained throughout the pet's life. Pet-selection counseling (detailed in Chapter 7) assists the client in choosing a pet that is appropriate for their life style and desires, although relinquishment has not been associated with lack of planning. Pet-selection counseling is also an educational tool to prevent behavioral problems and disorders from developing by assessing areas of concern or possible inappropriate expectations. New pet-owner counseling can occur immediately after a client obtains a pet and should include a systematic approach that includes the important points for behavior management and problem prevention. Every veterinary visit should include specific questions pertaining to behavioral health.

BOX 4.2: BEHAVIOR-RELATED QUESTIONS A TECHNICIAN SHOULD ASK AT *EVERY* APPOINTMENT.

	General behavior health assessment
	Is your pet having accidents in the house?
Is there anything your pet does not "like you to do," for example,	
	Hugging or restraining?
	Touching his/her collar or other body part?
	Brushing, bathing, nail trimming?
	Picking him/her up?
	Removing his/her food bowl or toy?
	Moving him when he/she is sleeping?
	Has your pet growled or hissed at anyone or anything lately?
	Does your pet readily interact with family members?
	Does your pet readily interact with strangers?
	Is there anything your pet seems afraid of?
	Has there been any destruction by your pet?
	How do you stop unwanted behavior?*
What type of training are you using to teach your pet? □ Food treats □ Clicker training □ Choke or pinch collar □ Shock	
If there was any behavior you would like to change in your pet, what would it be?	

*Note: This question could be smoothly incorporated into another question, for example: What did you do when you found the destruction? The goal is to determine if the owner is using punishment and to then educate them on the side effects and give them alternate methods for changing behavior.

The key is prevention when possible and early detection of pet behavior concerns before they have had a detrimental effect on the HAB. Inform pet owners of preventive behavioral services the hospital offers, including training classes and preferred educational sources as soon as possible. Puppy and kitten classes (described in detail in Chapter 7) are instrumental in strengthening the HAB. Classes also bond the client to the hospital and the staff. Early education can prevent problems from developing. High-risk puppies or kittens can be identified quickly and treatment prescribed.

All veterinary hospitals should either have a qualified trainer on staff (could also be the veterinary technician) or be associated with a qualified trainer. A qualified trainer is defined as an animal trainer who is certified from a standardized positive-based curriculum and is policed by an organization in which certification can be revoked if the trainer acts unprofessionally or outside the organization's code of ethics (Shaw, 2011).

> • A qualified trainer is defined as an animal trainer who is certified from a standardized positive-based curriculum and is policed by an organization in which certification can be revoked if the trainer acts unprofessionally or outside the organization's code of ethics.

Training classes (detailed in Chapter 7) should be based on positive training techniques and should not use or encourage punishment. Punishment almost always damages the HAB, has serious side effects (see Chapters 6 and 7), and usually does not work. Classes should be based on clear, concise, and consistent interactions. Classes should teach the client to look for what they want their pet to do, rather than focus on "wrong behavior" or "pack leadership" theories.

With the number of families sharing their homes and lives with pets, veterinary colleges must strive to incorporate and educate students on the importance of animal behavior. Currently, only one-third of veterinary colleges include animal behavior training in their curriculum (Sherman and Serpell, 2008). The goal for any veterinary professional should be more than just practicing medicine. Focusing on maintaining a healthy relationship and preserving the bond between clients and pets is the key. Clients make a commitment to their pets the day they bring them home. It is of upmost importance that they are educated on normal and abnormal behavior, counseled on appropriate training techniques/modifications, given proper resources, and in some cases, referral to an animal behaviorist. Offering behavioral services shows you value the relationship between pet and client and the importance of preserving the bond (Sherman and Serpell, 2008).

Behavioral problems and disorders chip away at the HAB if undetected or unaddressed. The research clearly shows that pets are less likely to suffer the consequences of relinquishment if up-to-date information from veterinary professionals is provided to pet owners. There may be no other area in veterinary medicine that technicians have such a significant role in keeping pets in their homes than by helping owners develop a strong HAB.

Animals with behavioral disorders and the people who love them

The relationship between a client and a pet with a serious affective behavioral disorder is one that is multidimensional and affects all members of the family unit. In this chapter, "behavioral disorder" is defined as psychological or behavioral patterns outside behavioral "norms" that usually have an affective aspect (Shaw, 2011). A "Behavior problem" in veterinary medicine is defined as the animal's behavior that causes a problem for the owner. The issues could be lack of training, conditioned unwanted behavior, a behavioral disorder, or a combination of issues. A veterinarian's diagnosis may be required.

- A "Behavior problem" in veterinary medicine is defined as the animal's behavior that causes a problem for the owner.

- The issues could be lack of training, conditioned unwanted behavior, a behavioral disorder, or a combination of issues. A veterinarian's diagnosis may be required.

- A "behavioral disorder" is defined as psychological or behavioral patterns outside behavioral "norms" that usually have an affective aspect and requires a diagnosis by a veterinarian.

There has been nearly nothing written on the intricacies of such a relationship. Clients have compared it to living with a child with an emotional disorder, a parent with Alzheimer's disease, or even living in an abusive relationship as a victim. One person wrote, "…I expected understanding but was blamed instead of supported. I was accused of being a weak [pet owner] and I endured lots of unwanted and inappropriate advice. These messages came from close friends, family members, [trainers and veterinary professionals]. The blame and judgment came from so many directions that it was hard to believe they weren't true. On top of this, I felt guilty that I somehow caused my [pet's] condition and I searched for explanations. Did I discipline too hard? Was

this genetics? Had there been abuse by someone and I didn't know about it?"

The aforementioned selection was only slightly modified from the book Raising Troubled Kids by Margaret Puckette. Ms. Puckette was writing about her child with an emotional disorder. By changing only a few words, the excerpt could easily be the words of a person living with a pet with a behavioral disorder. My references for this section have come from the experts – pet owners who have coexisted and loved an animal with significant and serious behavioral disorders (Anonymous, 2011).

The stigma

Stigma or stigmatizing occurs when shame and ridicule are placed on someone for breaking a societal "taboo." Stigma is manifested by bias, distrust, prejudgments, fear, embarrassment, and anger and lead to the stigmatized person having low self-esteem, isolation, and hopelessness. It is a barrier in the treatment of human mental health issues both from the patient and the family's standpoints and similarly felt among pet owners who live with a pet that has a serious behavioral disorder. One pet owner described the stigma she suffered when keeping her aggressive dog, "Family members and neighbors called him 'mean' or 'Cujo'." She reported feeling shameful and embarrassed but also felt guilty if she considered euthanizing him. A prevalent and common thread described by pet owners was a desperation that if "others could only see what he is like with us they would understand." Many felt as though they had caused their pet's disorder by being "bad pet owners" or that they "let their pet down" in some way.

The impact on the pet owner

Caregiver burden and caregiver strain are terms used to describe the problems, stress, and adverse events that affect the lives of significant others in a psychiatric patient's life. Clients living with a pet with a significant behavioral disorder have described similar stresses and difficulties (Table 4.1).

Clients have described feelings of hopelessness in finding help for their pet after being given advice to "not let him get away with that" and to be a stronger "pack leader" only to have such advice cause the pet's issues to worsen. Others were left feeling completely alone when they were told by a family member, friend, neighbor, trainer or veterinarian to "put the animal down" without giving them a diagnosis or explanation for the animal's behavior. They express shock, fear, and anger if they were injured by their pet both because of the injury and because of the emotional strife it caused in their family. Some describe a loss of trust and deep confusion. A common description is that "he is so loving and wonderful 90% of the time. Yet, there were times we were afraid of him. We never knew when his aggression would strike again. We were 'on guard' all of the time and we loved him at the same time." These exceptional pet owners are often willing to dramatically modify their own lives for the well-being of their pet, sometimes to the point it may not be entirely beneficial to their own well-being. One pet owner admits, "The unexpected is our enemy. I do not have my grandchildren spend the night. I rarely have visitors. I have specially built primary and secondary gates to manage any interactions that may occur. While I know of no one who lives in this manner, I have grown accustomed to it so there are no regrets on my choice for him to live out his life as it is today. I only regret the harsh treatment I administered early on without understanding his disorder."

Conclusion

The veterinary behavior technician must be the support system for clients who live with a pet with a serious behavioral disorder. Pet owners may struggle with conflicting advice from the media, trainers, neighbors, and family members. It is imperative they feel connected and confident with the veterinary behavior technicians. It is one of the most intimate, intense, and rewarding relationships a veterinary technician will have with a pet owner.

References

ADA 2010 Revised Requirements: Service Animals. (2011) U.S. Department of Justice, Civil Rights Division, Disability Rights Section.

AACAP (2004) Facts for families: conduct disorder **33**.

Anonymous (2011) *Client Essays*, J. Shaw, West Lafayette, IN.

Arluke, A. and Killeen, C. (2009) *Inside Animal Hoarding: The Case of Barbara Erickson*, Purdue University Press, West Lafayette, IN USA, pp. 167–220.

Baldry, A.C. (2005) Animal abuse among preadolescents directly and indirectly victimized at school and at home. *Criminal Behaviour Mental Health*, **15** (2), 97–110.

Beck, A.M. and Katcher, A.H. (2003) Future directions in human-animal bond research. *American Behavioral Scientist*, **47** (1), 79–93.

Bernstein, E.M. and Putnam, F.W. (1986) Development, reliability, and validity of a dissociation scale. *Journal of Nervous and Mental Disease*, **174** (12), 727–735.

Blazina, C., Boyra, G., Shen-Miller, D. and Springer-Link (Online service) (2011) *The Psychology of the Human–Animal Bond A Resource for Clinicians and Researchers*, Springer Science+Business Media, LLC., New York, NY.

Brown, S. and Katcher, A. (2001) Pet attachment and dissociation. *Society & Animals*, (9), 25–42.

Brown, S.E. and Katcher, A.H. (1997) The contribution of attachment to pets and attachment to nature to dissociation and absorption. *Dissociation*, **10** (2), 125–129.

Butler, K. (2004) *Therapy Dogs Today: Their Gifts, Our Obligation*, Funpuddle Publishing Associates, Norman, Oklahoma, USA.

Carlson, E.B., Putnam, F.W., Ross, C.A. *et al.* (1993) Validity of the dissociative experience scale in screening for multiple personality disorder: a multicenter study. *American Journal of Psychiatry*, **150**, 1030–1036.

Census, U. (2010) *U.S. Bureau of the Census*.

Davidson, H. (1998) What lawyers and judges should know about the link between child abuse and animal cruelty. *ABA Child Law Practice*, **17**, 60–63.

DeViney, D.L. (1983) The care of pets within child abusing families. *International Journal for the Study of Animal Problems*, **4**, 321–329.

Ensminger, J.J. (2010) *Service and Therapy Dogs in American Society*, Charles C. Thomas Publishing, IL, USA.

Evans, R.D. and Forsynth, C.J. (1998) Dogmen: the rationalization of deviance. *Society and Animals: Journal of Human Animal Studies*, **6** (3), 203–218.

Evans, R., Gauthler, D.K. and Forsyth, C.J. (1998) Dog fighting: symbolic expression and validation of masculinity. *Sex Roles*, **39** (11/12), 825–838.

Faver, C.A. and Strand, E.B. (2003) To leave or to stay?: Battered women's concern for vulnerable pets. *Journal of Interpersonal Violence*, **18** (12), 1367–1377.

Frick Benjamin, B. and Paul, J. (1993) Oppositional defiant disorder and conduct disorder: A meta-analytic review of factor analyses and cross-validation in a clinic sample. *Clinical Psychology Review*, **13** (4), 319–340.

Gibson, H. (2005) Dog fighting detailed discussion. Animal Legal and Historical Center.

Helpguide.org. (2010) Improving emotional health: strategies and tips for good mental health http://www.helpguide.org (accessed 28 September 2011).

Hering, C. (2008) Health benefits of companion animals. *Health Insights Today: A Service of the Cleveland College Foundation*, **1** (2), 1–4.

Hines, L.M. (2003) Historical perspectives on the human animal bond. *American Behavioral Scientist*, **47** (1), 7–15.

Kellert, S.R. and Felthous, A.R. (1985) Childhood cruelty toward animals among criminals and noncriminals. *Human Relations*, **38** (12), 1113–1129.

Levi-Strauss, C. (1966) Anthropology: its achievements and future. *Nature*, **209** (5018), 10–13.

Livingston, G. (2010) The new demography of American motherhood. Pew Research Center: A Social and Demographic Trends Report.

Luescher, A. and Martin, K.M. (2010) *Dogs! & Cats: Diagnosis and Treatment of Behavior Problems*, Purdue University, West Lafayette.

Luk, E.S.L., Staiger, P.K., Wong, L. and Mathai, J. (1999) Children who are cruel to animals: a revisit. *Australian and New Zealand Journal of Psychiatry*, **33** (1), 29–36.

Salman, M.D., Hutchinson, J.M., Ruch-Gallie, R. *et al.* (2000) Behavioral reasons for relinquishment of dogs and cats to 12 shelters. *Journal of Applied Animal Welfare Science*, **3** (2), 93–106.

McCurnin, D.M. (2010) *Clinical Textbook for Veterinary Technicians*, Saunders, Philadelphia.

Miller, P. (2001) *The Power of Positive Dog Training*, John Wiley & Sons, Inc., New York, NY.

Miniño, A. M. (2011) *Death in the United States, 2009*. NCHS data brief, no 64. Hyattsville, MD: National Center for Health Statistics. 2011.

Pachana, N.A., Massavelli, B.M. and Robleda-Gomez, S. (2011) A developmental psychological perspective on the human–animal bond, in *The Psychology of the Human–Animal Bond* (eds C. Blazina, G. Boyra and D. Shen-Miller), Springer, New York, pp. 151–165.

Patronek, G.J. (1997) Issues for veterinarians in recognizing and reporting animal neglect and abuse. *Society and Animals*, **5** (3), 267–280.

Patronek, G.J., Glickman, L.T., Beck, A.M. *et al.* (1996) Risk factors for relinquishment of dogs to an animal shelter. *Journal of the American Veterinary Medical Association*, **209** (3), 572–581.

Patronek, G.J. and Nathanson, J.N. (2009) A theoretical perspective to inform assessment and treatment strategies for animal hoarders. *Clinical Psychology Review*, **29** (3), 274–281.

Perez-Merz, L., Heide, K.M. and Silverman, I.J. (2001) Childhood cruelty to animals and subsequent violence against humans. *International Journal of Offender Therapy and Comparative Criminology*, **45** (5), 556.

Randour, M.L. and Hardiman, T. (2007) Creating synergy for gang prevention: taking a look at animal fighting and gangs, in *Proceedings of Persistently Safe Schools*, Hamilton Fish Institute, The George Washington University, Washington, DC, p. 199.

Salman, M.D., New, J.G. Jr., Scarlett, J.M. *et al.* (1998) Human and animal factors related to relinquishment of dogs and cats in 12 selected animal shelters in the United States. *Journal of Applied Animal Welfare Science*, **1** (3), 207–226.

Scarlett, J.M., Slaman, M., New, J. and Kass, P. (1999) Reasons for relinquishment of companion animals in U.S. animal shelters; selected health and personal issues. *Journal of Applied Animal Welfare Science*, **1** (1), 41–57.

Serpell, J. (1995) *The Domestic Dog: Its Evolution, Behaviour, And Interactions With People*, Cambridge University Press, Cambridge, NY.

Shaw, J. (2011) Should you or shouldn't you: when is a veterinarian's diagnosis required, in *Purdue University Veterinary Fall Conference*, Purdue University, W. Lafayette, IN.

Sherman, B.L. and Serpell, J.A. (2008) Training veterinary students in animal behavior to preserve the human–animal bond. *Journal of Veterinary Medical Education*, **35** (4), 496–502.

Siegel, J.M., Blazina, C., Boyra, G. and Shen-Miller, D. (2011) Pet ownership and health, in *The Psychology of the Human–Animal Bond*, Springer, New York, pp. 167–177.

Vaca-Guzman, M. and Arluke, A. (2005) Normalizing passive cruelty: the excuses and justifications of animal hoarders. *Anthrozoos: A Multidisciplinary Journal of The Interactions of People & Animals*, **18** (4), 338–357.

Walsh, F. (2009) Human–animal bonds II: the role of pets in family systems and family therapy. *Family Process*, **48** (4), 481–499.

5 Communication and connecting the animal behavior team

Julie K. Shaw[1] and Lindsey M. Fourez[2]

[1] TEAM Education in Animal Behavior, LLC, Spicewood, TX, USA

[2] Purdue Comparative Oncology Program, Purdue University, West Lafayette, IN, USA

Characteristics of a strong and empowered animal behavior technician–client–patient relationship begins with a technician who has the ability to communicate knowledge, demonstrate technical skill, and is able to teach in multiple different styles dependent on the style the patient and the client need at any particular moment. The communication relationship is comparable to that of a nurse–parent–child relationship. The

---

relationship is often laden with high emotion but also reaps deep and long-lasting rewards.

The animal behavior technician must also be able to connect and coordinate the behavior team to work together for the benefit of the pet owner and the pet.

A comparison between marriage and family therapist and the role of the animal behavior technician

Strong commonalities between the counseling aspects of animal behavior therapy and the field of marriage and family therapy (MFT) have been found (Canino *et al.*, 2007).

Four major parallels were found between marriage and family counseling and the role of an animal behavior technician.

(1) One of the most striking similarities between the work of the animal behavior team and emotionally focused MFTs involves how change occurs in the context of treatment. Both professions seek to change the emotional experience of the clients, although in veterinary behavioral medicine the goal is often to also change the emotional experience of the pet along with that of the pet owner's. Couples, for instance, often find themselves in a destructive interaction cycle that repeats itself in times of stress. In comparison, pet owners may have developed a general negativity toward their pet. The content of the problem is irrelevant until a more positive interaction can be developed. For instance, restructuring the emotional process of the owner toward understanding their pet is not directly attempting to get back at them when destruction occurs when left alone, but rather their pet is having a panic attack that they will not return home. This type of restructuring can dramatically change the emotional experience for the pet owner.

Assisting the client in developing clear and predictable communication skills and stopping punishment-type techniques can be the foundation for changing the emotional state of the animal.

(2) There are also similarities in the methods for obtaining information from the client. A detailed history, including input from all pertinent family members, is obtained in both disciplines. The idea is predicated on the belief that all people in the family system are affected by the problem, regardless of how individual in nature the problem may appear. It is important to determine if a specific event triggered the call for an appointment and if the

current stress is underlying the presenting problem or is only a symptom of it. The simple question of "what triggered you to seek help now?" will often obtain the required information. The answer may be that the pet owners only recently found there were services to assist with their pet's disorder or they may have been a sudden change in their life style, a change in the family dynamics (birth of a child, divorce, etc.), or a more serious incident of the behavior.

(3) Similar difficulties and barriers encountered with clients are found between MFT and veterinary animal behavior. In general, clients enter a therapy room with some level of anxiety about the process they are about to undertake. Frequently, pet owners believe they have "caused" the problem to their pet and feel deep shame or guilt, causing a reluctance to impart information. This fear may come from the concern that they will be blamed or that they may be told to euthanize their pet. In order to build a rapport with clients, the technician must gain their trust. Trust is gained by effectively and genuinely opening up to the client, and in turn, the client begins to feel safe and becomes open. It is helpful if the technician perceives that these concerns may be an issue to directly communicate to the pet owner that you are not going to tell them to euthanize their pet but that you are there to assist them and that withholding information will make it more difficult for you to assist them. Gaining the trust of the pet owner is imperative. At no point is it useful to place blame on the pet owner. They are seeking your help now, and regardless of the information they were given in the past, that should be the focus.

Asking the client to change how they currently interact with their pet involves significant effort on the part of the client and includes asking them to take risk into unfamiliar territory. It is critical that the veterinary technician creates a safe, non-judgmental, and positive environment with the owner. The veterinary technician's assistance can be critical for the positive outcome of the case by instructing the owner not only as to how he or she can successfully implement the veterinarian's prescribed treatment plan into their daily lives but also to ensure that the owner understands specifically how the prescribed techniques will modify the pet's behavior. The veterinary technician may feel resistance from the client if the client feels coerced into bringing their pet for treatment. Such situations may occur if the client was given an ultimatum by the legal system, other family member, or another authoritative figure.

Resistance may be exhibited when clients who continually disagree and protest make excuses or show no effort to implement the therapeutic recommendations or terminate treatment prematurely (Egan, 2002). This result can occur if the veterinary behavior team places guilt or blame on the client or implies that the owner is the sole cause of the problem (Hetts, 1999). Clients who are resistant appear to be those who believe they are not entering into the therapeutic process voluntarily, but resistance can be counteracted by identifying and pointing out areas their pet is showing fear and anxiety, often without the owner's knowledge. Fear and anxiety on the owner's part can be decreased by giving them choices and input into the creation of the treatment plan, therefore empowering the owner and creating a team effort. In addition, it is helpful to let the clients know that their fears and concerns are normal and to be expected. Letting clients know that you have seen the problem before and that there is treatment is often enough to initiate the process of change.

(4) Presenting problems seen in marriage and family counseling and animal behavior consultations are similar. Anxiety-related behavioral disorders and problems (lack of training or conditioned unwanted behaviors in pets) are the two common problems that seem to cut across the field of animal behavior and MFT. MFTs, in particular, report that anxiety and child behavior problems are among the five most commonly seen problems in the therapy room (Northey, 2002).

Communication

Communication skills have to be taught, learned, applied, and then adapted to fit one's personal style. When information is inadequately presented to the client, trust is lost, and the client becomes stressed and anxious (Chun *et al.*, 2009).

Nonverbal communication

Just as a veterinary behavior technician must accurately read the body language of their patient, they must also be adept at interpreting that of the pet owner. Eighty percent of communication with another individual is given through nonverbal cues, whereas only 7–20% of the message is actually sent through words (Durrance and Lagoni, 1998; Carson, 2007).

Often, body language can give direct insight into the status of the human–animal bond (HAB). Observe whether the pet owner leans away from their pet or are constantly reaching to touch the pet.

The technician must then combine what they see in nonverbal with verbal communication to determine if both verbal and nonverbal cues match up. If the pet owner appears open to your suggestions and is sending the correct words and vocal cues, but is standing with arms crossed against the body, a mixed message is sent (Durrance and Lagoni, 1998). Attending to both verbal and nonverbal cues is critical to interpreting the full scope of the pet owner's thoughts.

Nonverbal communication includes essentially all forms of communication other than words, such as facial expressions, body postures, tone of voice, eye contact, gestures, and hand movements.

When working with a pet owner, it is important to pick up on closed body language. For example, if the pet owner's arms are crossed against their chest and are diverting their eyes, most likely they are having feelings of conflict to what you are saying. Likewise, it is important to be aware of your own body language and the messages you are conveying back to the owner (Durrance and Lagoni, 1998).

There will be times when speaking with a client that their nonverbal and verbal communication differs from each other. Research has shown that when words are not compatible with nonverbal cues, the receiver should give more focus to the nonverbal cues. Mixed communication can often be seen when we say things we believe others want to hear. For instance, Ms. Smith might tell you Fluffy has been acting fine, but her body language (tone of voice, lack of eye contact, and slumped posture) speaks quite differently. In this case, dismissing such nonverbal cues may bring about feelings of carelessness and lack of empathy. By noticing a pet owner's mismatched communication, you convey good listening skills and can evoke feelings of trust.

Nonverbal cues can be placed into four categories: kinesics, proxemics, paralanguage, and autonomic shifts. *Kinesics* focuses on body gestures, movement, and position. Facial expressions and touch can also be placed in this group. *Proxemics* pertains to personal space and on how the environment is setup. If the clinic or even the examination room is not welcoming, the client will automatically put up a barrier. *Paralanguage* focuses on how the voice is controlled. This is the category in which the focus is put on the tone, pace, volume, and emphasis. Research shows that when information is given in a soft and slower pace than normal, it will be taken as soothing to the receiver. The last category is *autonomic shifts*. These are items that are out of our control, such as blushing, sweating, or increased breathing. If autonomic shifts occur, the client may be upset, and recovery mode should start immediately. The four categories of nonverbal communication should be used to help determine if the pet owner feels safe. If a client becomes extremely uncomfortable, they may go into a "fight or flight" agenda (Carson, 2007).

If a client starts into the "fight or flight" mode, damage control should take place quickly. A client in the fight mode may have a tense stance, clenched teeth and fists, and narrow eyes. If a client is entering the flight mode, they will have increased body tension, push or step back, change in voice volume, increase in breathing rate, and change in facial color. These are the clients who will start to create barriers and hold on to the animal tighter (Carson, 2007). If a client starts into "fight or flight," the goal is to get them back to a safe place quickly.

Clients can be brought back to the safety zone by perceiving and addressing any mismatched information. Pet owners have often researched their presenting problem on the internet, and there is a chance the information you are presenting is not the same as that previously discovered by the client, therefore causing confusion.

It is important to understand that when a client is upset, it is not a reflection of how they feel about you personally. In this situation, the STOP format can be beneficial (Ryan, 2005) (Figure 5.1).

Verbal communication

The effectiveness of verbal communication depends on the words chosen, emphasis, grammar, tone, and pace (Durrance and Lagoni, 1998). There are eight communication techniques required for proper verbal communication. The first is *acknowledging*. This is the act of noticing someone and making a person feel they exist. Examples include saying, "I understand," "Is that right?", and so on. The second technique is *normalizing*. This allows one to acknowledge and let them know that there is an understanding of previous experiences and gives them credibility. The third technique is giving *permission*. This helps people perform what they feel needs to be done. Fourth is asking *appropriate questions* of a person. This technique allows one to get the information needed. Technique number five is *paraphrasing* what has been discussed. In a conversation, this helps let the person talking know that the listener understands what has been said. The sixth technique is *self-disclosing* to a client. Sharing a personal story or analogy with a client helps make a connection. With this technique, the client knows that you have been through a similar experience and that you know what they are feeling. The seventh technique is *gentle confrontation*. This technique is used to point out a problem or inconsistencies in a statement. Sometimes, when a client is upset or angry, this technique can be used to let them recognize their limits. The final technique is *immediacy*. Immediacy is a combination of gentle confrontation and self-disclosure. It is often used in an emergency situation when large amounts of information are being given quickly (Durrance and Lagoni, 1998).

Road blocks to verbal communication

Do not take an adversarial role when communicating with the pet owner. When people feel that their beliefs

S = Signal — Observe your own non verbal body language and signals you are sending

T = Take control of your emotions — Change negative thoughts to positive thoughts to change your emotions

O = Opposite — Do the opposite of your current signals

P = Practice — Continue to practice until STOP becomes part of your communication style

Figure 5.1 STOP when responding to an upset client.

or attitudes are being attacked, they become uncomfortable and defensive, closing down communication. Avoid direct threats such as "If you don't stop 'Fluffy's' aggression, she will likely have to be euthanized." Do not be judgmental or blaming such as "'Fluffy's' aggression is because of the way you have trained her"; this will not create a team-building atmosphere. "Commanding" a person or dog creates a "do-it-or-else" atmosphere, which is not optimum for the learning process. A good teacher understands that although the pet owner's current attitude may differ from what you are attempting to teach, it is likely only transient. Simply accept the pet owner's current perceptions as information and continue to build rapport with them (Ryan, 2005).

Active listening

Much of our life is spent listening; yet to be a skilled listener takes practice. Listeners usually interpret what they hear through a protective filter formed through life experiences; therefore, no two people hear things exactly the same (Ryan, 2005). Active listening focuses on the emotional content of the conversation. By asking questions, paraphrasing, and using open body language, you encourage clients to further discuss those feelings. Necessary silences and minimal encouragers are techniques used in active listening. Necessary silence allows clients to vent their feelings or gather their thoughts. Minimal encouragers are used to keep the conversation going. Minimal encouragers can be head nods, eye blinks, or a simple "yes," "uh-huh," or "I see" to let the client know you are listening and an active part of the conversation (Durrance and Lagoni, 1998).

Establishing an alliance with the family (pet owner and significant family members) in a noncritical manner is frequently a key to the success of the case. A partnership relationship style provides an equal separation of the power between the client and the veterinary behavior team (Gray and Moffett, 2010). This technique gives control to the client by allowing them to openly discuss and choose aspects of the treatment plan.

In the past, owners may have been blamed for the issues their pet was having rather than being reinforced for seeking help to alleviate the issue. Listen to the family's experiences and specific areas of stress. Often the patient's owners have been put into a position of being damned if they do too much or too little. They may have restricted taking the pet outside to avoid conflicts but were then told that they needed to socialize their pet more (Abosh and Collins, 1996). They may have attended many training classes and read many books only to find that the training they were taught and the

books they read were outdated and may have worsened the problem.

Areas of stress should be acknowledged during the creation of the treatment plan. For instance, if one family member indicates they are frightened of the pet, that person may be asked to ignore the patient completely until the follow-up appointment. Or, they may be asked to toss treats from a distance when another person is clicker training the patient. Finding a safe indirect interaction can be the first step in repairing the HAB. In some cases, it may be recommended that the patient be boarded for a time to give the family respite. In some cases in which the HAB has been seriously damaged, this respite gives the family time to adjust to not having the pet in the home and can be the first step in the grief process, although some owners may feel "relieved" with the pet out of the home and then feel remorse for the feelings of relief.

Connective communication techniques

The four-habits communication model

Pet owners are less concerned with how much their pet's medical caregivers know than with how much they care (Stein *et al.*, 1998). The four-habits model is a tool that can be applied and used to perfect communication skills and focuses on relationship-centered care. The goal of the four-habits model is to establish rapport and build trust rapidly, expedite the effective exchange of information, demonstrate concern and care, and increase compliance.

The model has four main goals that are established when applied correctly. The first is that one builds a rapport with the client, thus ensuring a higher level of trust with the behavior team that helps move the proper exchange of information. It makes it easier to discuss issues with clients, giving more accurate information in the end. Another goal is that as a professional, the four-habits model teaches us to show care and concern for the client and the patient. The last goal is to increase compliance, therefore increasing the chances for a positive outcome (Frankel and Stein, 1999; Adams and Frankel, 2007). See Table 5.1 for a modified guide of the four-habits model for client communication between the behavior team during a behavior consultation.

Validation

Validation occurs when the veterinary behavior team truly understands what the clients are experiencing and gives them permission to feel upset, angry, and

Table 5.1 Modified four-habits model for client communication between the entire behavior team in a behavior consultation.

Invest in the beginning Skill	Task	Example
Create rapport quickly	Introduce the behavior team to everyone in the room	Explain roles in the appointment
	Acknowledge any wait	
	Convey knowledge of patient's history by commenting on previous visit or problem	
	Attend to client and pet's comfort	Include a water bowl and blanket for the patient.
	Make a social comment or ask a nonmedical question to put the client at ease	Let the client know "there is nothing 'Fluffy' can do 'wrong' here."
	Adjust your language, pace, and posture to that of the client's	
Elicit client's concerns	Start with open-ended questions	
	Repeat concerns back to check understanding and prioritize the client's concerns	"I understand you are most concerned about 'Fluffy's' aggression to children but also her urinating in the house, is that correct?
Plan the visit with the client	Let the client know what to expect	"The doctor will get more information from you while I work with 'Fluffy'. Once we have the full history, our behavior team will create your treatment plan, and I will show you some training techniques"
Elicit the client's perspectives		
Ask for the client's thoughts	Determine the status of the HAB, including all family member's input	"How do you feel about 'Fluffy?'"
Ask for a specific goal	Determine if the client's expectations are appropriate	"If we could improve the aggression by 50%, would that be enough?"
Explore the impact on the client's life		"How are YOU doing?"
Demonstrate empathy		
Be open to the client's emotions	Assess the client's changes in body language and voice tone	"How do you feel about what we have talked about so far?"
	Look for opportunities to use brief empathic comments or gestures	"Living with an animal with a serious behavior disorder is very difficult and can be very emotionally draining."
Make at least one empathic statement	Name a likely emotion the client may be feeling	"It is understandable if you are afraid of 'Fluffy'."
	Compliment the client on efforts to address problem	"It is obvious how much you love 'Fluffy'."
Convey empathy nonverbally	Use a pause, touch, or facial expression to convey your understanding and empathy	
Be aware of your own reactions	Be genuine in your own emotional response	
	Take a brief break if necessary	
Invest in the end		
Deliver diagnostic information	Frame diagnosis in terms of the client's original concerns	"We will address 'Fluffy's' general anxiety issues first, which will also help with her aggression and accidents in the house, does this make sense to you?"
	Test client's comprehension	
Provide education	Explain rationale for tests and treatments	"To prevent 'Fluffy' from continuing to practice her unwanted behaviors while we work on the issue, we would like you to avoid triggers … "
	Review possible side effects and expected course of recovery	
	Recommend management techniques	
	Provide written materials and refer to other resources	

CHAPTER 5

Table 5.1 (*Continued*)

Invest in the beginning Skill	Task	Example
Involve client in making decisions Complete the visit	Discuss treatment goals and realistic expectations for progress Explore options, listening for the patient's preferences Assess patient's ability and motivation to carry out plan Ask for additional questions and concerns Assess satisfaction Reassure patient of ongoing care	"I understand ignoring 'Fluffy's' attention seeking will be difficult but this is only temporary while we work on her issues." "What do you feel will be the most difficult aspect of 'Fluffy's' treatment plan for you to follow?" "How do you feel about what we have talked about?" "We will see you back in 4 weeks, in the mean time, we will be following up with you and your trainer."

Modified from Frankel and Stein (1999).

so on. The pet owner should be told there is nothing wrong, shameful, or irrational about their emotional responses to this situation. A veterinarian or veterinary technician might say, "This must be very difficult for you. It has to be exhausting to be on guard and worried. Those feelings are quite understandable." During the interview process, the client may admit to hitting their animal when it injured them or a family member. This statement is frequently presented with intense feelings of guilt. The veterinarian or veterinary technician can alleviate this guilt by normalizing with a statement such as, "That is quite a normal and understandable response." Validation helps build trust between the client and the behavior team.

Normalizing

As stated earlier in Chapter 4, clients often feel alone and alienated. Many times they have not found others who have dealt with the specific problem their pet is facing before, and they desperately want to hear, "We have seen this problem before and there is hope." Simply knowing that they are not alone can change the course of the consultation and is likely to give the client relief and open them to potential treatment strategies.

Guiding the conversation

Sometimes it becomes necessary to interrupt a client's story. This should not be thought of as interrupting as much as guiding the conversation to the pertinent information and is a critical therapeutic skill (Canino *et al.*, 2007). Guiding the conversation can be done is such a way that it does not feel like an interruption. Saying something such as, "Hold on to that thought, we will come back to it. Please tell me more about … " or "Back up a second, tell me more about the first time he growled

at you." Usually, such statements are not perceived as impolite but a way to obtain the specific information needed.

Reframing

Two common communication issues that can significantly contribute to relationship issues between pet owners and their pet are inaccurate owner interpretations of behavior and unrealistic expectations (McCurnin, 2010).

Anthropomorphic interpretations distract from the needed objective observations required to accurately assess a situation, and unrealistic expectations create a scenario for failure and a weak HAB by setting up both the animal and client for the failure, although it may be necessary to reframe some comments in order to obtain a better understanding of the problem. However, many pet owner interpretations may simply be ignored but noted and addressed later in the education process (Table 5.2).

The dominance theory

The dominance theory may be the greatest interpretative miscommunication in companion animal behavior. The dominance theory was originally based on studies performed on wolf packs in the 1940s. It was extrapolated that dogs had social hierarchies comparable to wolves. The adapted theory went as far as to assume that a human family replaces a dog pack. It was theorized that a dog tries to gain the top position over family members and may become aggressive to lower ranking "members of the pack."

There were three significant flaws in the early research.

CHAPTER 5

Table 5.2 Reframing anthropomorphic interpretations.

Client statement	Technician's response	Client's rephrasing	Technician's reframing[a]
He hates men	What does he do that tells you he does not like men?	He backs up and growls	So he is worried about men and feels he has to defend himself
He knows he should not get into the trash	What does he do that tells you he "knows" he should not get into the trash?	He runs away when I come into the room, and the trash is on the floor	So, he has learned when trash is on the floor you may be upset
He gets mad if I try to move him	What does he do when you try to move him?	He growls at us	First let us make sure he is not in pain, then we can teach him to move to the place you want him to without creating conflict
He tries to dominate me when I brush him	What does that look like?	He tries to get away from me when I brush him	So, he is uncomfortable with brushing
He knows I do not like it when he gets on the couch	What does he do that tells you he knows the couch is off limits?	He puts his ears back and growls when I approach him	So, he expects a conflict when he is on the couch and he does not know what to do
He knows what I want him to do, he is just being stubborn	What makes you believe he is stubborn?	He would not do what I want him to do	It is likely he does not understand what you want because something has gone wrong in the training process
He is a very dominant dog	What does that look like?	He walks in front of me when we go on walks	Has he been taught loose leash walking?
He pees on the floor when he is mad at me for leaving him	What makes you believe he is angry at you?	He does not like it when I leave and paces and pants when I am getting dressed for work, and he only does it when I leave	He is likely so upset and anxious when you leave that he cannot control himself. Can you imagine how afraid he must be to lose control of his bladder?
He knows what he did wrong because he looks guilty	What does "guilty" look like?	He puts his ears back, tucks his tail, and hides from me	So he suspects you are upset and he does not know what you will do next so he is afraid
He tries to dominate us when we punish him	When do you need to punish him?	When he has something we do not want him to have	It sounds like he is afraid and unsure what is expected of him. Let us teach him he does not have to be afraid when he has something and then we will teach him to not pick up certain objects
We have spoiled her and that is why she would not listen to us	Can you give me an example of when she acts "spoiled"?	She climbs on the dinner table no matter how many times we tell her not to	Let us control the times she is near the table unsupervised and teach her to go to a mat
She is bossy	What does she do when she is "bossy"?	She barks at me when I tell her to sit	Barking can be a sign of frustration. Let us reteach the sit and see if we can decrease her frustration
He is protecting me that is why he is aggressive	What does that look like?	When a stranger approaches, he growls and stands behind me	It sounds as though he may be unsure of strangers and feels safer when you are nearby or he may be more confident that you will protect him and be his "back up" support system

[a]Responses may be phrased in a question format in the attempt to gain agreement from the pet owner. In addition, many pet owner interpretations may simply be ignored but noted in the education process.

(1) The initial wolf studies were short-term and only focused on about 1% of a wolf's life, namely hunting (Murie and Etats-Unis. National Park, 1944). Wild life biologist, Dr. David Mech, an internationally recognized expert on wolves, points out that the notion of "alpha wolf" and the struggle to be "top dog" were based on observations of captive groups of unrelated wolves. These artificial social groups bear little resemblance to a pack of free-living wolves that (except for the breeding pair) are all related to one another. The idea that individuals in a family of wolves are engaged in constant daily struggles to best one another, and that our dogs do the same with us, is simply not true (Mech, 2008).

(2) Sweeping conclusions were made from this misinformation and then generalized to dogs, ignoring 15,000 years of domestication, and then generalized again to the human–dog relationship. Veterinarian Ian Dunbar made the comparison that trying to understand dogs better by looking at wolf behavior is comparable to humans attempting to improve their parenting skills by observing primates.

(3) The researchers observed what are now known to be ritualistic displays and misinterpreted them into forcible dominance displays. For example, researchers determined that a higher ranking wolf forcibly pins a "subordinate" wolf to the ground. We now know that the "subordinate" wolf is not forced to the ground but voluntarily assumes the position as part of ritualized appeasement behavior – a method of avoiding conflict.

This dominance theory has been over used, complicates the relationship we have with dogs, and puts pet owners in an adversarial role. Pet owners are led to believe that their dog is trying to "take over" and therefore "must not be allowed to get away with things."

In the past, puppies were considered "dominant" when they demanded petting, pushed through doorways, jumped up to greet people, or guarded objects. It is now understood that when a puppy "demands petting" or paws at the owner, it is simply performing a conditioned behavior. The puppy is rewarded for pawing when the owner gives it attention. Pushing through a door way is simply an indication that sitting at the door has not been taught – it is an issue of lack of training. Jumping on people is a greeting behavior and is conditioned by people responding to the behavior with touch and attention. Guarding of a resource is almost always initially fear or anxiety related but becomes conditioned through avoidance conditioning. The puppy then becomes more offensive after experiencing the success of getting out of the stressful situation and eventually no longer shows anxiousness. Guarding of a resource can be an early indication that a puppy is at risk of developing conflict-induced aggression (Box 5.1).

BOX 5.1: RISK FACTORS FOR DEVELOPING OWNER-DIRECTED AGGRESSION (CONFLICT-INDUCED AGGRESSION).

Risk factors

Suffered a serious illness under 4 months of age
Not walked off property regularly
Higher level of excitement, reactivity, and fearfulness
Inappropriate or overly aggressive play
Guarding (objects, food, or space)
Handling issues
Shows conflict behaviors

Guy *et al.*, (2001c).

An alternate explanation is that whenever the dog is uncertain or uncomfortable in a situation (i.e., conflict situation), it has learned to use aggression to avoid the situation (i.e., avoidance conditioning). The dog becomes less fearful because it learns how to avoid the fear-provoking situation. The aggression has nothing to do with the debunked "dominance theory."

The "dominance theory" often damages the HAB because owners believe that their puppy views them as a lower ranking "pack member." Owners often feel they need to practice techniques such as "scruff shaking," "alpha roll overs," and other domination techniques to control their puppy. These techniques increase anxiety and fear for both the owner and the puppy and are counterproductive in the treatment process. Owners are often relieved and compliant to the treatment plan when they understand that the puppy is not trying to "dominate" them but is anxious and uncertain (Shaw, 2005).

Empathy

Empathy is the ability to have a deep emotional understanding of another's feelings and experiences. The ability to empathize both with the patient and with the pet owner is the greatest attribute of the veterinary behavior technician and one of the most challenging skills to obtain.

CHAPTER 5

> • Seek first to understand then to be understood. Stephen Covey

Ancient Toltec wisdom may give us the most simplified principles for clear empathetic communication. The Toltec tradition is about freedom from a belief system, in other words, not being attached to any particular point of view (Rosenthal, 2005). Being able to perceive and understand a client's perspective allows you to "walk in the shoes" of the client. Attempting to empathize with the pet includes understanding the deep fear and confusion that often create or add to a pet's behavior disorder. Empathy for the pet allows the technician to see the pet in a light other than as an aggressive or fearful animal.

Empathy builds trust and creates a platform for effective communication and relationship development. Developing the ability to empathize requires the ability to "step back" from our own emotions and beliefs to let the other's emotions and view point in. Letting go of your own perspective, even temporarily, requires courage on your part but is essential in developing the ability to sincerely empathize with others.

Empathy and understanding for the client carry over to the patient. Philosopher Marcha C. Nussbaum said that as we learn to imagine what another creature might feel in response to various events and we begin to identify with the other creature, we learn something about ourselves. Being able to identify and empathize with the fear and anxiety many of our patients exhibit is the first step in modifying their behavior. When a pet is described as a "mean dog" or a "mean cat," the label ends the process to genuinely empathize. Recognizing that the animal is trying to protect itself from the stimulus (you) and emphasizing with them changes your motivation and enhances your ability to teach both the animal and the client. When we understand the needs that motivate our own and other's behavior we have no enemies. Marshall Rosenberb

> • When we understand the needs that motivate our own and other's behavior we have no enemies.
>
> Marshall Rosenberb

The following four Toltec principles are the foundation for genuine empathetic and unambiguous communication (Figure 5.2).

Teaching

A veterinary animal behavior technician is a teacher, a leader, and a mentor to the pet owners. The following are attributes of an excellent teacher.

Enthusiasm and passion are contagious to whomever you teach. If you love what you do, it will show. *Kindness and humility* will guide your teaching away from condescending actions or remarks. Understanding that there is no "one way" to perform things creates an open learning environment for both the student and the teacher. *Be patient and flexible.* If your student is not "getting it," it means you need to be comfortable enough with the material to modify your teaching technique for that specific learner. Being able to modify "on the run" also keeps the material fresh and interesting for you. A sense of humor will keep what you are teaching light and fun. Remember to laugh at yourself and at your own mistakes. This often helps the student to relax and understand that making a mistake is learning. *Make each student feel special and important.* Shaping human behavior is no different from shaping a pet's behavior. Find something to reinforce that is heading toward the goal behavior (Ryan, 2005).

Learning styles

As stated previously, teaching style should be modified for the pet owner's learning style. The following are common simplified learning styles.

Listeners – Listeners like to be told what to do. They find lectures and presentations helpful. They are the typical classroom-style learners.

Readers – Readers often get frustrated in a lecture style of teaching. Readers prefer to peruse notes and think about things at their own pace. In a lecture-type setting, they will likely only partially listen and instead read ahead in the notes. If they do not understand something that was said, they are likely to stop listening and instead read what is written.

Writers – Writers learn by making notes in their own words. Note taking allows them think about what they know before writing the information. To assist the writer-type learners, pause to give them time to write their thoughts and "catch up." It is also helpful for this type of learners to give them pertinent information in writing, with space for them to add their own notes.

Talkers – Talkers need to question and discuss the information being presented until they are sure it has been placed into their long-term memory. Talkers are most helped by frequently pausing for questions

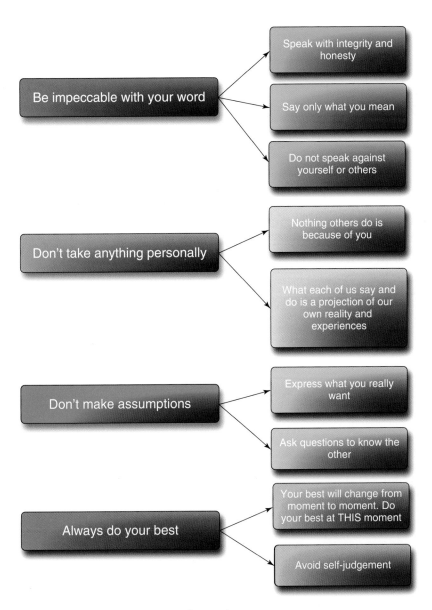

Figure 5.2 Toltec principles for empathetic communication and interactions.

and allowing them to interrupt when questions arise. They often perform best in a group discussion setting.

Watchers – Watchers like to see demonstrations on both what works and what does not. They then try to imitate. Watchers prefer videos and live demonstrations.

Doers – Doers become impatient with lectures. They prefer to "do" and find out for themselves what works and what does not. To assist "doers," give them exercises to practice and create role-playing demonstrations for them (Straker, 2012).

TAGteach

TAGteach (McKeon, 2012) is a package of tools that emphasizes the use of positive reinforcement and incorporates several well-established behavioral principles and practices. Although the purpose of TAGteach is to improve skill acquisition for the student, its first benefit

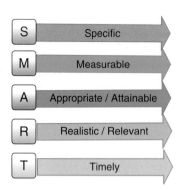

Figure 5.3 Smart learning goals.

goes to the teacher. Teachers quickly learn to identify, highlight, and reinforce vital skills for the student and deliver information in a learner-accessible manner. When teaching the pet owner specific goals, it is important to keep the learning goals specific, measurable, attainable, realistic, and timely (Meyer, 2003; Cornell, 2012) (Figure 5.3).

The Focus Funnel™

Analogous to a common household funnel, the job of the Focus Funnel is to channel and reduce. The Focus Funnel encourages teachers to distill potentially confusing information into critical sound bites that can be easily absorbed by students. It starts with "the lesson." The teacher gives a lesson containing the largest amount of material, including all information pertinent to learning a skill. Next, the teacher delivers "the directions." The directions contain only information vital to the performance of the skill. Finally, immediately before the student performs the new skill, the teacher gives the student a single goal or "Tag Point" that when performed, will be marked with an audible marker (Figure 5.4).

The Tag Point™

The Tag Point is uniquely constructed to be the pivotal point of focus for the student and the teacher. Tag Points support a positive student–teacher relationship by clearly stating a single criterion for success (Box 5.2).

BOX 5.2:

Tag Points – WOOF

What you want
One thing at a time
Observable and measurable
Five words or less

http://www.tagteach.com.

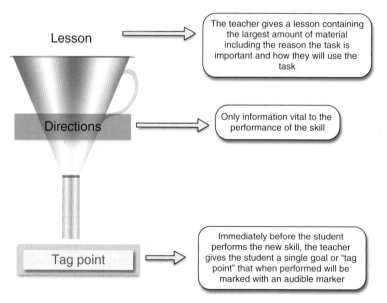

Figure 5.4 The Focus Funnel™ is used to channel and reduce information.

The focus point is analogous to a Tag Point. It is phrased in the same manner but is referred to as a *focus point* rather than a Tag Point. This can be used when the learner will not be audibly tagged by an observer, but instead the learner focuses on the task and determines on their own if they have met the criteria.

The tag

After the teacher delivers the Tag Point, the student performs the skill. The teacher marks the moment the Tag Point is achieved with an audible sound. The audible mark always means success. Most students are reinforced by success. Therefore, the audible mark becomes reinforcing. Using a short sharp sound such as a clicker or a tone from a cell phone as a marker is preferred over verbal marks such as "yes" or "good." The pure sound is easily processed by the student and reduces the emotions associated with the human voice. The more distractions eliminated during the actual moments before, during, and after learning, the more focus we get from our students. If the teacher notices something else within the skill that needs to be improved, it can be made into a different Tag Point or discussed at a later time. Success is solely contingent on the performance of the designated Tag Point.

An example of using the Focus Funnel in veterinary medicine might be the following:

The lesson is that dogs often communicate with body language. Some of the natural friendly behaviors humans express toward dogs can actually be perceived as a threat. For example, people often greet dogs by looking directly at them, walking toward, and leaning over them. All of these behaviors would be interpreted as a threat if between two dogs.

The directions are that when meeting a dog instead of looking directly at the dog, glance at it then look away.

The Tag Point or focus point is to look at your feet.

Success makes us feel confident. Success makes us want to do it again. Use the Focus Funnel, Tag Points, and an audible marker as tools to quantify and highlight success for you and your students.

The communication cycle

Treating and preventing behavior disorders requires a team approach that includes the veterinary technician as the "case manager," the veterinarian who diagnoses, prescribes, and gives a prognosis, and a qualified trainer who works in the field with the pet owner. A list of included forms for expediting the communication cycle is included in Table 5.3 and the Appendix.

Table 5.3 Form utilization.

Form	Who uses	How to use
Behavior problem list + refer to Triage Table 1.4	Completed during first contact with pet owner (veterinary technician/trainer)	Used at first contact to triage and determine if the next contact should be with hospital's qualified trainer (could also be the veterinary technician) or be seen by the veterinarian
Field assessment	Completed by "veterinary technician/ qualified trainer working with the pet owner "in the field"	Completed and submitted to the veterinary hospital when the qualified trainer sees the pet owner in the field and suspects the issue may be a behavioral disorder rather than a training issue
Field follow-up form	Completed by the veterinary technician/trainer	Completed by the qualified trainer after seeing a patient referred to them by the veterinary hospital
History Part A – behavior consultation	Completed by the veterinarian technician or pet owner	Completed before the behavior consultation
History Part B – behavior consultation	Completed by the veterinarian	Completed during the behavior consultation
Observation chart	Completed by the veterinary technician during the initial consultation	Create a second observation chart to be used to determine progress at the follow-up appointment
Plan of care	Completed by the veterinarian	Plan for the veterinary technician/trainer to assist the pet owner with application of the prescribed treatment plan
Follow-up behavior consultation form	Completed by the veterinarian	Completed by the veterinarian after a follow-up behavior consultation

CHAPTER 5

The veterinary technician is the key to the communication cycle by being in contact with the entire team to keep everyone in the loop. When a client calls in with a "behavior problem," it is the veterinary technician who should perform a phone assessment and triage the case. The technician will determine from the communication whether the next contact should be a consultation with the veterinarian or a qualified trainer. If it is initially determined that the "behavior problem" is likely a lack of training or a conditioned unwanted behavior it is referred to the hospital's qualified trainer. It is imperative that the veterinary technician and the qualified trainer have an open and clear communication. If the trainer determines that the initial phone assessment was correct and the issue is training or lack of it, the pet owner will remain with the trainer, but the trainer will send a follow-up report to the veterinary technician on the patient's training progress. If the trainer determines that the issue is more complex than first anticipated, then the patient is referred back to the veterinarian for a diagnosis and treatment plan. At that point, the veterinarian may diagnose a behavioral disorder and along with the input from the technician and trainer create a treatment plan or choose to refer the case to a veterinary behaviorist.

If a treatment plan is prescribed, a Plan of Care (see Plan of Care in Appendix 4) should be submitted to the technician or trainer who will be working with the pet owner. The trainer or veterinary technician working with the patient and pet owner then sends follow-up reports back to the veterinary technician (case manager) who then reports follow-up progress to the veterinarian, and the treatment plan is adjusted as discussed by the team (Figure 5.5).

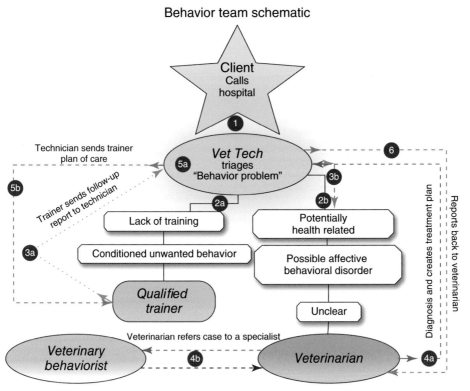

Figure 5.5 1. Client makes the first contact with the veterinary technician. 2a. The veterinary technician assesses the situation and suspects a training issue and sends to the veterinary hospital's qualified trainer. 2b. The veterinary technician assesses the situation and determines case needs to be seen by the veterinarian. 3a. The trainer sends follow-up report to the veterinary technician on patient's training progress. 3b. The trainer determines the issue is more complex than first anticipated, and patient is referred to the veterinarian for a diagnosis and treatment plan. 4a. The veterinarian provides diagnosis and creates treatment plan or 4b. The veterinarian refers the case to veterinary behaviorist. 5a. The veterinary technician assists the client in applying the prescribed treatment plan. 5b. Plan of care is sent to the trainer to continue to assist the client with the treatment plan. 6. The veterinary technician reports follow-up progress to veterinarian, and the treatment plan is adjusted as needed.

Assessments

Getting an informal impression or evaluation of the situation is the first step in triaging and differentiating a behavioral problem from a behavioral disorder (see Table 1.2).

Preventive care: preventive care refers to the measures taken to prevent a behavioral disorder from occurring rather than curing or treating the symptoms of an existing disorder. It is the primary role for veterinary technicians.

> - Preventive care: preventive care refers to the measures taken to prevent a behavioral disorder from occurring rather than curing or treating the symptoms of an existing disorder.
> - It is the primary role for veterinary technicians.

Intervention care: intervention care refers to measures taken to improve or alter an existing behavioral disorder. Intervention requires a veterinarian's diagnosis and treatment plan.

> - Intervention care: intervention care refers to measures taken to improve or alter an existing behavioral disorder. Intervention requires a veterinarian's diagnosis and treatment plan.

Initial phone assessment

Often, the first contact from the pet owner pertaining to their pet's behavior will be a phone call to the veterinary hospital. The first phone call is the time to begin building the team approach and bonding the pet owner to the team. During the initial phone assessment, the veterinary technician should obtain brief but specific information to determine the further steps to be taken. The phone assessment should include the following areas.

Signalment and family orientation

Age of the pet – The age of the pet may help determine the duration of learning history that has occurred. If the issue is aggression, the duration the animal has been "practicing" the aggression may help determine the animal's confidence level. Young animals usually show conflict behaviors before a bite, whereas older ones have developed their own coping skills (i.e., aggression or flight) and practiced them for many years and may

no longer demonstrate conflict behaviors because they are no longer in conflict.

Another consideration regarding the age of the pet is the need to rule out medical contributing factors. In general, an adult or senior pet that has an acute change in behavior is indicative of a medical issue.

Breed – The breed of the animal is important for detecting breed predispositions, such as chasing and herding behaviors. The size of the animal may also have an impact on the level of triage needed. For example, giant breeds of dogs can inflict more significant damage than toy breeds; therefore, the situation can have a more immediate need.

Where the pet was obtained, age obtained, and when the animal was taken from the litter – Early history will give insight into socialization history and early communication skills learned or not toward conspecifics.

Family orientation and other pets in the household – The family orientation, age of children, number of children, and other pets in the household will impact the pet's learning history. Children can increase the opportunities for learning unwanted behaviors and will also impact the risk associated with aggression issues.

Identify high-risk factors

Research from the Ontario Veterinary College (Guy *et al.*, 2001a–c) identified risk factors for puppies developing aggression toward family members, which should be considered "red flags" during phone assessments (see Box 5.1).

Description and prioritized problem list

The veterinary technician should complete a "problem list" (form in Appendix 5) (Table 5.4). The "problems" are a list of pet owner complaints, not diagnosis.

Ask the pet owner to describe their primary behavior concern and then describe the last incident, including what happened before, during, and after the event. The description the pet owner gives should be comparable to playing a movie. Asking questions such as, "What did that look like?" and "What did you do after the behavior occurred?" will give insight into the behavior and steer the conversation away from interpretational descriptions. For example, "He hates it when it storms" is not as helpful as, "When it begins to storm 'Fluffy' hides under the bed and shakes. I pull her out from under the bed and cuddle her," which provides the technician with much more pertinent information (see Table 5.2).

It is helpful to know what initiated the call, especially when the behavior has been ongoing. Inquiring about event changes is one way of assessing the extent to

Table 5.4 Behavior problem list.

Eliminative	Social	Ingestive
□ Incontinence	□ Barking/howling/whining	□ Anorexia
□ Diarrhea/vomiting	□ Rolling in unsavory items	□ Chewing objects
□ House soiling	□ Jumps up on people	□ Coprophagia
□ Urine marking	□ Demands attention	□ Compulsive eating
□ Urination on pheromones	□ Demands touch	□ Compulsive drinking
□ Other _____	□ Aggressive to owners	□ Eating grass/plants
	□ Aggressive to strangers	□ Eating garbage
Grooming	□ Aggressive to dogs/same household	□ Pica
	□ Aggressive to strange dogs	□ Prey catching
□ Licking self	□ Aggressive to other animals	□ Car chasing
□ Sucking on self	□ Other _____	□ Light/shadow chasing
□ Chewing on self		□ Stealing food
□ Scratching self		□ Fly snapping
□ Checking hind end		□ Air/mouth licking
□ Other _____		□ Other _____
Temperament related	**Reproduction**	**Locomotory**
□ Depressed inappetent	□ Cannibalism	□ Circling/whirling
□ Hyperexcitable/active	□ False pregnancy	□ Tail biting
□ Hyperreactive	□ Masturbation	□ Pacing, figure 8s
□ Nervous/anxious	□ Mounting people	□ Digging
□ Fear of thunder	□ Mounting animals	□ Lameness/cond.
□ Fear of loud noises, e.g., thunder	□ Self nursing	□ Roaming
□ Fear of people	□ Other _____	□ Scratching objects
□ Fear of situations		□ Freezing
□ Fear of objects/animals		□ Other _____
□ Other _____		

Comments:

which the pet owner and the pet may be in crisis. A specific recent event may have prompted the call for an appointment. A pet's behavior may have been managed until a recent life change (pregnancy, divorce, extended family addition, etc.) or a significant episode may have caused an escalation in concern. Regardless, it is important to find out if the current issue is acute or a chronic problem. Specific information can help pinpoint whether the stress is underlying the presenting problem or is only a symptom of it (Canino *et al.*, 2007).

Asking the question, "What have you done to treat the problem?" gives the technician insight into the possible frustration level of the pet owner and can determine whether the pet owner is using techniques, including punishment, which could cause the issue to worsen or put the pet owner in a dangerous situation. The pet owner may say, "We've tried everything!" or "I know I'm making it worse …" In these cases, the technician

should be supportive and instruct them how to safely interact until the issue can be addressed.

Specific questions to ask pertaining to aggression
During the phone assessment, it is imperative to determine whether the pet owner is in danger of being injured. Asking specifically about past bite history, including number of bites, and whether the bites were inhibited is critical. Information as to if the pet bites once and leaves or continues to aggress during an episode should be obtained. The technician should assist the owner in identifying potential warning signs before the aggression occurs. Pet owners should be asked if they are aware of known triggers for fearful or aggressive behavior, and when those triggers can be identified, they should be avoided until the pet can be seen for a full behavior consultation. If targets cannot be identified or if there are many triggering factors, the

pet owner should be asked to interact with the pet as little as possible and in a cue-response-reward format when interaction must occur (see Chapter 8). The goal is to keep the pet owner safe until the consultation and to prevent further deterioration of the HAB.

Status of the HAB

Possibly, the most critical area to obtain information is the status of the HAB. A seriously damaged HAB should be treated as in an emergency situation. Regardless of whether the problem is suspected to be a training issue or behavioral disorder, once the HAB is damaged, it can be difficult to treat the problem. Asking the pet owner how they "feel about their pet" and whether they are afraid of their pet can give critical insight to the current relationship. The technician should also inquire about the relationship with other family members involved with the pet and how their attitudes may affect the current situation.

Assessment in the field

The qualified trainer associated with your veterinary hospital (the qualified trainer could also be the veterinary technician) may be the first contact for the pet owner. When this occurs and the trainer suspects the pet's issues may be based on an affective behavioral disorder, the trainer may either refer the client immediately to the veterinarian or provide a field assessment and then submit their assessment to the veterinary behavior team (see Appendix 27 for a sample field assessment) (Table 5.5).

Parts of a behavior history

A thorough history must be taken to give appropriate and proper recommendations. Without a proper history, wrong advice may be given, and compliance will be low.

It is diagnostically helpful to break the history down into 3 parts: *signalment and general management history*, including husbandry, *general temperament evaluation*, and *detailed information pertaining to the specific issues*. When discussing specific issues, information concerning when and where the behavior occurs, what triggers the behavior, what behavior is shown, including body language and facial expressions, who or what is the target of the behavior, how people react to the behavior, and how the animal acts and looks after the behavior is obtained. Specific information should also be obtained as to the severity, frequency, and what the pet owners have done in attempts to change the behavior.

After obtaining specific details relating to the presenting complaint, clients should be asked to describe the very first time the problem occurred to assess the development of the problem. The clients are also asked to describe in detail the three most recent incidences of the behavior (see Appendix 1 for sample history forms).

During the appointment, the veterinary technician should complete an observation form. A second observation form can be completed at follow-up appointments to assess progress (see Technical observation form in Appendix 10) (Table 5.6).

Follow-up reports

Follow-up training and behavior modification reports should be sent to the behavior team on a monthly basis or as needed. If major changes in the treatment plan

Table 5.5 A field assessment should include the following.

Content	Details
Owner's prioritized behavioral concerns	This list should include both training issues and behavioral disorder concerns
General signalment and family orientation	Include changes in family orientation and status changes (divorce, etc.)
Problem history	Include pertinent information the veterinary behavior team should know when making their diagnosis and treatment plan, including previously attempted treatment and training techniques
Medical conditions or concerns	Known medications or gross health concerns as reported by the owner (lameness, pain, etc.)
Assessment meeting observations	Include pertinent family interactions, observations, and environmental concerns
Plan training and management suggestions	Include goals, training techniques, training tools, and exercises recommended
Status of the HAB	Note any damage or breaks in the HAB. Comments made by the family such as, "we cannot take much more" or "we are ready to give up" are critical when the behavior team considers a treatment plan
Specific concerns	This section should include the trainers concerns pertaining to potential compliance issues, lack of progress or anxiety/aggression issues, which may have an affective basis, including lack of impulse control or difficulty learning

CHAPTER 5

Table 5.6 Veterinary technician's observations during a behavior consultation.

	Start of appointment	15 min	30 min	60 min	End of appointment
Treats	0	Chicken	Anything	Anything	Anything
Treat proximity	0	From owner	From floor 3 ft from owner	Technician's hand	Technician's hand
Interactions	Next to owner	Attention seeking to owner	Walking around room	Greeting people in room	Greeting new people who enter
Trainability (1–10)	0	2	6	8	10
General behavior	Growling	Occasionally growling	Interested in technician	Wagging tail	Sleeping
Restrictions	Muzzle and tie down	Muzzle removed	Allowed off tie down, dragging leash	Off leash	Off leash

Significant events during appointment
Charged door when a noise occurred outside the examination room

Treats – type of treat taken.
Proximity – where took treats (owner's hand, floor, technician's hand, etc.).
Interactions – does the pet interact with others? Interactions with owner?
General behavior – general comments about behavior during appointment.
Restrictions – note any restrictions used during the appointment.
Significant events – note any reactions to stimuli or general comments.
This form can be used to access progress when the patient returns for a follow-up appointment.

are considered, changes should be discussed before implementation. In a poll conducted on the Veterinary Information Network, veterinarians indicated that it was imperative their treatment plans not be changed by trainers in the field without first discussing those changes (Shaw, 2011).

In the same regard, the trainer should be alerted to follow-up appointments at the veterinary hospital and any changes in the treatment plan on a consistent and regular basis (see Follow-up communication form in Appendix 11).

During follow-up appointments, it is helpful to ask the pet owner to rate the problem on a scale of 1–10 (10 being the worst the problem has ever been) to what the problem is currently. The goal is to see a minimum of a 50% improvement at the follow-up appointment. A scale system is helpful for the behavior team and the pet owner to objectively analyze behavior improvements.

Acquiring a behavior history and improving pet owner compliance
Question styles
Clients will commonly not give objective interpretations of their pet's behavior but instead their rationalized interpretations. Therefore, it is important to ask open- and close-ended questions to distill the information you need. Repeat the information back to the client in a simplified form to verify through reflective listening, the information they have presented. Sometimes, leading questions may be needed. Later, the question can be asked in reverse, giving the clients an opportunity to contradict themselves or provide additional insight.

Closed-ended questions are those that can be answered with a yes or no or a single word or a short phrase. Closed-ended questions are comparable to multiple-choice questions. For example, "Is 'Fluffy' aggressive to strangers?" is a close-ended question. Closed-ended questions place the control of the conversation with the questioner. They give facts and are easy and quick to answer.

Open-ended questions require the pet owner to answer with more information and are comparable to essay questions. Open-ended questions require the pet owner to think, reflect, and offer opinions and feelings and put the respondent in control of the conversation. When asking open-ended questions, you will not only need to guide the conversation, but also leave openings for the client to digress somewhat so you "can read between the lines." For example, "Whom is 'Fluffy's'

Table 5.7 Examples of open- and closed-ended questions.

Closed-ended questions	Usage	Example
	Opening question to begin a conversation	"Did you have a nice drive?" "Isn't the weather nice?"
	Testing understanding	"So, you would like to focus on 'Fluffy's' urination in the house today?"
	Setting up a desired frame of mind	"Do you feel better about the current issue you are having with 'Fluffy'?"
	Getting closure of a final agreement	"You can walk 'Fluffy' twice daily, correct?
Open-ended questions	**Usage**	**Example**
	Follow-up from a closed question	"Are there any other issues you would like to discuss today?"
	To find out more about the client's needs	"How is 'Fluffy's' behavior affecting your family?"
	Assisting clients in understanding the extent of the problem	"How do you feel 'Fluffy's' fear affects your daily activities?"
	Getting the client to trust you	"How are you feeling about 'Fluffy' these days?"

Modified from Straker (2002–2012).

aggression directed toward?" pet owner's answer, "He is mostly aggressive to my husband." By reading between the lines, this statement could be interpreted to mean, he is aggressive to the husband most of time but also other people at other times (Table 5.7).

Reflecting is communicating back what you have heard. Reflection is used at a point in the conversation in which a large amount of information has been presented and is intended to help summarize the information to make sure that all information has been provided. Reflection can also be used to get back on track, if a client starts to stray from the specific information being sought.

Improving compliance

In veterinary medicine, the definition of compliance is how consistent and accurate a pet owner completes their pet's prescribed regimen. When there is a lack of compliance, there is an increase in frustration both from the client and from the behavior team.

A study looking at owner compliance found that spending too little time with clients caused a decrease in compliance (Shaw, 2007).

American Animal Hospital Association (AAHA) also performed a study looking at owner compliance with six basic health care recommendations and found that noncompliance occurred when veterinarians failed to communicate clearly or provide clear recommendations. Both studies indicate that compliance is enhanced when trust and rapport are established with clients. It has also been found that clients are more willing to follow directions when playing an active role in the decision-making process (Shaw, 2007).

Compliance enhancers

Empathy – Allow the pet owner to be frustrated or angry at their pet's behavior. Acknowledge and reinforce what they have done so far to improve the issue. Let them know you have seen similar cases and give examples of your past experiences.

*Appropriate and clear goal*s – Ask the owners for their specific goals, what degree of improvement would they be happy with, and what degree of improvement could they live with. Consider the pet owner's limitations, and do not blame them for those limitations. Determine the pet owner's level of commitment to work on the issue. If there are multiple problems to be addressed, set priorities for treatment with the pet owner's input. If certain issues must be addressed ahead of the pet owner's priorities (for example, decreasing anxiety before addressing barking), explain to the pet owner why it is necessary to proceed in the prescribed order (i.e., decreasing the anxiety may also decrease reactivity and barking).

Seeing progress quickly – Owners are more likely to comply with a treatment plan if they see subtle improvement quickly. Simply teaching their pet to target or learn a cue can improve the pet owner's enthusiasm in applying the treatment plan.

Keep explanations and the treatment plan simple and in point form – Small steps are important when providing large amounts of information to clients. Giving small amounts of information intermittently decreases the chance of overwhelming the pet owner. Overwhelmed pet owners do not feel safe (Abood, 2007). Be logical and only provide what is completely necessary. Ask the clients if they understand why points of the treatment plan are important (i.e., you are ignoring attention-seeking behaviors so we can decrease hyper-excitablity) and have them repeat the key points back. Ask the owners what aspect of the treatment plan they feel will be the most difficult to apply and problem solve or modify as needed.

Implement the treatment in steps – Start with simple management modifications and training before going into time-consuming and complex behavior modification techniques. Let the pet owners know that this is only the first step in the treatment plan, and more steps will be added in follow-up appointments.

Provide a written discharge and instructions – Include handouts and recommended reading for pet owners to review at their leisure once they have had time to digest the information they have received during the consultation.

Establish realistic expectations for progress – A working rule of thumb is that it takes equally as long to treat a problem as it took to become established. Emphasize the quick improvements that are being seen (i.e., response during the appointment to training). Remind owners that conditioned behaviors may worsen as they go through extinction bursts, and that means the behavior is on its way to improving.

Have the pet owners keep a diary so that progress can be clearly seen – Dealing with an animal with a behavioral disorder on a daily basis can make it difficult for the pet owner to see progress. A behavior diary can be helpful by noting significant stimuli, medications added, and other relevant daily activities. Using a graph format, the pet owner can observe progress that might not be obvious on a daily basis (see Behavior Diary in Appendix 12).

Stay in touch with the pet owner – Follow-up care by the veterinary technician is critical. Checking in with the pet owner a few days after the appointment to clarify the treatment plan will reinforce them that they are not alone. The veterinary technician is the case manager and should also stay in contact with the qualified trainer who is assisting the client "in the field."

Charge enough – Free or under-priced advice is not valued (Luescher and Martin, 2010).

The technician is the key in improving pet owner compliance to behavior treatment plans. Spending appropriate time with clients, providing explanations and understanding, answering questions, and allowing collaboration enhance owner compliance and build healthy relationships.

Grief counseling

The relationship we have with our pet overlaps many comparable human relationships such as friend, significant other, family member, and child. "This is not to say that even the most bonded person believes his or her pet is human. Pets seem to occupy an overlapping but different space from humans in a family. Even people who think of their pets as children know this is not literally true. In part, they are identifying their pets as family members by the way in which pets function within the household" (Cohen, 2002).

The ultimate goal of grief counseling is to assist the pet owner in the grieving process so the grief can become a positive experience, with the end result being a hope for the future.

The "normal" grief process

This section discusses what is considered "normal" or noncomplex grief, which is defined as grief that begins to fade and subside into adequate coping mechanisms within 6 months.

Grief: an individual's inner emotional feelings occurring because of a loss.

> - *Grief*: an individual's inner emotional feelings occurring because of a loss.

Mourning: outward, social expression of the loss. Often the mourning process is dictated by societal norms and impacts. The process of mourning allows a person to move through the grief process and when inhibited can delay the grief process. Ceremony helps you to know what to do when you do not know what to do.

> - *Mourning*: outward, social expression of the loss. Often the mourning process is dictated by societal norms and impacts.
> - The process of mourning allows a person to move through the grief process and when inhibited can delay the grief process.
> - Ceremony helps you to know what to do when you do not know what to do.

Bereavement: the state of events or loss that causes grief.

> • *Bereavement*: the state of events or loss that causes grief.

Grief is a very private and individual process; no two people travel through grief following exactly the same path. Grief is often discussed as occurring in stages, whereas in reality, it occurs more in waves or cycles that come and go depending on triggers in the environment. There are numerous grief paradigms (Table 5.8). In this section, the five stages of coping with dying by Elizabeth Kubler-Ross: denial, anger, bargaining, depression, and acceptance are historically the most commonly used paradigm, although they are being used erroneously in this application as they were developed using information from dying cancer patients rather than survivors of a lost one. Newer clinical approaches include both a more postmodern individualizing of loss and a rejection of predictable stages. "Different individuals grieve in different ways, and counselors should be aware of the diversity of such ways if they are to assist clients to follow their path of grief" (Walter, 1996).

The grief model whether you choose to use it will depend on the pet owner and your comfort.

Types of grievers

Intuitive grievers experience grief at an affective level. They work through grief by expressing their deep emotional pain by crying, shouting, and so on. *Instrumental grievers* are more likely to demonstrate their grief in cognitive and physical terms (exercising, talking about their thoughts, etc.) rather than demonstrating intense emotion. They process their thoughts, ruminating and revisiting memories. Because instrumental grievers do not outwardly show intense emotion, it is important their grief is not overlooked. *Intuitive–instrumental grievers* experience a combination of both styles, although one style may be more pronounced, depending on their own personality type and attachment to the pet (Cordaro, 2012).

Complex grief

The grief felt when a pet is diagnosed with a behavioral disorder or is eventually euthanized because of it is multifaceted and complex. There has been no research in any mental health or veterinary science journals specifically pertaining to grief directly associated with pet owners living with pets with behavioral disorders (Luiz Adrian *et al.*, 2009). Owing to the complexities and the stigma associated, it can be ascertained that the grief associated in such a situation is complex and convoluted.

Disenfranchised grief

Disenfranchised grief occurs when a loss is not acknowledged or supported by societal norms. In the case of disenfranchised grief, the bereaved feel unsupported and are unable to openly mourn; therefore, the grief process may be delayed. Common disenfranchised losses include pet loss, death of a loved one by suicide, or a death of a loved one because of AIDS (Worden, 1991). Most pet owners will likely struggle with some degree of disenfranchised grief as an empathetic failure, making them less likely to share the authenticity of emotional pain (Cordaro, 2012).

The society has not acknowledged the relationship we have with pets as a true relationship and has proscribed pet-related bereavement as unacceptable. Instead, the society prescribes that pet owners "swiftly overcome grief reactions and replace the deceased pet." Consequently, the implicit norm that is endorsed is that the bonds forged between people and companion pets do not have the same depth and meaning as bonds between people; therefore, the grief felt when a pet dies would not be as intense as when another person dies. It is not recognized as a true loss (Cordaro, 2012).

An extension of disenfranchised grief occurs when the person mourning finds it difficult to discuss the loss because of stigmatization (Worden, 1991). Stigmatization was mentioned in Chapter 4 in regard to treating an animal with a behavioral disorder but also occurs when an animal is euthanized because of a behavioral disorder. Pet owners are often caught in a complex paradox. Many are criticized for treating the animal "when they could just get another pet," but also if they choose not to treat the disorder or end treatment, they may be ostracized because they "could have done more, he was a healthy dog". When they do euthanize for the disorder, they are left without support. It is often a no-win situation for pet owners, leaving them alone to grieve without the benefit of being allowed to mourn the loss.

Pet owners may not reach out to friends or family members because they fear the stigma placed on them and the pet. It is therefore critical for the pet owner to know that the veterinary technician will support them in whatever decisions they make, with no judgments. By building a strong, safe relationship with the pet owner, the technician can give them the needed solace and comfort they may not be able to find elsewhere. If this is not the case, the pet owner may choose euthanasia and do so in a secret manner, never making

Table 5.8 Common grief models.

Kubler-Ross stages of grief	
Denial	"This cannot be happening"
Anger	"Why is this happening? This must be the trainer's fault"
Bargaining	"Maybe if we try a new medication or a different dosage things will get better"
Depression	"This hurts too much, I am overwhelmed with sadness"
Acceptance	"I have done everything I can, and I know that I am giving her a gift of love by letting her go"
The five stages of grief	
Numbness and denial	Numbness or shock can help cushion the blow as you adjust to the loss. This stage can last a few hours, days, or even a few weeks
Yearning and anger	The numbness wears off, and the painful realization of the loss hits full-force; you will ache missing your pet. You may be angry and have regrets
Emotional despair, sadness, and withdrawal	The storm of intense emotions of the second stage gives way to a period of heavy sadness, silence, and withdrawal from family and friends
Reorganization	Reorganization and the beginning of positive emotions. Over time, sadness will lessen, and you will start to perceive your life in a more positive light, although bouts of grief and sadness will persist
Letting go and moving on	The final phase of this model is to let go off your need for the lost pet and begin to move on with your life. Sadness will lessen greatly and you will begin to think of the future
The seven stages of grief	
Shock and denial	You may deny the reality of the loss at some level. Shock provides emotional protection from being overwhelmed
Pain and guilt	As the shock wears off, it is replaced with the suffering of unbelievable pain. You may have feelings of guilt or remorse, life feels chaotic and frightening
Anger and bargaining	Frustration leads to anger, you may lash out and blame others. You may bargain, "I would give up anything to have him back"
Depression, reflection, loneliness	A sad period of reflection, the true magnitude of the loss sets in. You may isolate yourself to focus on memories
Upward turn	As you start to adjust to life without your pet and begin to move on
Reconstruction and working through	As you become more functional, your mind starts working again
Acceptance and hope	You learn to accept and deal with the reality of your situation. You will be "different" but able to begin to think about the future
The new grief stages	
Shock	Shock and numbness set in to protect your mind from being overwhelmed. It may feel as though you are sleepwalking, not fully in reality and unable to make the simplest of decisions.
	Allow family and friends to give support. Begin mourning rituals
Suffering	As the shock wears off, the pain begins. This is a time of emotional upheaval and extreme pain emotionally and physically
	The hallmarks of this phase are rapid mood swings, intense emotions, and loss of control over your psyche. You may even feel like you are losing your sanity
	This is not only the time the most emotional support is needed, but also the time friends and family begin to get on with their lives
	Late in this stage you will begin to exist again but feel lonely and depressed, alternating between intense grief; the "roller coaster" of grief. Expect fluid and unpredictable changes in emotion. Do not fight the emotions, allow them to be
	This is the active grieving stage. Yield to the grief; experience it fully and openly in your own way
Recovery	Acceptance and full recovery do not happen overnight. Your depression and despair will just slowly begin to dissipate
	Although not the end of the pain, you begin to learn to function with the pain in your life. You begin to reconnect to life and remember what "happy" felt like
	The ability to function and more immediate life demands start to take precedence
	The benefit of grief may be seen – you have a new appreciation for life and a new-found ability to live life in the moment

contact with the veterinary hospital or staff again because they feel they will be judged or that they are bad pet owners. If they feel safe and not judged, the choice of euthanasia can be seen as a gift, continuing and deepening the bond with the veterinary hospital and veterinary professionals.

Grieving the pet they thought they had

Families living with a pet with a serious behavioral disorder will grieve; some have compared the grief experience as being analogous to death of the pet they thought they had and accepting the pet they do have. Grief associated with accepting that their pet has a serious behavioral disorder can be difficult because it lacks finality comparable to any chronic health disorder.

Unlike grief owing to death, this type of grief is complex and ongoing. The diagnosis of a serious behavioral disorder may bring initial relief and hope to the pet owner, relief that the problem has been seen before and they are not to blame and hope the issue can be treated. Such feelings may only be temporary, as they realize their pet's behavioral disorder is likely lifelong and will therefore have a direct impact on their family. As clinical signs of the behavioral disorder may lessen, pet owners may cling to the hope that the disorder will spontaneously remit (Abosh and Collins, 1996). When an animal is diagnosed with an affective behavioral disorder (with a likely brain chemical imbalance), the pet owner must vacillate between attempting to resolve the loss while also adapting to the difficulties their pet's issues impact on their lives. Such grief may not resolve over time but may intensify as the pet owner is confronted with the reality that their pet may always need some degree of management and may be limited in which activities they can participate. The cyclic and ongoing nature of the grief is a result of periodic durations in which the animal is reported to be "wonderful 90% of the time" followed by episodes of the behavioral disorder (aggression, panic, compulsions, etc.). This same type of grief has been reported by parents when their child or family member is diagnosed with a mental illness and is still highly unrecognized in human medicine by grief counselors (MacGregor, 1994). The grief is described as complicated and nonfinite. During this stage of grief, the pet owner has not only lost their pet, but also lost the emotionally healthy pet they thought they had.

Families are affected in ways that include coping with symptoms of the disorder, increased responsibilities, disruption of family life, inability to get help, and the social stigma associated with behavioral disorder (Richardson *et al.*, 2011). This type of grief can resurface at the same intensity as it did at diagnosis when a perceived "set back" occurs and is therefore surface-similar to the "chronic sorrow" of parents of emotionally or mentally challenged children.

Choosing to euthanize because of a behavioral disorder

The specific type of grief discussed in this section is when a physically healthy pet is euthanized when a pet owner is unable to continue to treat or manage a pet with a behavioral disorder.

In these situations, one or more of the following behavioral disorders is likely involved:
1. Aggression
2. Unresolved inappropriate elimination
3. Severe separation anxiety
4. Severe thunderstorm phobia
5. Compulsive disorders – especially self-mutilation (Hetts, 1999)

Denial/shock

Denial occurs when the current situation is too unbearable to emotionally accept. Shock follows, which is a numbness and detachment. Denial and shock are protection mechanisms as the griever prepares to move further into the grief process. An appropriate analogy is that shock is comparable to ice covering a raging river (the river being pending grief). Shock allows our psyches to prepare for dealing with the raging river below.

When a pet owner is suddenly presented with information they were not expecting, they may be unable to immediately digest the information presented. Be patient and repeat yourself during the process. The pet owner will likely need to contemplate what they have heard. It is helpful for other family members or friends to be present to also hear the information being presented so that it can be reiterated to the pet owner later. Giving an option for a second opinion may also aid in the clients absorption of the information.

Anger

A pet owner's anger is often directed toward persons or situations that they believe caused or exasperated their pet's issues. They may blame veterinarians, trainers, breeders, pet stores, or others they believe they obtained outdated or incorrect information from.

It is important to focus on what can be done rather than what has happened in the past that cannot be changed. Emphasizing past experiences is information for the future, and simply listening to the pet owner without exasperating their anger is helpful. Anger directed toward you is not personal; it is simply part of the pet owner's grief experience (see Figure 5.1).

Bargaining

As pet owners begin to accept their pet's behavioral disorder and deal with the future, they may begin to bargain, looking for "other options" or ways out of their current circumstance.

Rehoming versus euthanasia

When aggression is directed toward family members, it is generally not a situation in which the pet is rehomeable or adoptable. It is not fair to rehome the pet and have a new family become attached to the pet. Likely, the new family will become the recipient of aggression in similar situations and have to struggle with the decision to rehome or euthanize. This does not benefit the HAB or the welfare of the pet. It places another family at risk of injury and heartbreak. Often, attempts to correct the problem are inappropriate (positive punishment), and this negatively affects the welfare of the pet. Euthanasia would be a responsible decision in this situation. It would be the best decision from a public health standpoint and for the welfare of the pet. Not all companion animals make good pets and enjoy human companionship.

Exceptions may include the following: aggression directed only toward children living in the home or another pet in the home. In this situation, the pet could be rehomed to a child-free or pet-free home, with the new pet owner fully aware of the issue and agreeable to keeping the pet away from children and other animals.

Guilt

While anger is directed toward someone or something, guilt is anger directed at oneself. Holding onto guilty feelings can keep an owner from moving on or having quality relationships with future pets.

Guilt is present in any grief experience but may be exaggerated for pet owners by their heightened sense of responsibility for their pet comparable to that for the well-being of a child. Pet owners often believe they contributed to their pet's disorder by not noticing the extreme symptoms of anxiety, choosing the wrong trainer, or by not being a strong "pack leaders" (see section titled **The dominance theory** earlier in this chapter). Often, after explaining to the pet owner that they are not the direct cause of the disorder, they continue to believe that somehow they should have been able to prevent it. The feeling of powerlessness to deal with the problem exasperates this type of unrealistic guilt. Allowing the pet owner to have an active involvement as a member of the treatment team can give them a bit of empowerment and relief from this type of guilt. Pet owners who feel listened to and supported and receive accurate and up-to-date information feel empowered and may move to take action with a treatment plan or consider other options.

The notion of pet owners being "bad pet owners" if their animal must be euthanized because of a behavioral disorder creates a scenario of grief and guilt that can be overwhelming. Pet owners may have feelings of guilt because of perceived inadequacy as pet owners and feelings of complicity in the development of their pet's disorder. The loss of an animal because of a behavioral disorder can shake a pet owner's belief in themselves as "good" pet owners. Family members may blame each other, causing family tension. "There are no bad dogs, only bad pet owners" is a very hurtful and blaming statement, and in fact, likely to be untrue.

- "There are no bad dogs, only bad pet owners" is a very hurtful and blaming statement, and in fact, likely to be untrue.

Receiving a diagnosis can alleviate the pet owner's feelings of guilt that they directly caused their pet's behavioral disorder. When a pet owner feels guilty, ask them to state exactly what they specifically feel guilty about. Remind them what they have done in attempt to treat the problem. Acknowledge that the difficult decisions they are making take deep love and courage only a very brave, selfless, and compassionate pet owner can make (Table 5.9).

Table 5.9 Common guilt-ridden statements made by pet owners with responses.

Statement	Response
"I did not do enough to help her"	"You have done everything you can to help her. You have done more than most people could have ever achieved. You have given her the happiest moments of her life and for that I know she is deeply grateful"
"People think I am crazy for keeping him"	"They do not see the wonderful moments, the times where he is happy and relaxed with you. They simply do not know him as you do and therefore cannot understand"
"I created the problem, it is my fault"	"Your pet was most likely born with a physical brain chemistry disorder. There are training techniques and communication styles that can increase anxiety, but you did not create your pet's behavior disorder"
"I made the problem worse"	"You cannot do what you do not know. I have done many things to my past pets that I now wish I could go back and change because I have better and newer knowledge. But all we can do is move forward with the up-to-date information we know. 'Fluffy' taught us lessons that we will take with us into the future"

- Guilt and pet owner self-forgiveness
  1. Identify the reasons you must consider choosing euthanasia.
  2. Accept the fact it is your responsibility to make this decision.
  3. Acknowledge the pain and guilt you may be feeling.
  4. Identify precisely what you feel guilty about.
  5. Compassionately listen to your desire to avoid this decision.
  6. Love yourself and know that you are innocent of any wrong-doing.
  7. Know that it takes tremendous love to consider taking an action that will release your pet from his suffering, while it leaves you with so much pain.

(Peterson, 1997)

It can be hypothesized that pet owners who have euthanized a pet due to a behavioral disorder may experience prolonged guilt, although there has to date been no research produced on the subject.

Anticipatory grief and acceptance

Anticipatory grief occurs **before** the death of the pet and is the beginning stage of coming to terms and accepting euthanasia as the appropriate option (Cordaro, 2012). The pet owner may begin to ask specific questions such as, "How would we 'do it'?", "Would you be there with us?" This is a critical point for the veterinary technician to gain the confidence of the pet owner. Letting them know the details of the process and the steps that would be taken to make sure their pet is comfortable and

unafraid, working with the pet owner to make decisions as to who they would like being in the room, and so on help the pet owner feel in control.

The resolution and acceptance of the loss can be characterized not by forgetting the loss but by being able to remember the pet with a source of warmth and pleasure rather than pain (Wright, 2007–2011). Something that can only happen after the anticipation of death can be accepted (Walter, 1996).

Breaking the bond

When the "bad times" begin to dramatically subtract from the "good times" and the stress from dealing with potentially dangerous or unpredictable circumstances outweigh the comfort the pet gives to the pet owners are signs the bond has become unhealthy, and gentle breaking of the bond may need to occur. In general, it is not our role to tell a pet owner when they should choose euthanasia for their pet (Hetts, 1999). Choosing euthanasia, specifically in regard to a behavioral disorder, is a very complex and personal decision. It is the role of the technician to support and guide the pet owner in whatever decision they make, whether that is treatment or ending the pet's life. The decision to end the pet's life needs to be that of the pet owner's and not made solely on your recommendation.

Coming to terms with such a decision is a process. It is your job to guide the pet owner through the process side by side rather than as an authoritative figure. When a pet owner asks, "What would you do?" they are asking for your guidance, validation, and knowledge that you will not judge them but will support them. I frequently reiterate, "That is a very personal decision and I will support you in whatever decision you make."

Determining the current level of attachment

Understanding the depth of the emotional bond, the role of the pet in the pet owner's life, and the quality of the pet owner's social support system will help understand and predict the depth of the pet owner's grief (Cordaro, 2012).

Exceptionally strong and complex attachments may occur in the following situations.

- The pet was rescued from near-death or a traumatic life experience.
- The pet owner believes the pet got them through an intensely difficult experience or time in their life.
- The pet owner had the pet through childhood.
- When the pet owner has had little outside support in their life and believes their pet to be their main support systems.
- Service animals that have assisted a physically, mentally, or emotionally challenged individual.
- The pet owner is deeply anthropomorphic toward their pet.
- The pet owner views their pet as a symbolic link to a person they have lost.
- When the pet owner has invested a great deal of time, financial resources, and effort into the treatment of their pet. This can be especially the case when dealing with long-term behavioral disorders or other health-related disorders (Lagoni *et al.*, 1994).

Once the HAB has been damaged, it is very difficult, if not impossible, to repair. Some pet owners have made the comparison of living in an abusive relationship. "I can't trust him." "He's good most of the time but if I do the 'wrong' thing everything can change. It is like walking on egg shells." "I can't completely relax even when things are going well." These comments are likely an indication the pet owner is feeling significant caregiver strain (see Table 4.1 and Appendix 6).

In cases in which the pet owner is not ready to consider euthanasia as an option, it will be the task of the behavior team to guide the pet owner slowly and at their pace. Many pet owners need time and the knowledge that they have done everything they can before considering euthanasia as an option. Setting a time frame to revisit and reaccess is often the key to the pet owner accepting the thought of euthanasia. Knowing they have tried all treatment possible helps alleviate guilt. Creating goals agreed on and setting a time frame (2–4 weeks) to evaluate progress and whether goals have been reached give the pet owner time to step back and have a method for determining progress or lack of it.

A person's reluctance to choose euthanasia for their pet may stem from their own personal past experiences, which do not have a direct correlation with the current circumstance. For instance, a family member may have developed a mental illness or been taken off life support. In these cases, additional professional help may be needed.

Pet owners may desperately feel the need to be validated, asking questions such as, "What would you do?" My response in these situations is honest and direct, "This problem would be very difficult for me to live with in my own home." Often, hearing that a professional who deals with such issues on a daily basis would also find the situation difficult is a clear validation to the pet owner that they have done enough.

The veterinarian should give the medical, diagnostic, and prognostic reports; the technician can then translate that information into "real life information." Showing concern for the pet owner's emotional, physical, and mental health well-being by saying, "I'm worried about you." "How are you doing? This must be incredibly stressful for you." gives permission for the pet owner to release emotions that are not being expressed.

The technician can emphasize that the behavior team's goal is to promote and protect the HAB and to help create healthy relationships between pets and people. Acknowledge the importance of the pet and its positive qualities. "This is very difficult because 'Fluffy' is such a wonderful companion much of the time." The technician may find it appropriate to say, "'Fluffy' loves you and does not want to injure you, but her brain chemistry disorder makes it difficult for her to control her behaviors. We've tried everything medically and behaviorally possible to decrease her fear, and we are running out of options. I'm concerned for her quality of life and your quality of life. How do you feel about what I've said?" The pet owner may not be able to respond or be too emotional to respond. The technician should reiterate, "We are here for you and 'Fluffy,' and we will continue to support you regardless of any decision you make. You will not be judged in any way but fully supported."

If the pet owner introduces thoughts of euthanasia before the treatment team is anticipating it, they should not be discouraged. It is an indication, regardless of the pet's issue, that the HAB is tenuous or severed. At this point, the veterinarian must make the decision whether to encourage treatment or support the pet owner. This may be a point in which either the treatment plan is accelerated using every tool available or the treatment may be simplified, while the pet owner makes a decision whether to continue. It is tragic when a pet owner is already in the grieving process and loosening their attachment to the pet, encouraged to continue trying, only to be later heading down the same path in the future. Much has to be determined by listening to the pet owner, and in some cases, specifically asking them how they "feel" about the pet. The depth of the damage to the HAB will likely correlate with lack of compliance to the treatment plan.

When considering euthanasia, the following points should be considered:

- Rarely does a decision have to be made at this moment; allow the pet owner time. Sometimes, recommending respite by boarding the pet will give the pet owner time to continue to consider their life without the pet.
- No decision is perfect. If in the least bit unsure of their decision, the pet owner should be encouraged to postpone the decision.
- The decision should not be made in anger or desperation.
- The pet owner should not act or refrain from acting because of what they believe others will think.
- The pet owner should be able to acknowledge and recognize all they have done for their pet, and let it be enough.

It is an indication the pet owner may be moving toward accepting euthanasia as an option when they are able to

- accept the pet is mentally and emotionally suffering, and see evidence that treatment has failed;
- reach the point at which holding on becomes more painful than letting go and the pet owner has come to accept that euthanasia is a loving way to end the pet's suffering; and
- accept their responsibility in the decision without excessive guilt.

"Choosing euthanasia would be a responsible and humane decision." Dr. Andrew Luescher, DVM, DACVB, PhD in response to an owner considering euthanasia.

- "Choosing euthanasia would be a responsible and humane decision."

Dr. Andrew Luescher, DVM, DACVB, PhD in response to an owner considering euthanasia.

All three areas must be dealt with before a pet owner can accept euthanasia with peace (Peterson, 1997). "Letting go is not giving up, it is a deliberate decision to end suffering." Peterson (1997)

- "Letting go is not giving up, it is a deliberate decision to end suffering."

Peterson (1997)

The decision

Once the decision for euthanasia has been made, it means the process of creating a special event can begin. The last weeks or days with the pet can be turned into a gift and become filled with positive memories. The pet owner should be encouraged early in the process to begin creating a tribute to their pet. Possibilities could include writing a letter to their pet, constructing a memory book with photos, and keeping a journal about their grief. Some pet owners find it helpful to save tufts of hair and clay paw prints. The technician should follow the pet owner's lead and monitor their needs.

After euthanasia, some form of sentiment and condolence to the pet owner should be arranged. Often, a card is passed among staff members and doctors, allowing for them to share fond memories of the pet, words of testament, and empathy to the client for their loss. Clients are deeply touched by the heartfelt words and appreciate the care and support provided by the practice.

After the loss

As with suicide and other disenfranchised grief situations, often the first question is, "What should we tell people about how 'Fido' died?" Euthanizing a pet because of a mental or behavioral disorder is complex and difficult to grasp for many people. Acceptance, a final stage in grieving, can be difficult to obtain because of the bewilderment and sometimes lack of definite answers to "Why did this happen." Among others blaming the pet owners, the most cutting blame can come from the pet owner themselves. It is common for the pet owner to remember every mistake they made with their pet, every harsh word, and wonder if "that" is what caused the behavioral disorder. Most will have done the best they could with what they had at the time, which is all we can expect of others or ourselves.

The pet owner will need to make a decision as to with whom and how much they share about their pet's death. In reality, if the pet was euthanized because of a serious behavioral disorder, then the animal suffered from the physical problem of having a neurochemical brain disorder.

There is a stigma when euthanasia occurs because of a behavioral disorder comparable to the stigma people feel when a family member has committed suicide; therefore, it is not uncommon for people to be uncomfortable when they find the pet has been euthanized, specifically for a behavioral reason. People may say nothing in fear of saying the wrong thing. Some may blame the pet owner for their animal "parenting" skills. When asked,

"How did your pet die?" the answer could simply be, "He had a brain chemistry imbalance that could not be medically corrected." Most behavioral disorders are likely a combination of life experience (or lack of it) and a physical organic brain chemistry disorder.

> • Most behavior disorders are likely a combination of life experience (or lack of it) and a physical organic brain chemistry disorder.

Pet owners need to be encouraged that they are good people and good pet owners who have suffered a tragedy.

Pet owners may be told by family or friends to "get over it". If what they mean is that the pet owner will eventually begin moving forward, that will occur in time. If they mean the pet owner should forget the loss, they will not. A pet wiggles its way into a place in our hearts that needed filling. When that pet is no longer present, the space is filled with memories. The pain will recede, eventually to an ache and finally to soft memories (Wolfelt, 2004).

Successful grief counseling will have an impact on future HABs. Assisting the client through their own private grief path with no judgments, only honest empathy, will bond the pet owner to the technician and the veterinary hospital. When performed properly, grief counseling means growth for all involved (Table 5.10).

Relief

Feeling guilty for feeling happy is called *recovery guilt*. A sense of relief may occur after the euthanasia, followed by guilt or shame for feeling that relief. Living with an animal with a behavioral disorder can be extremely stressful. The constant worry and anxiety are gone, and the pet owner may now be filled with both relief and guilt for feeling that relief. The relief comes because not only is the pet owner's stress gone but also because the suffering of their pet is also now relieved.

After care – additional support

Signs of abnormal complicated grief (traumatic or prolonged grief) include a powerful pining for the deceased, great difficulty moving on, a sense that life is meaningless, bitterness, and anger pertaining to the loss and last longer than 6 months. Other characteristics of complicated grief may include avoiding all reminders of the death, inability to trust others since the death, bitterness and anger related to the loss, difficulty moving on with life, numbness since the loss, and feelings that life is meaningless since the loss (Ozgul, 2004).

Pet owners may focus on wanting to change the past, mulling over what "should have" been done differently. When looking at the past becomes exaggerated or excessive, the process of grief may be delayed. Some may hold onto the grief as "punishment" for "letting the animal down." There may come a time when the veterinary practice is ineffective or ill-equipped in providing support to a grieving client. Similarly, clients faced with extreme depression and feelings of hopelessness would

Table 5.10 Managing grief after the decision to euthanize.

Strategy	Definition	Example
Catharsis	Coaxing client to express emotions	"I will be just outside the door if you would like to talk."
Empathizing	Identifying with the client's experience	"What you are going through is incredibly difficult and courageous. You are not letting 'Fluffy' go because it is what you want, you are doing it because it will end 'Fluffy's' suffering. She never has to be afraid again. What a brave and loving thing you are doing"
Sympathizing	Expressing an emotion for the owner. May include using "body language" or gestures to convey emotional support	Sitting quietly with the client, holding their hand, not being rushed
Reassurance	Talking to instill confidence	"It is very clear how much you love 'Fluffy' and she knows that. This is your last and greatest act of love to her"
Redirecting	Encouraging owners to focus on the positive aspects of their relationship with their pet	"What was 'Fluffy' like as a kitten/puppy? What is your favorite memory?"
Comforting touch	Touching the owner's shoulder and the pet	Pet "Fluffy" and show your own compassion and comforting touch to both the pet owner and the pet

Modified from Morris (2012).

better benefit from additional counseling services or support groups.

Clients may confide in you their feelings of not being able to go on without their pet. In these instances, it is absolutely imperative that the pet owner is referred to appropriate and more aggressive help. Clients should not feel ashamed for the feelings they are having. However, concern for their well-being must be expressed so that additional resources can be recommended.

It is important to have a list of resources readily available. Provide clients with a phone list of counselors and support group hotlines as well as recommended grieving books and valid online resources. Many veterinary universities offer pet-loss support and counseling services.

When equipped with the right resources, you can find comfort in knowing that you are providing your clients with the proper services and support they need to help them through their loss.

Conclusion

> * The capacity to love, requires the necessity to mourn.
>
> Wolfelt (2004)

Strengthening, protecting, and promoting the HAB should be the primary goal of veterinary medicine. Relieving the sufferings of animals and their owners also includes alleviating emotional and mental sufferings. There will be times when removing a pet from its home either by rehoming or through euthanasia will be the appropriate and most prudent decision to protect future HABs. If we allow pet owners to continue a destructive relationship with their pet, possibly allowing a family member or child to be seriously injured, thus teaching that family member or child to fear animals and they then teach their own children to fear animals, we have done a great disservice to the pet owner and to the HAB and have failed.

Guiding a pet owner through the grief process associated with living with a pet with a serious behavioral disorder is not only a complex, but also a deeply bonding process. "Considering pet loss as a normative grief process is not only an indication to bereaved pet owners that their loss is valued, but also an initial step toward reinstating within our society a stigmatized grief" (Cohen, 2002). When the grief process associated with the treatment of behavioral disorders and euthanasia is skillfully, honestly, and sensitively supported, it can be a profound

experience for both the pet owner and the veterinary professional. Assisting a pet owner into and through the grief process should be seen as an absolute and ultimate honor.

> * Assisting a pet owner into and through the grief process should be seen as an absolute and ultimate honor.

References

Abood, S.K. (2007) Increasing adherence in practice: making your clients partners in care. *Veterinary Clinics of North America: Small Animal Practice*, **37** (1), 151–164.

Abosh, B. and Collins, A. (1996) *Mental Illness in the Family : Issues and Trends*, University of Toronto Press, Toronto.

Adams, C.L. and Frankel, R.M. (2007) It may be a dog's life but the relationship with her owners is also key to her health and well being: communication in veterinary medicine. *Veterinary Clinics of North America: Small Animal Practice*, **37** (1), 1–17.

Canino, J., Shaw, J. and Beck, A.M. (2007) A look at the role of marriage and family therapy skills within the context of animal behavior therapy. *Journal of Veterinary Behavior: Clinical Applications and Research*, **2** (1), 15–22.

Carson, C.A. (2007) Nonverbal communication in veterinary practice. *Veterinary Clinics of North America: Small Animal Practice*, **37** (1), 49–63.

Chun, R., Schafer, S., Lotta, C.C. *et al.* (2009) Didactic and experimental training to teach communication skills: the university of wisconsin-madison school of veterinary medicine collaborative experience. *Journal of Veterinary Medical Education*, **36** (2), 196–201.

Cohen, S.P. (2002) Can pets function as family members? *Western Journal of Nursing Research*, **24** (6), 621.

Cordaro, M. (2012) Pet loss and disenfranchised grief: implications for mental health counseling practice. *Journal of Mental Health Counseling*, **34** (4), 283–294.

Cornell, K. (2012) 5 Steps to effective feedback. *Exceptional Veterinary Team*, **4** (1), 37–40.

Durrance, D. and Lagoni, L. (1998) *Connecting with Clients: Practical Communication for 10 Common Situations*, American Animal Hospital Association Press, Lakewood, CO, USA.

Egan, G. (2002) *The Skilled Helper: A Problem-Management and Opportunity-Development Approach to Helping*, Pacific Grove, California, Brooks/Cole.

Frankel, R.M. and Stein, T. (1999) Getting the most out of the clinical encounter: the four habits model. *Permanente Journal*, **3** (3), 79–88.

Gray, C. and Moffett, J. (2010) *Handbook of Veterinary Communication Skills*, Wiley-Blackwell, New Jersey, USA.

CHAPTER 5

Guy, N.C., Luescher, U.A., Dohoo, S.E. *et al.* (2001a) A case series of biting dogs: characteristics of the dogs, their behaviour, and their victims. *Applied Animal Behaviour Science*, **74** (1), 43–57.

Guy, N.C., Luescher, U.A., Dohoo, S.E. *et al.* (2001b) Demographic and aggressive characteristics of dogs in a general veterinary caseload. *Applied Animal Behaviour Science*, **74** (1), 15–28.

Guy, N.C., Luescher, U.A., Dohoo, S.E. *et al.* (2001c) Risk factors for dog bites to owners in a general veterinary caseload. *Applied Animal Behaviour Science*, **74** (1), 29–42.

Hetts, S. (1999) *Pet Behavior Protocols: What to Say, What to Do, When to Refer*, AAHA Press, Lakewood, CO.

Lagoni, L., Hetts, S. and Butler, C. (1994) *The Human–Animal Bond and Grief*, W.B. Saunders, Philadelphia, PA.

Luescher, A. and Martin, K.M. (2010) *Dogs! & Cats: Diagnosis and Treatment of Behavior Problems*, Purdue University, Lafayette, IN.

Luiz Adrian, J.A., Deliramich, A.N. and Frueh, B.C. (2009) Complicated grief and posttraumatic stress disorder in humans' response to the death of pets/animals. *Bulletin of the Menninger Clinic*, **73** (3), 176–187.

MacGregor, P. (1994) Grief: the unrecognized parental response to mental illness in a child. *Social Work*, **39** (2), 160–166.

McCurnin, D.M. (2010) *Clinical Textbook for Veterinary Technicians*, Saunders, Philadelphia.

McKeon, T. (2012) TagTeach International. Available from http://www.tagteach.com (accessed 7 November 2012).

Mech, L. D. (2008) Whatever happened to the term Alpha wolf. *International Wolf Magazine*, Winter: 4–8.

Meyer, P.J. (2003) *Attitude is Everything: If You Want to Succeed Above and Beyond*, The Meyer Resource Group Incorporated, Scotts Valley, CA.

Morris, P. (2012) Managing pet owners' guilt and grief in veterinary euthanasia encounters. *Journal of Contemporary Ethnography*, **41** (3), 337–365.

Murie, A. and Etats-Unis. National park (1944) *The Wolves of Mount McKinley*, U.S. Government Printing Office, Washington.

Northey, W. (2002) Characteristics and clinical practices of marriage and family therapists: a national survey. *Journal of Marital & Family Therapy*, **28** (4), 487–494.

Ozgul, S. (2004) Parental grief and serious mental illness: a narrative. (cover story). *Australian & New Zealand Journal of Family Therapy*, **25** (4), 183–187.

Peterson, L.M. (1997) *Surviving The Heartbreak Of Choosing Death For Your Pet*, Greentree Publishing, Las Vegas, Nev..

Richardson, M., Cobham, V., Murray, J. and McDermott, B. (2011) Parents' grief in the context of adult child mental illness: a qualitative review. *Clinical Child & Family Psychology Review*, **14** (1), 28–43.

Rosenthal, S.A. (2005) *The Complete Idiot's Guide to Toltec Wisdom*, Alpha Books, New York, NY.

Ryan, T. (2005) *Coaching People to Train Their Dogs*. Sequim, WA, Legacy Canine Behavior and Training.

Shaw, J. (2007) Is it acceptable for people to be paid to adhere to medication? No. *BMJ*, **335** (7613), 233.

Shaw, J. (2011) A Poll to Determine Veterinarians' Current Role Expectation of Dog Trainers. ACVB/AVSAB Veterinary Behavior Symposium, St. Louis, MO.

Shaw, J. L., A (2005) Problem puppies: new theories on dominance. *Veterinary Technician* **26**(7), 499–502.

Stein, T., Nagy, V.T. and Jacobs, L. (1998) Caring for patients one conversation at a time. *Permanente Journal*, **2** (4), 62–68.

Straker, D. (September 19, 2012) Six Learning Styles. http://www.changingminds.org (accessed 26 October 2012).

Straker, D. (2002–2012) Open and Closed Questions. (accessed 26 October 2012).

Walter, T. (1996) A new model of grief: bereavement and biography. *Mortality*, **1** (1), 7–25.

Wolfelt, A.D. (2004) *When Your Pet Dies : A Guide To Mourning, Remembering & Healing*, Companion ; Gazelle, Fort Collins, Colo.; Lancaster.

Worden, J.W. (1991) *Grief Counseling and Grief Therapy : A Handbook for the Mental Health Practitioner*, Springer Publishing Company, New York.

Wright, J. (2007–2011) The Stages of Grief: Understanding the Grief Cycle. http://www.recover-from-grief.com/new-grief-stages.html (accessed 3 November 2013)

6 Learning and behavior modification

Virginia L. Price

Saint Petersburg College, St Petersburg, FL, USA

CHAPTER MENU

Learning can be defined as the permanent change in the behavior of an animal after being exposed to a stimulus (Barker, 2001). Although the changes may not be apparent immediately, as seen in latent learning (see Tolman and Honzik, 1930 for more details about latent learning in rats), they are nevertheless real changes that affect behavior. Animals learn throughout their lifetime beginning in the uterus. They learn when a person is teaching them behaviors and when they are interacting with their environment or other animals. They even learn while watching people or other animals. Learning is a full-time pursuit for all animals. The flexibility of the animal brain is just becoming apparent in today's research. From research on animal cognition to animal perception, our knowledge about animals has grown tremendously. Because this is a growing area of science, it is vital to keep current by reading new information.

- Learning is a full-time pursuit for all animals.
- The flexibility of the animal brain is just becoming apparent in today's research.

This chapter discusses some of the innate and environmental effects on learning and different ways that animals learn. Behavior modification techniques using these types of learning are defined. In Chapter 8, the practical uses of these techniques are discussed. No book chapter can capture completely the complexity of animal learning. Students should read a variety of sources and use critical thinking to create their own ideas on how animals learn.

- Students should read a variety of sources and use critical thinking to create their own ideas on how animals learn.

Genetics and learning

"Genetics has profound effects on an animal's behavior." (Grandin and Deesing, 1998, p. 24). Different species and breeds of animals perform species- and breed-specific behaviors because of differences in their genetic codes. Lorenz (1965) spent many years studying

---

Canine and Feline Behavior for Veterinary Technicians and Nurses, First Edition. Edited by Julie K. Shaw and Debbie Martin.
© 2015 John Wiley & Sons, Inc. Published 2015 by John Wiley & Sons, Inc.
Companion Website: www.wiley.com/go/shaw/behavior

innate behaviors he called fixed action patterns. Animals performed these behaviors or behavioral chains after being exposed to a specific stimulus in their environment called a *sign stimulus*. For example, parent birds feed baby birds that display the red interior of their mouths. Cats exhibit a pattern of predatory behavior after seeing or hearing a prey animal. Behaviors can be thought of as being on a continuum from innate to learned, with behaviors being either innate, learned, or a combination of the two (Lorenz, 1965). Behaviors generally believed to be reflexes can be affected by the environment through chemical or contextual input. Environmental influences do not always mean learning; they can be nutritional or chemical influences.

> • Behaviors can be thought of as being on a continuum from innate to learned, with behaviors being either innate, learned, or a combination of the two (Lorenz, 1965).

Although it would be orderly for all behaviors to be adaptive, this cannot be the case. The basis for evolution is a large number of diverse offspring from which the environment selects the fittest individuals using natural selection (Darwin, 1859). Skinner (1966) discussed how behaviors may appear, although they are counterproductive for an animal. These behaviors are less likely to be passed on to future generations, but they may be passed on if the animal has enough adaptive behaviors to survive long enough to reproduce. It is this capability, reproduction, which judges whether the animal is fit, as in the survival of the fittest, not aggression and not hierarchical placement.

> • It is this capability, reproduction, which judges whether the animal is fit, as in the survival of the fittest, not aggression and not hierarchical placement.

Expressed behaviors may appear the same in different animals, but they can still be formed through different combinations of conditioned and unconditioned learning (Krushinskii, 1960). These behaviors although developed in a variety of ways, still appear the same when elicited. Fixed behavior patterns or behavioral units are the end result, but the environment and other stimuli affect the exact form this pattern takes. These fixed patterns are governed by natural selection

(Krushinskii, 1960). The ability of animals to behave in varied ways and yet still arrive at the same behavioral outcome is beneficial for them. Flexibility allows animals to take advantage of different situations and arrive at the same ends by different means. By allowing conditioned and unconditioned reflexes (behaviors) to be combined, the nervous system becomes more sensitive to the stimuli it encounters (Krushinskii, 1960).

Hormones are substances the body secretes that chemically instruct its systems to perform specific actions. Male sex hormones are associated with the genetic code that instructs the fetus to become male; the lack of these hormones allows the fetus to remain female. This change alone may affect many things later in the animal's life, as animals that are masculinized *in utero* may learn and behave differently than those that are not.

The study on dogs by Krushinskii (1960) showed that male dogs more often exhibited active defense reflexes than female dogs, and the former had a stronger nervous system (not defined), but there were no sex differences found in excitability. In a study on learning abilities in dogs, sex differences varied by breed (Serpell and Hsu, 2005). While female dogs in two dog breeds exhibited better learning abilities, male dogs in other dog breeds performed better in learning tasks. Interestingly, the same study found that conformation show dogs exhibited lower learning ability than field trial dogs in two different breeds. In a study of male and female dog puppies, Beckoff (1974) found no differences in play behavior besides the male Beagles mounting during play, whereas the female dogs did not. In comparison, Hart (1995) found that male dogs showed more dominance (the term dominance was not defined) and aggression toward the owner than female dogs. It is interesting that these two traits were found together in male dogs, as they may be assessing the same trait; the term dominance is no longer used to describe behaviors or traits. Female dogs were found to be more easily trained for obedience and house training. In research, comparing the behavior of Beagle male dogs, female dogs, and female dogs that were treated with testosterone propionate (a fast acting shortest estered testosterone product available), male dogs were found to maintain a resource (bone) more often than both the types of female dogs (Beach *et al.*, 1982). Female dogs treated with the hormone were more likely to maintain the resource than those untreated. Using shelter dogs, Wells and Hepper (1999) found that female dogs spent less time looking at people than male dogs did, and both sexes of dogs looked and barked at male humans more than they did toward female humans. In cats, Barry and Crowell-Davis (1999) found no differences in behavior owing to sex except that female cats did not allorub other cats, and male cats did allorub both sexes. Allorubbing is seen when a cat rubs its head, side, and/or tail on another cat, object, or person. The functions of this behavior include scent exchange as well as a pleasurable tactile sensation (Crowell-Davis *et al.*, 2004).

Sexual differences in behavior can be created by environmental factors. People place a great deal of importance on sexual differences, and change in an animal's behavior can be affected by a person's beliefs about how sex affects behavior. People may reinforce unruly behavior in male animals, believing it is normal behavior in male animals. Conversely, they may reinforce quiet, calm behavior in female animals, believing it to be their nature. These manipulations of an animal's behavior may not be conscious. Confirmation bias may affect the behaviors reported by owners or scientists. There could be a bias inherent in the questions scientists ask about sex differences in behavior, which then affects the knowledge we have to draw from. Because behavior is generally a combination of genetic and environmental effects, sexual differences seen in behavior may also be because of the environmental differences.

> • Sexual differences in behavior can be created by environmental factors.

> • Because behavior is generally a combination of genetic and environmental effects, sexual differences seen in behavior may also be because of the environmental differences.

Animals are generally better able to learn certain types of behaviors because of the manner in which their brains and bodies are organized. Prey animals learn to categorize predators by the methods of their predation, and we know this because they exhibit prey-specific alarm calls. Vervet monkeys gave three specific predator alarm calls: one for flying predators (eagles), one for snakes, and yet another one for leopards (Seyfarth *et al.*, 1980). Brains are naturally structured to classify and categorize sensory input. This is a time-saving feature of the nervous system used for species survival.

The organization of these classifications is based on genetic coding, although it is modified throughout an animal's life through its experience. Support for this is seen in working dogs in which their natural behavior through breeding may be to herd sheep and through experience may learn to also herd cattle, geese, or human children.

> • The organization of these classifications is based on genetic coding, although it is modified throughout an animal's life through its experience.

In an ongoing study on domesticating fur foxes, the foxes were bred by selecting for tameness. Consequently, other characteristics, physical and neurochemical, were also modified (Belyaev, 1979). These modifications had even more effect on the animal's behavior through learning. As the foxes were bred to be tamed, it changed their neurochemistry, allowing them to feel more comfortable with people. They solicited people for attention. This behavior was reinforced eliciting more attention-seeking behavior from the foxes. We observe similar behavior patterns in other domesticated species. Domesticated species have longer socialization periods and less reactivity to environmental stimuli because of a change in their hypothalamus–pituitary–adrenal axis resulting from domestication, otherwise known as *selection for the ability to be easily tamed*. Their natural behaviors allow for their easy taming, which then allows for a cascade of learning associated with tame behaviors.

> • Domesticated species have longer socialization periods and less reactivity to environmental stimuli because of a change in their hypothalamus–pituitary–adrenal axis resulting from domestication, otherwise known as *selection for the ability to be easily tamed.*

CHAPTER 6

Animals selected through natural or artificial selection to perform behaviors will tend to better perform these behaviors over generations through this selection process. Evidence of this is seen in wild animals when they take advantage of an environmental niche and is also seen in domestic animals. Wild animals may take advantage of a rainforest or a desert environment, whereas domestic animals may instead take advantage of a farm yard or household environment. Through selection processes, natural or artificial, the animals become better able to take advantage of their niche. We can witness this evolution in action as our dog and cat populations surpass the numbers seen in their closest wild relations, showing their superior fitness.

Animals may feel intrinsic reinforcement for species- or breed-specific behaviors (Coppinger and Coppinger, 2001 reported about this phenomenon in dogs). For example, scent hounds appear to feel good when they are tracking a scent, and because of this reinforcement, they are more likely than are dogs from other breed groups to spend time tracking scent, thus perfecting this behavior through learning. They may also have better ability to track scent because of the configuration of their olfactory system. All domestic animals use their olfactory systems to a greater capacity than humans do, and evidence for this lies in the amount of brain space used to evaluate olfactory sensations and the amount of neural tissue in the nose collecting the sensory input. Research in this area is very exciting and will lead us to a better understanding of animal behavior (see Overall and Arnold, 2007 – in dogs).

Alleles (Figure 6.1) are the variations of a gene that produce different characteristics in living beings (National Human Genome Research Institute, n.d.). One way in which alleles are involved in variations in behaviors is through the differences in the physical shapes of the animals they help to build (Coppinger and Coppinger, 2001). This idea is simplified immensely as genes create proteins, not animal shapes or behaviors, but these small building blocks are where these differences are seen at the most basic level. The Coppingers wrote that huskies are known for their sled-pulling ability, which is largely because of their compact shape, whereas Alaskan Malamutes are too large to pull a sled far without overheating. Cats, owing to their shape, size, and sensory abilities, are excellent small rodent hunters. They have the sensory ability to detect and the physical ability to stealthy stalk and kill their prey. Hemmer (1990) also noted that coat density and body size can inhibit behavior of all types by creating hyperthermia on even minor activity. This is another example of how phenotype may affect behavior and learning.

> • One way in which alleles are involved in variations in behaviors is through the differences in the physical shapes of the animals they help to build (Coppinger and Coppinger, 2001).

Allelic differences between individuals, breeds, and species allow for differences in the genetic onset, offset, and rate of behaviors; these differences are not in chromosome numbers, shapes, or the placement of genes along the chromosomes (Coppinger and Coppinger, 1996, 1998) but instead are in when the gene turns on or off during the animal's ontogeny (development). Some alleles turn on and off genes at different stages of an animal's life, permitting the onset and offset of behaviors during maturation (Trut, 1999 – domesticated foxes). Other alleles manage the rate of behavior or the thresholds needed to elicit a behavior. Of course, there are no single alleles or genes that control a specific behavior; behavior is more complex than that. Genes make proteins. Proteins link with other proteins to build the animal's physical and mental characteristics. These characteristics allow behaviors to tend to clump in specific individuals that share common genetics and environments.

Besides having a genetic configuration that naturally reinforces a behavior and the correct body shape to allow for a behavior, the gene(s) that allows for that behavior must be turned on before the finished behavior pattern can be produced by the animal. There is no use trying to train an animal for a behavior unless they are capable of learning it. No one would even try to train a neonate to pull a sled. Neonates are not able to perform this behavior; they cannot even walk yet. In time they will be running, but for now, they must pull themselves along by their forelimbs. Later in their ontogeny, they will begin to walk and then run. Once they are running, we can then start teaching them to pull a sled. And if they were well-bred, sled-pulling huskies, they could, with practice, become very good at it. Many behaviors in animals are affected by the onset and offset of genes during ontogeny. Behavior changes throughout an animal's life both because of genetic changes and because of environmental influences (Estep, 1996).

> • Besides having a genetic configuration that naturally reinforces a behavior and the correct body shape to allow for a behavior, the gene(s) that allows for that behavior must be turned on before the finished behavior pattern can be produced by the animal.

Temperament was found to be a heritable trait in dogs (Scott and Fuller, 1965); a dog's temperament is at least in part passed on by its parents. There is evidence that temperaments in cats are also heritable (McCune, 1995; Estep, 1996). Heritability is only an accurate measure

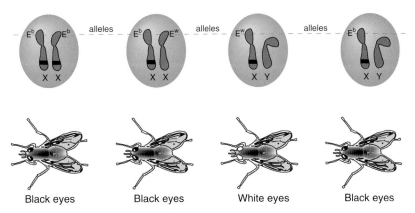

Black eyes   Black eyes   White eyes   Black eyes

Figure 6.1 An example of alleles. Courtesy: National Human Genome Research Institute. For detailed definitions of genetic terms go to: http://www.genome.gov/glossary/index.cfm?id=4.

for the group of animals represented in a study. Genes from these animals may or may not be representative of the larger population. The definition of heritability is a shared genome. Consequently, it cannot be assumed that animals outside of the study group share the same genome. Generalization to animal populations at large should be tempered accordingly. Readers are cautioned to keep this in mind when analyzing evidence of heritability in various studies. Although temperament is not a group of specific behaviors, it is a stable way of behaving across time and context. An animal's temperament accounts for its uniqueness (Hall, 1941). Temperament, including issues such as emotional reactivity, anxiety, and fearfulness, affects learning.

- Although temperament is not a group of specific behaviors, it is a stable way of behaving across time and context.

Scaring or hurting animals does not help them learn. It contributes to behavioral shut down (learned helplessness) and avoidance of the trainer. In a study using two groups of police dogs, one group was previously trained without using shock but nonetheless using harsh techniques, and the other group was previously trained using shock collars; Schilder and van der Borg (2004) found that the dogs trained with shock exhibited significantly more signs of fear in the presence of their trainers. These dogs were not being shocked during the study, yet one of the dogs still exhibited the effects of learning with shock after not being shocked during training for a year and a half. These dogs made an association between the

trainers who previously shocked them and the shock. They also made associations between the environment in which they were previously shocked and the shock and between the behavioral context when they were previously shocked and the shock. These dogs exhibited fear, stress, and conflict while in the context of previous shocks (being near the trainer, obedience work, and decoy work). This supports the idea that using shock collars to train dogs may cause long-term negative effects on behavior in the given context.

Emotional reactivity is part of an animal's temperament. It is a measure of how much of an emotional reaction an animal has to a stimulus and how long it takes for them to return to homeostasis (normalcy) after being exposed to the stimulus. Emotional reactivity is a heritable trait, and animals with increased emotional reactivity may have more trouble learning specific tasks (Scott and Fuller, 1965 – dogs). Although there is evidence of reactivity levels being heritable, the environment exerts a large effect on this measure. A reduction in emotional reactivity can be realized by reduced stress in the mother during pregnancy, allowing normal mother–offspring interactions after parturition and handling of the neonate by people (Boissy, 1998).

- Emotional reactivity is a heritable trait, and animals with increased emotional reactivity may have more trouble learning specific tasks (Scott and Fuller, 1965 – dogs).

High reactivity in Rhesus macaques was found to be reduced when affected young monkeys were fostered by nurturing mothers (Suomi, 1997). This illustrates how genes and the environment combine to affect reactivity. Others found that rat's deficits (anxiety, neophobia, and poor performance in learning and special memory tasks) because of social isolation could be reversed using enrichment (Hellemans *et al.*, 2004). Evidence of the effects of fear or over emotionality on learning can also be found in the study by Fuller and Clark (1966) that used chlorpromazine, a tranquilizer, to enable Beagle puppies to learn an attachment to handlers, whereas the puppies not given the tranquilizer were unable to form similar attachments. There is much data to support these parameters. However, many people still believe that it is best to isolate neonates from human handling or to bottle-raise singleton offspring. Veterinary technicians need to educate animal owners and breeders on these issues to ensure they contribute to creating less reactive animals in the future by promoting the appropriate handling of neonates and by fostering litters on a mother animal or at the very least allowing these neonates access to adult conspecifics.

> • Veterinary technicians need to educate animal owners and breeders on these issues to ensure they contribute to creating less reactive animals in the future by promoting the appropriate handling of neonates and by fostering litters on a mother animal or at the very least allowing these neonates access to adult conspecifics.

An example of how genes can affect behavior in dog breeds was found in the types of defense behaviors exhibited by three dog breeds. Defense behaviors in dogs can be classified as either active or passive defense. Active defense is characterized as lunging and biting, whereas passive defense is characterized by escape behaviors. Escape behaviors are the fight, flight, or freeze seen during sympathetic nervous system arousal. Passive and active defense behavior tendencies in dogs are inherited; however, through breeding studies, the environment was found to influence passive defense more readily than active (Krushinskii, 1960). Dogs that were raised in isolation were more likely to exhibit passive defense as long as they were not the product of two dogs with only active defense. German shepherd dogs were more likely to show this trait than were Airedale terriers. Although Airedale terriers were able to be induced into showing passive defense if reared in isolation, they did not show this trait at the same rate as German shepherd dogs did. Doberman Pinschers were not able to be induced into showing passive defense, even when raised in isolation. It is more common today to find Doberman Pinschers that exhibit passive defense, illustrating how these behaviors can shift over time because of selective breeding. Another caution while reading this information is to remember that breeds are a local phenomenon that may or may not reflect the behaviors seen in breeds of the same type in a different location. For example, Labrador retrievers from England may be calmer than Labrador retrievers from the United States.

> • Another caution while reading this information is to remember that breeds are a local phenomenon that may or may not reflect the behaviors seen in breeds of the same type in a different location.

Perception is how the animal's brain interprets the sensory input they attend to. There are specific ways in which animals perceive sensations because of the organization of their sensory organs, the brain structures that interpret them, and the environment the animals live in (see Gibson, 1958 for a discussion on perception in animals). The effects of perception on learning are large, as it influences how sensory input will be used at the most basic level by setting up parameters for other sensations to be measured against (Goldstone, 1998). Wells and Hepper (2006) found that dogs exposed to an odor *in utero* preferred that odor to another or no odor. This supports the hypothesis that even *in utero*, an animal's perception is affecting its learning. Food preferences may also be partially determined *in utero* by sensory input. The chemical composition of the amniotic fluid includes chemicals from the mother animal's diet as does chemicals in the milk (Thorne, 1995). This is a mechanism by which animals could learn food preferences from their mother.

In an initially perplexing example, Vervet monkeys were able to use secondary vocal signals to warn about predators but were not able to use secondary visual signals (Cheney and Seyfarth, 1992). In this study, monkeys used alarm calls from various bird species to look for predators, but if they saw the physical trail of a python, they did not look for the snake. The explanation given by the authors involved the consistency of the signal being paired with the predator. Alarm calls of birds were usually paired immediately with the visual image of the predator, whereas the visual signs of the snake were often seen without a snake in proximity. This speaks to one of the main principles of classical conditioning – a conditioned stimulus (CS) (python) must be paired consistently with an unconditioned stimulus (US) (python trail) for the animal to emit the conditioned response (CR) (python alarm call).

Attention is a vital aspect of learning. What the animal perceives is affected by the filtering of sensations they are exposed to through the mechanism of attention. Only the stimuli that are noticed can be used for learning purposes. Cats were found to be able to learn a behavior proceeded by a cue; only if that cue was first presented at an intensity level high enough to gain attention could the cats then learn to attend to it at a much less intense level (Bourassa and Weiden, 1985). This lower level of intensity did not produce learning if used at this less intense level initially. Although this shows that attention is important for learning to occur, it also shows that attention thresholds can be modified by learning. For example, dogs trained using yelled cues can later be trained to perform behaviors using whispered cues. There is some evidence that attention need not be conscious for learning to occur (Debner and Jacoby, 1994 – in humans).

The way in which animals think about the function of stimuli they perceive can also constrain their learning. These constraints of thinking about things are called *affordances*. Affordances were described by Michaels and Carello (1981) as ways in which perceived objects can be used by the perceiver. A hawk that sees a snake may perceive a prey item, whereas a rat that sees a snake may perceive a predator. These different perceptions are both correct, yet they elicit different behaviors. The hawk will dive toward the snake in order to kill and eat it, whereas the rat will jump back and run away from the snake before it can strike.

Humans are often constrained by their perceptions of an object. Riddles take advantage of this tendency using the mainstream perceptions of an object to purposefully misdirect us from the solution. Dogs were shown to be misled by their own affordances when repeatedly trying to reach a goal by a previously functional route. In their minds, that route was the only one that led to the goal, leaving dogs to ignore other possible solutions. These dogs continued for six trials to attempt the unfruitful route without any attempts at alternate routes, and only after they observed another person or dog reach the goal

by an alternate route did they attempt it (Pongrácz *et al.*, 2001).

Paradoxically, learning has a large effect on perception. Perception changes with practice (Gibson, 1958). Learning about the environment affects what animals perceive. Animals are able to modify their perception to better assess their specific environment (Goldstone, 1998 – humans). With experience, a rat may learn how to kill snakes for a meal, and after being exposed to a riddle's solution, humans are rarely fooled again.

> • Learning about the environment affects what animals perceive.

Effect of domestication on learning

Domestication has been defined as the "process by which captive animals adapt to man and the environment he provides" (Price, 1998, p. 31). While Ducos (1978, p. 54) defined it as, "… when living animals are integrated as objects into the socioeconomic organization of the human group, in the sense that, while living, those animals are objects for ownership, inheritance, exchange, trade, etc., as are the other objects (or persons) with which human groups have something to do. Living conditions are among the consequences of domestication, not the mark of it." No matter how domestication is defined, it has come to mean animals that live in restricted environments compared to their wild counterparts. The restriction of the environment may be because of the environmental qualities available to the animal as well as the changes to sensory organs of the animals through the process of domestication. These animals depend on humans for artificial selection instead of depending on natural selection as seen in wild animals, and they depend on humans for the satisfaction of their needs.

Domestic animals as a group have common characteristics allowing them to be more easily domesticated than other wild animals. These characteristics include individuals with significantly smaller brain sizes and the ability to reproduce in captive groups; the increase in sexual behavior is accomplished through the stress reduction seen because of the animals' lower reactivity (Hemmer, 1990). Lower reactivity and less sensitivity to environmental stimuli are connected. They are the ways in which animals are able to cope with the changes that domestication brings. These changes contribute to the behavioral differences seen between similar wild and domestic animals. Behavioral differences found between domestic and wild animals are largely ones of quantity through changes seen in the thresholds needed to elicit behaviors (Price, 1999).

> • Domestic animals as a group have common characteristics allowing them to be more easily domesticated than other wild animals.

Increased diversity of appearance in domestic animals is supported through decreased natural selection (relaxed selection) as well as artificial selection for desired traits; this diversity includes ones in size, proportion, color, horns, coat type, and skin type (Hemmer, 1990). These variations become abundantly clear when observing the appearance of domestic animals in comparison with their wild counterparts. Changes in appearance can affect behavior and learning through homeostasis along with other mechanisms.

Domestic animals have smaller brains than their nearest wild relatives (Coppinger and Coppinger, 2001 – dogs; Hemmer, 1990 – dogs and cats; Williams *et al.*, 1993 – cats). The smaller domesticated brain has a smaller neocortex in particular. This reduction in the size of the neocortex causes a reduction in storage capacity and information processing, which is the basis of the lessening of external stimulus reactions observed in domestic animals (Hemmer, 1990). This reduction was no longer seen in breeds selected for behavioral specialization. In these breeds, animals' brain sizes increase with the complexity of the task at hand through artificial selection for increased memory and learning ability (Hemmer, 1990). Differences in neocortex size between dog breeds and individuals within these breeds likely correlate with the level of social complexity seen in groups of these dogs. Dogs with smaller neocortexes are likely to exhibit less complex social interactions, whereas those with larger neocortexes are likely to exhibit the opposite strategy. Support for this was found in a study by Goodwin *et al.*, (1997), in which they found that dog breeds that were morphologically similar to wolves exhibited more complex visual communication patterns than those that were less morphologically similar to wolves. These differences would be especially interesting if

we knew that external morphological differences represented differences in neocortexes. In a research by Belyaev (1979 – in foxes), changes in signaling through selection for tame behavior was found to correlate with changes in neurotransmitters. This hints at brain changes correlating with at least visual signaling.

> • Domestic animals have smaller brains than their nearest wild relatives.

Domesticated cats have a reduced brain size when compared to their wild counterparts, and Siamese cats showed an additional reduction in brain size of 5–10% from the average domestic cat (Hemmer, 1990). As seen with domesticated dogs, the reduction in genetic variation correlated readily with the reduction in brain size, particularly the neocortex. Hemmer (1990) noted that the predatory behavior of domestic cat was dissociated by domestication. The cats displayed this dissociation by exhibiting an increase in play behavior paired with a decrease in the killing of prey items along with the behavior of depositing dead uneaten prey animals in conspicuous places for people to find.

The selection for reduced reaction to environmental stimuli, attenuation of behavior, and reduced reactivity are not only correlated to a reduction in brain sizes but also correlated to the reduction in sensitivity of the sensory organs (visual, auditory, and olfactory; Hemmer, 1990). This reduced sensitivity seen in domestic animal's sensory organs is likely to accentuate the reduction of brain size by reducing the sensory input the brain receives. In humans, there is evidence of a correlation between sensory and cognitive decline because of aging, but the mechanism and cause for this affect are not yet known (Li and Lindenberger, 2003).

The reduced environmental awareness and reactivity of domestic animals enhance their learning ability in controlled situations because they are less distracted by their surroundings than are wild animals (Hemmer, 1990). Although Hemmer found wolves to be superior in problem-solving tasks, dogs excelled at trained tasks. Wolves appeared more focused on the goal of the directed activities, whereas dogs seemed more focused on the task itself. Dogs could be taught to persist at tasks when failure rates were high (Figure 6.2), whereas this type of persistence seemed to be inhibited in wolves (Hemmer, 1990).

Incredibly, there is evidence that dogs have cognitive abilities that wolves and even primates lack. In two different studies, dogs were found to communicate in

Figure 6.2 Canine persists in behavior with a food storage device.

ways that wolves and/or primates did not, by following a human gaze or gesture (Hare *et al.*, 2002; Miklósi *et al.*, 2003). Perhaps, domesticated animals do not need large brains to communicate well with people. Instead, large brains may be necessary for cooperative behaviors, hunting strategies, or complex problem solving. For example, although wolves hunt in highly cooperative packs, domesticated dogs mainly scavenge for food (Boitani *et al.*, 1995; Macdonald and Carr, 1995).

Coat color affects behavior through the common pathway shared by pigments (melanins) and neurotransmitters (catecholamines) (Hemmer, 1990). Generally, less pigment corresponds to less behavior. The behaviors affected include activity level, reactivity, and environmental appreciation; corresponding with this information, albino animals generally exhibit lower activity levels and less flight response (Hemmer, 1990). A reduction in sensory input (visual and olfactory) in albino animals may cause more fright responses or fearful aggression because their awareness of a stimulus may occur only when it is very close to them. Human interest in the unusual looking animal drove the change from wild-type coat colors to the wide variety of colors found today. Selection for unusual colors was a starting point for domestication and the changes seen in behavior and physiology (Hemmer, 1990).

- Coat color affects behavior through the common pathway shared by pigments (melanins) and neurotransmitters (catecholamines) (Hemmer, 1990).

Because domestic animals bond easily with humans owing to a lengthened socialization period (Scott and McCray, 1967 – dogs; Trut, 1999 – domesticated foxes), it is more common for them to pay attention to people and learn from them than it is for wild species. Topál *et al.*, (1998) found that dogs formed attachments with people that were similar to the child–parent human relationship by adapting the Ainsworth Strange Situation test for use in dogs. If dogs formed a secure attachment with a person, they were better able to explore and play in the person's presence. The findings using dogs were similar to the ones found for mothers and toddlers in a research conducted by Ainsworth (1979). In a related study, Topál *et al.*, (2005) found that dogs, but not wolves, formed attachments to humans. These differences were explained by the effects domestication has had on dogs. An animal's relationship with other animals or people may influence their learning by influencing their attention or applications of behaviors.

- An animal's relationship with other animals or people may influence their learning by influencing their attention or applications of behaviors.

Although Topál *et al.*, (1997) found dogs that were bonded to a person were less likely to problem solve without help from that person, they reasoned it had more to do with the relationship between the dog and the person than the dogs being cognitively challenged. These dogs looked to their owner for information to quickly solve problems instead of using trial and error learning analogous to what wolves did (Miklósi *et al.*, 2003). The dog–human partnership helped the dog solve the problem quickly.

In another study, Pongrácz *et al.*, (2005) found that a dog learned from a stranger or their owner equally well to find a new route around a barrier. Conversely, Gent (2006) found that dogs learned more effectively when familiar with the person they observed, although familiarity did not affect learning when watching another dog. Pongrácz *et al.*, (2008) found that other characteristics in dogs, ones that led to differentiated social relationships between dogs, affected whether dogs learned from another dog's behavior. In their study, dogs that were determined to be dominant over other dogs in their home environment (using owner questionnaires) showed significantly less social learning than that exhibited by dogs that were determined to be submissive when the demonstrator was a dog. These differences in learning were not found when

CHAPTER 6

a person was the demonstrator. It is not clear how the relationship between a dog and a person affects learning in dogs, but we are starting to collect the clues through these studies. There is little evidence available on how relationships between cats and people affect their learning, but it was established that cats can find food when a person points to its location (Miklósi et al., 2005).

Animals that are less reactive to environmental stimuli have smaller adrenal glands. Now that domestic animals are bred with smaller adrenal glands, they are less reactive to stimuli, but this also means that they cannot respond well to drastic changes in the environment. They are dependent on the environment remaining somewhat consistent through the manipulation of humans for their survival. This is illustrated by the lack of adequate predatory avoidance behavior in most domesticated species (Price, 1999). Domestic cats and dogs are frequent prey items for birds of prey as well as wild canids.

> • Now that domestic animals are bred with smaller adrenal glands, they are less reactive to stimuli, but this also means that they cannot respond well to drastic changes in the environment. They are dependent on the environment remaining somewhat consistent through the manipulation of humans for their survival.

Effects of nutrition on learning

Nutrition of the fetus and the neonate affects the development of the neurological system, which affects learning at the most basic level. The creation of myelin sheaths on the outside of nerves is affected by the nutrition consumed by the animal. These sheaths affect the speed of neural transmissions throughout the body. Brain and neural growth are also affected by adequate protein and calories. If there are not enough of these nutrients in the diet, the animal will not be able to create the neural framework necessary to carry the nerve impulses quickly and efficiently throughout the body to the brain. When animals are deprived from obtaining the needed nutrition, the brain is affected in all regions, with the cerebellum showing the most effect (Wiggins and Fuller, 1978).

> • When animals are deprived from obtaining the needed nutrition, the brain is affected in all regions, with the cerebellum showing the most effect (Wiggins and Fuller, 1978).

If the animal starves during the first few weeks of life, during glial cell multiplication (0–14 days in rats) and rapid myelin synthesis (0–20 days in rats), the animal cannot recover these losses even after eating normally for a year (Wiggins and Fuller, 1978). Children with these nutritional deficits exhibited reduced exploratory behavior and developmental lags in the following domains: motor, hearing and speech, social–personal, problem solving, eye–hand coordination, categorization, integration of information from different sensory systems, and temporal integration of information (Cravioto and DeLicarie, 1975). Communication and language development showed the worst effects and the least recovery after the child began receiving good nutrition. Cravioto and DeLicarie (1975) reported in their study (Zimmerman, 1973) using monkeys the main deficits found were in tasks using attention and observation. Taking this evidence into account, early malnutrition in animals is likely to cause permanent damage to areas of the nervous system that controls attention, observation, and the synthesis of information from different sensory systems. Damage to these systems could then cause problems with species-specific and general learning of social and communication behaviors. A lack of proficiencies in these systems could also contribute to an increase in aggression.

> • Taking this evidence into account, early malnutrition in animals is likely to cause permanent damage to areas of the nervous system that controls attention, observation, and the synthesis of information from different sensory systems.

What an animal eats during its later development will also affect its ability to learn. There are a few pet foods that contain docosahexaenoic acid (DHA), an omega-3 fatty acid found in fish oil, which has been found to enhance learning in animals (Horrocks and Yeo, 1999). Specifically, dogs were found to have enhanced learning when DHA was included in their diet (Reynolds *et al.*, 2005 and Kelley *et al.*, 2004 as cited by Bauer, 2006).

Early environment and learning

The environment in which the animal develops sets up the systems by which they learn. Even the time spent by the fetus *in utero* affects learning. The senses of animals provide the stimuli by which they learn about their environment throughout life. Learning about their environment is serious business for animals that want to live long enough to reproduce.

> • The senses of animals provide the stimuli by which they learn about their environment throughout life.

Tactile stimuli or touch is vital for normal development. Neonates have highly developed tactile sensation systems (Caulfield, 2000). They are set up to use tactile stimulations to learn about their environment, and these stimulations affect the development of their nervous systems. Premature human infants were found to have fewer neurological deficits if they received "stimulating" tactile stimulation (Weiss *et al.*, 2004). Animals without normal maternal interactions develop abnormal neurological systems, including increased neural cell death and an increased stress response (Zhang *et al.*, 2002). At least some of the responses that were affected by maternal deprivation can be reversed using tactile stimulus (van Oers *et al.*, 1998 – in rats; Weiss *et al.*, 2004 – in human infants). There is also evidence that handling during a neonates' development will enhance learning ability through the reduction of reactivity (Fox, 1970, see Morton, 1968 for more information). All these evidence support the importance of the tactile sense for normal neurological development and for learning about the animal's environment.

> • Animals without normal maternal interactions develop abnormal neurological systems, including increased neural cell death and an increased stress response (Zhang *et al.*, 2002).

Sounds can affect learning by their ability to orient an animal toward a stimulus. Once the animal focuses on the stimulus, they can learn about it. Animals can also learn about sound. They can make associations with different sounds and can learn to attend to the different characteristics of sound. Changes to an animal's behavior in response to sound can be indications of neural changes in the auditory cortex (Blake *et al.*, 2002 – monkeys). Often, people use auditory cues to elicit behaviors in animals. Animals are able to discriminate between auditory cues but may not be as accurate as we believe they are.

Visual stimuli are likely to affect learning in various ways. Both the dog's and the cat's visual systems are geared toward high visual contrast in low light situations and moving visual stimuli (Miller, 2001). Fukuzawa *et al.*, (2005) found that visual cues are important ones for dogs, and dogs used these visual cues in combination with the verbal cues used by people. When only the verbal cues were used, the dogs were significantly less likely to perform the cued behavior than when both visual and verbal cues were present. Dogs were found to be sensitive to the gaze of humans when the person was giving a cue for a behavior (Virányi *et al.*, 2004). This was demonstrated by the dog being significantly more likely to perform a behavior if the person giving the cue was looking at the dog than if the person was looking somewhere else or if they were behind a screen.

Animals learn how to learn by being exposed to different environmental stimuli and by having problems to solve (Overall, 2009). When an animal is provided with all its physical needs and its environment remains static, it is less likely to develop the skills necessary to learn efficiently. Animals in barren environments have smaller brains and less plastic neurological systems (Bennett *et al.*, 1964 – rats). These animals can develop stereotypic behaviors (Mason *et al.*, 2007). They may have a reduced or altered appreciation of pain (Melzak and Scott, 1957 – dogs). They may also be more difficult to train than animals with a more enriched past. Mice raised in an impoverished environment were slower to learn a maze than those with an enriched environment (Iso *et al.*, 2007). Although there is some evidence in mice that being raised in complex social environments predicts complex social skills not increased learning ability (D'Andrea *et al.*, 2007). In this study, social learning was not investigated.

CHAPTER 6

The increase of fear responses during the seventh or eighth week of development (Scott and Fuller, 1965 – dogs; Karsh, 1983 – cats) weakens the animal's curiosity about new experiences, objects, and individuals. The animal now learns and remembers which stimuli are reinforcing and which are punishing. As the learning rate about the environment decreases, the sensitive period called *socialization* slowly comes to a close. The socialization period is one of accelerated learning in which the animal learns much about its relationships with other animals as well as about its environment. This is not the only time during an animal's life that they learn about the environment or other animals. This type of learning continues throughout the animal's life; it is the accelerated rate of learning that slows. This explains why animals exposed to a rich social environment when young show increased social abilities throughout their lives (D'Andrea *et al.*, 2007 – mice).

> • Animals exposed to a rich social environment when young show increased social abilities throughout their lives.

Habituation and sensitization

Habituation and sensitization are simple forms of nonassociative learning in which an animal learns to either ignore or attend closely to a stimulus. They are not making associations between two stimuli. Instead, during habituation, an animal learns that a stimulus is not important and stops noticing it. Habituation occurs after repeated exposures. This is not something someone does to an animal such as a behavior modification technique such as desensitization. Instead, this is a way in which an animal learns. The animal figures out over time whether the stimulus is dangerous. Animals habituate to wearing a collar just as humans habituate to wearing a watch.

Sensitization is seen when an animal becomes more aware of a stimulus after repeated exposures. These stimuli may be loud, painful, or frightening in other ways to the animal. Once an animal is sensitized to a stimulus, it is more difficult to desensitize them to it. Animals can become sensitized to thunder as do people. It startles them causing fear. They learn to listen for the scary sound of thunder. They may also learn to associate other stimuli with thunder through higher order conditioning seen in classical conditioning.

There is an evolutionary basis to nonassociative learning through natural selection. It is adaptive for animals to learn which stimuli are harmful and which are not. It is also adaptive for animals to become used to stimuli that will not harm them. Being in a constant state of fear is not beneficial to any animal; it is vital that they learn through repeated exposures which stimuli are truly dangerous and which are not.

> • Being in a constant state of fear is not beneficial to any animal; it is vital that they learn through repeated exposures which stimuli are truly dangerous and which are not.

For a stimulus to elicit habituation or sensitization, the animal must notice it. The animal's attention on the stimulus is necessary for them to learn about it. The rate of presentation will affect the animal's ability to learn about it. If the stimulus is presented often, the animal can learn more quickly about it. Even after habituation has occurred if the stimulus is not presented to the animal for a long time, the animal may react to it as if it were novel. This is called *spontaneous recovery*. Spontaneous recovery occurs in all types of learning. It is as if everything the animal has learned is stored waiting for the proper time to present itself. If new learning is not used, the animal can revert back to earlier learning.

> • Spontaneous recovery: even after habituation has occurred if the stimulus is not presented to the animal for a long time, the animal may react to it as if it were novel.

The intensity of the stimulus will affect the animal's reaction to it. Loud sounds are more likely to cause sensitization than habituation as are any intense stimuli. The more severe the stimulus is the more likely it will cause the animal to become sensitized to it. Habituation is more probable if the stimulus is innocuous or harmless. Of course, this judgment is made from the animal's perspective.

The temperament of an animal affects how they make judgments about the environment surrounding them. If the animal is highly reactive and fearful, it will judge more stimuli to be dangerous and thus will become sensitized to them. Although an animal's temperament is largely present at birth, it can and is modified through-out life by experience. During an animal's socialization period, they can be exposed to many stimuli, creating a broad basis of exposure to many objects, experiences, sounds, and living things. This allows them to have the best chance of being able to habituate to the stimuli commonly found in their environment throughout their life.

> • Although an animal's temperament is largely present at birth, it can and is modified throughout life by experience.

Behavior modification using habituation

The following are the behavior modification techniques that use habituation as their basis. Because animals are able to learn that a stimulus is not harmful, we are able to use these types of behavior modification to change how they respond to different stimuli.

Flooding is a technique that places the animal near the feared stimulus or in the feared situation until they no longer react with fear. This can be a useful technique if the animal is not very afraid of the stimulus or situation. If the animal is affected greatly by the stimulus, they can become more fearful by using this technique. Flooding can cause intense fear and stress for the animal (Figure 6.3). A great example of flooding is the television show Fear Factor. Contestants are placed so that they cannot escape, then something they fear (rats, spiders, or cockroaches) are put on them. Of course, in the show, the contestants rarely feel better about the source of their fear after competing. Similarly, animals can become more fearful of the stimulus after using this technique. Reactions to flooding can include attempting to flee the procedure or becoming aggressive while trying to flee. The animal may even be injured while trying to escape. If they are not exposed to the feared stimulus until the fear is completely gone, they will continue to associate the stimulus with danger.

Desensitization is another method of habituating an animal to a feared stimulus. Box 6.1 provides defini-tions for human psychological terms for desensitization. These techniques are modified when working with nonverbal patients. With desensitization, the stimulus is broken down into its components and modified to lower its intensity. Then, these components are ranked from the least to the most feared component. A plan is made in which the animal will be exposed to the least feared aspects of the stimulus first. Then, over time

Figure 6.3 A Greyhound, Buck, showing signs of stress because of flooding. He is afraid of the light-colored floor tiles.

and as the animal learns to become used to it, each component of the stimulus is presented. With repeated exposure, the animal learns to habituate to each part of the stimulus. Because the components are presented independently and because the intensity is modified to increase the speed of habituation, the animal learns how to cope with the stimulus without the intense anxiety flooding can elicit.

> **BOX 6.1: PSYCHOLOGICAL TERMS FOR DESENSITIZATION.**
>
> • Systematic desensitization – A person imagines the situation or object of their fear while relaxing. The fear-producing stimuli are put into a list according to their fear-producing properties. The person begins imagining the least feared item and works up to the most feared item.
> • *In vivo* desensitization – A person is exposed to the situa-tion or object of their fear while relaxing. All other aspects of this behavior modification technique are the same as systematic desensitization.

Using the example of a human's fear of spiders, we can list the frightening components as size, speed of movement, proximity, and hairiness. It would depend on the individual how these components were ranked. Each component can be modified in some way to make the spider initially less scary. For example, we could start off with a very small, bald, dead spider contained in a sealed jar 10 feet away from the subject. This stimulus is small (size), cannot move because of death and is contained (speed of movement), is not hairy, and is far away (proximity). After the subject is relaxed with this stimulus, we could modify one of the characteristics of the spider. We could use a very small, live, bald spider contained in a sealed jar 10 feet away from the subject. We would continue in this way until the subject could pick up a very large, hairy, fast moving, live spider without fear.

Desensitization is often used with classical counter conditioning. This combination of techniques allows the animal to learn a new emotional response through classical conditioning (associations) while habituating to the stimulus.

> • Desensitization is often used with classical counter conditioning. This combination of techniques allows the animal to learn a new emotional response through classical conditioning (associations) while habituating to the stimulus.

Attention focusing and relaxation exercises can enhance the results of these techniques. Animals can be taught to focus on another stimulus besides the feared one. However, an animal will not be able to perform this if they are very afraid. The relationship the animal has with the person conducting the behavior modification may affect the process. If the animal is able to learn to focus on another stimulus, then they are learning to ignore the feared one.

Relaxation can be measured by observing behaviors or by measuring physiological parameters (Poppen, 1988). There is a relaxation protocol in the text by Overall (1997) on behavioral medicine encouraging owners to reinforce relaxed postures such as ear, jaw, and head positions as well as general relaxed posture. Once the animal is relaxing more frequently, the behavior can be put on cue and asked for in different situations. Refer to Chapter 8 for teaching relaxation.

Operant conditioning

Learning in which a behavior is affected by its consequences is called *operant conditioning* (Box 6.2). This type of learning is seen in animals when they associate performing a specific behavior with some sort of benefit or detriment. Operant conditioning is classified as an associative type of learning (Skinner, 1966). When a behavior is followed by something the animal wants, the behavior will strengthen; conversely, if the behavior is followed by something the animal fears or dislikes, the behavior will weaken. Weakening of behavior can also be seen when the behavior is followed by nothing. Operant conditioning is used when training animals to perform behaviors, as it primarily deals with voluntary behaviors. It is also the type of learning involved when a behavior is weakened using punishment. This type of learning is not synonymous with positive reinforcement training, as punishment is part of operant conditioning.

> • Learning in which a behavior is affected by its consequences is called *operant conditioning*.

BOX 6.2: DIFFERENT TERMS FOR OPERANT CONDITIONING.

- Skinnerian learning
- Trial and error learning
- Instrumental learning – some slight differences
- Type 2 conditioning
- Type R conditioning

Teaching an animal to come by giving it some sort of reinforcer, such as a food treat, each time it comes to you is one example of operant conditioning. Another example using punishment is when an animal's behavior of jumping into a bathtub is weakened if the bathtub contains water. Of course, the animal would have to dislike being in water for this to weaken the behavior. The stimulus following the behavior does not have to be something a person or other animal does to them. Instead, it can be a natural consequence of the animal's behavior. If an animal tries to eat a bee, they will be stung, probably teaching them to stop eating bees in the future. There are other factors that can affect this type of learning. They are discussed later in this section.

Operant conditioning is occurring all the time throughout an animal's life. They learn through trial and error which behaviors bring them stimuli they want and which bring them stimuli they dislike. All types of training use operant conditioning, and animals use operant conditioning when not being trained. The stimuli affecting an animal's behavior can be a variety of food, touches, sounds, activities, and odors. It is up to the individual animal whether a stimulus is reinforcement or punishment. Both reinforcement and punishment must occur within 2 s of the behavior and before the performance of another behavior or their effect on the behavior will be weakened tremendously (Skinner, 1966). Animals that appear to look guilty during ill-timed punishments are likely showing appeasement behaviors in response to anger exhibited by the person punishing them. Animals that did not perform the unwanted behavior will also show these behaviors. This supports the hypothesis that when an animal exhibits behaviors judged to be guilt by a person, they are no more likely to have committed the unwanted behavior than an animal that does not exhibit these behaviors.

> • It is up to the individual animal whether a stimulus is reinforcement or punishment.

Reinforcement has a functional definition. It must fulfill the function of strengthening a behavior for it to be labeled a reinforcer. All reinforcers are stimuli the animal wants, but it depends on the animal which stimuli are reinforcers for them. For example, my dog Scarlet finds broccoli extremely reinforcing, whereas my dog Lily does not. Lily is better reinforced using bread. Although both my dogs prefer food reinforcers, other dogs may prefer some sort of touch or play.

> • Reinforcement has a functional definition. It must fulfill the function of strengthening a behavior for it to be labeled a reinforcer. All reinforcers are stimuli the animal wants, but it depends on the animal which stimuli are reinforcers for them.

There are two types of reinforcements used in operant conditioning: negative and positive reinforcement. When you read these terms, you may think negative means bad and positive means good, but in this case, that would be incorrect. When referring to these behavior principles think about the mathematical symbols of subtraction (−) for negative and addition (+) for positive (Table 6.1).

Negative reinforcement takes away a stimulus when a behavior happens, causing the behavior to strengthen. Think about the types of things you would work to have removed. You might want someone to stop yelling at you, hitting you, or shocking you. If you performed a behavior and one of these stimuli stopped, your behavior would be reinforced through negative reinforcement.

A common example of negative reinforcement seen in a veterinary hospital is when a person approaches a "cage-aggressive" animal. If the animal lunges at the approaching person causing the person to back up, the animal will learn lunging behavior removes the scary person. Consequently, the behavior of lunging at the person will strengthen. The cue for this behavior is the person approaching the cage. Although the cage-aggressive behavior was initially performed in response to fear of the person, over time and repeated performances, the animal will become very confident using this behavior and will appear to be confident instead of fearful.

Positive reinforcement involves adding a stimulus the animal wants immediately after or during a behavior they are performing. Adding this stimulus strengthens the behavior that precedes it. You may hear people say they use positive reinforcement training, but if they use any type of punishment during training, they are actually using operant conditioning instead of only positive reinforcement.

If I teach my cat to jump onto a box and give her a food treat when she does so, I am using positive reinforcement to train this behavior. Animals can be taught an almost endless variety of behaviors and complex behavioral chains using positive reinforcement. This type of training is very forgiving. You can make mistakes, and the worst that can happen is you confuse the animal or teach an unwanted behavior. Using this technique you are more likely to strengthen the bond you have with an animal.

Reinforcers are often primary or unconditioned reinforcers. This means that the animal did not have to learn that these stimuli are good to receive. Examples

Table 6.1 Reinforcement and punishment.

Effect on behavior	Adding something	Taking something away
The behavior strengthens	Positive (+) reinforcement	Negative (−) reinforcement
Behavior of asking for candy is strengthened	Parent presents candy dish when child asks for candy	Parent squeezes the child's hand until they ask for candy
The behavior weakens	Positive (+) punishment	Negative (−) punishment
Behavior of asking for candy is weakened	Child is spanked for asking for candy	Candy dish is removed when the child asks for candy

of primary reinforcers are food, water, and temperature changes that enhance homeostasis. Reinforcers can also be learned through classical conditioning. These reinforcers are called *secondary or conditioned reinforcers*. They are associated through repeated pairings with a primary reinforcer or they can be associated with a previously associated secondary reinforcer. Examples of secondary reinforcers are toys and praise. Some training techniques use a conditioned reinforcer such as clicker training. The click sound is a secondary or conditioned reinforcer because once taught, that click means a treat is coming; the click is associated with a forthcoming food reward.

Theoretically, if you want to weaken a behavior, you could use punishment. Punishment is also defined functionally. A stimulus is only a punishment if when it is applied immediately after or during a behavior that behavior weakens. No matter how punishing you think a stimulus is, it is not a punishment unless it weakens the behavior it follows. You may come home each day to a dog that greets you by jumping on you. You may yell at this dog each day "no" or "get down," but these are not punishments for your dog because each day he continues to jump on you to greet you. For yelling to be a punishment for this dog, his behavior of jumping to greet you must weaken over time. Honestly, when you observe animals and notice the stimuli they find reinforcing (e.g., dogs eating cat feces), it is no wonder we are baffled at what they find punishing. When working with other species, you must suspend your own preferences and try to imagine the animal's sensory preferences. You can verify your ideas by watching their body language and keeping track of their behavior. Body language denoting pleasure is a likely sign of reinforcement, whereas body language denoting fear or avoidance is a likely sign of punishment. Counting behaviors to assess their strengthening or weakening can also be a reliable technique for judging whether a stimulus is reinforcement or punishment.

> - A stimulus is only a punishment if when it is applied immediately after or during a behavior that behavior weakens.

There are two types of punishments that mirror the two types of reinforcements: positive and negative punishment. Positive (+) still means we are adding something, and negative (−) still means we are removing something.

Positive punishment is being used when a stimulus is added either during or immediately after a behavior is performed, and the behavior is weakened. If the behavior does not weaken, then whatever you are doing is not punishment for that animal. If punishment is going to weaken a behavior, it does so within one or two trials. Continuing to use the same technique after no weakening of the behavior is observed is fruitless and potentially damaging to the human–animal bond. The types of stimuli used as punishment are all things the animal wants to avoid or escape from. Using positive punishment, especially if you are present during the punishment, can cause the animal to associate you with the aversive stimulus. Your presence can become a conditioned punisher. This can undermine any trust you have built with the animal. Other objects in the environment as well as contexts can also be associated with punishment. Keep in mind what the animal may learn if you decide to use punishment. If you use loud sounds as punishment, the animal may learn that loud sounds are punishing and may generalize that fear to a variety of loud sounds.

> - Continuing to use the same technique after no weakening of the behavior is observed is fruitless and potentially damaging to the human–animal bond.

When a stimulus is removed as a consequence of a behavior and the behavior weakens, negative punishment is being used. These stimuli would be something the animal wants. An example of negative punishment is when a person leaves the room when an animal performs an attention-seeking behavior. Because the animal wants attention and attention from the person is removed, as long as the behavior weakens, this would be considered negative punishment.

Animals can learn to associate stimuli with punishment through classical conditioning. When a stimulus is consistently associated with punishment, it becomes a conditioned or secondary punishment. A disapproving look or verbal reprimand can become a conditioned punishment. Even an owner coming home can become a conditioned punishment if coming home is consistently associated with another punishment. Primary or unconditioned punishments cause discomfort or fear. Examples of primary punishments are electric shocks and hitting.

Punishment is difficult to use properly, and even if it is used properly, it does not teach the animal to perform the desired behavior. I may want my dog to greet my friends by sitting. I can punish his jumping to greet behavior for years; it will never teach him to sit to greet people. The animal is left trying to figure out what behavior is wanted. This can cause conflict and frustration. An inconsistent punishment can also be thought of as an intermittent reinforcer because the behavior will sometimes continue to be reinforced. When this happens, the behavior will be strengthened not weakened. Using an intermittent reinforcer also leads to behavior that is the most difficult to extinguish (Skinner, 1966). Other techniques that can be used to change behavior are discussed in the section titled **Behavior modification using operant conditioning**.

Positive punishment and negative reinforcement are two completely different behavior principles, although they are often confused. A behavior must be weakened for a principle to be called a punishment. A behavior is strengthened when using negative reinforcement. There are some common characteristics of these two principles. Both positive punishment and negative reinforcement involve an adverse stimulus. These aversive stimuli produce fear and/or discomfort for the animal. Positive punishment adds the stimulus, whereas negative reinforcement removes the stimulus. Using these two principles, positive punishment and negative reinforcement, can cause some unintended side effects. Side effects can include avoidance, aggression, and behavioral suppression.

Cues are signals animals associate with performing a corresponding behavior. Some cues are intentional, and others are not. Animals may attend to a different cue than which we have intended. For example, a cat may use an owner waking up as a cue to meow, and the owner may reinforce this behavior with food. The owner may not be aware their behavior of waking up is a cue for the meow behavior. They may also not be aware of reinforcing meowing by feeding their cat. Animals learn to perform behaviors associated with a cue. This cue precedes the behavior, and the animal learns that if they perform the behavior after the cue, they are likely to be reinforced for it. A cue is also called a *discriminative stimulus* (D^s). These stimuli help the animal to discriminate when they will be reinforced for a behavior and when they will not. Once the animal reliably performs the behavior on cue, the behavior can be said to be under stimulus control (Box 6.3).

> **BOX 6.3: CHARACTERISTICS OF STIMULUS CONTROL.**
>
> Characteristics of stimulus control
> 1. Responds to the cue correctly a minimum of 80% of the time
> 2. Does not offer the behavior (in training session) without the cue
> 3. Does not perform a different behavior in response to the cue
> 4. Does not perform this behavior in response to a different cue

Motivation encompasses the individual differences in how animals respond to stimuli in specific contexts. There are many principles that can help us understand why animals are motivated to behave in differing ways even when exposed to the exact same stimuli.

Although animals are afraid of novel items, neophobia, in their environment, they are also fascinated by them, neophilia (Grandin and Deesing, 1998). This fascination of animals for new stimuli can be used to teach them to habituate to a variety of objects and manipulations. The use of force when introducing novel items is associated with increased fear, whereas if animals are left alone with a novel item, they will frequently approach it faster (Grandin and Deesing, 1998). Instead of restraining an animal and putting the otoscope into their ear, we could let them approach and explore the otoscope on their own terms first. We could make a pleasant association between the otoscope and something the animal likes: a treat or petting. After they are comfortable with it, we could then place it in their ear without incident. All pieces of equipment used on animals in veterinary practices could be introduced in this manner, making the animals more comfortable and making procedures go smoothly.

> • Animals should be allowed to explore veterinary equipment on their own terms. The equipment should be associated with something the animal likes. This will help the animal become comfortable and more accepting of the procedures.

Under laboratory conditions, animals were shown to behaviorally conform to the theory of operant conditioning, but once the animals came out into the complexity of the everyday world, instincts or innate behaviors began to show effects on learned behavior. These discrepancies in learning theory were already showing themselves in the autoshaping behavior of pigeons pecking a light for food reinforcements (Brown and Jenkins, 1968). It is a normal species-specific behavior that pigeons peck for food. In the study by Brown and Jenkins, they were taught to expect food to appear in a food dish after a light in their enclosure was illuminated. They learned this association quickly. But after many repeated trials, the pigeons began pecking the light when it was lit as if pecking produced the food. They had begun to behave toward the light as if it were food. Along with other innate behaviors, animals have species-specific behaviors affecting food gathering, and these behaviors were shown to affect behaviors learned through operant conditioning (Breland and Breland, 1961). Known as *instinctual drift*, this effect modifies learned behaviors to become more analogous to naturally occurring food-gathering behaviors. It seems the animal begins to associate the learned behavior with the food reinforcer. This association then changes the way they behave when presented with the cue for the learned behavior.

In a training scenario for a fair, the Brelands attempted to teach chickens to stand still on a platform to receive a food reinforcer. The chickens did so for a short time but eventually began to scratch at the surface it was standing on as if it was scratching for food. Although this behavior did not earn the chickens a reinforcer, was more difficult, and took more energy than standing still, the chickens persisted with the scratching behavior. This evidence goes against Skinnerian theories on how organisms learn and behave. When training an

animal, the natural behavioral tendencies of the animal must be taken into consideration. It seems a waste of time to teach an animal behaviors counter to their species-specific behaviors, as the learned behavior will be modified by these instincts over time.

> • When training an animal, the natural behavioral tendencies of the animal must be taken into consideration.

Through natural selection, animals' drives have been refined to reinforce a set of behaviors used to keep them alive long enough to allow them to reproduce. A drive can be defined as a force that energizes an animal to perform a behavior; diminishing or eliminating this force is reinforcing (Hull, 1943). Some of the drives recognized in animals are eating, drinking, performing reproductive behaviors, and seeking a comfortable environmental temperature.

It seems logical for animals to be motivated to drink when they are thirsty, whereas animals that have just drank their fill are no longer motivated to do so. It follows logically that food would be a reinforcer for a hungry animal, but what about running being a reinforcer for drinking behavior? If running is a restricted activity for an animal and the animal must drink to be able to run, the behavior of running becomes the reinforcer for drinking. Experiments with rats showed the same animals in different experimental contexts drank water for the opportunity to run and ran for the opportunity to drink (Premack, 1962). This paradoxical law of behavior is called the *Premack Principle*. Animals will perform a less profitable behavior to be able to perform a more profitable behavior; they will perform an unrestricted behavior in order to be able to perform a restricted behavior (Premack, 1962). It can help us explain why animals seem determined to perform one behavior for the opportunity to perform a restricted behavior. A dog may bolt out the door for the opportunity to run the neighborhood, whereas a cat may swim across a river for an opportunity to rest in a warm barn. In the dog example, the more restricted the access to the neighborhood is, the harder the dog will work to escape out the door. Likewise, the cat will work harder to swim the river if a warm resting place is difficult to find.

Animals become accustomed to performing certain behaviors or chains of behaviors to satisfy their drives or for other reinforcers. These habits of behavior can be assessed according to their strength, which depends on how many times the animal has been reinforced for performing them (Hull, 1943). Habit strength affects how long it takes for animals to unlearn behaviors and learn alternate ones. Reinforcement can be manipulated through the use of different reinforcement schedules (Ferster and Skinner, 1957) (Table 6.2). There are two main categories of reinforcement schedules: ratio and interval. Ratio reinforcements reinforce behavior after they are performed a certain number of times, whereas interval reinforcement schedules reinforce a behavior when it is performed after a certain amount of time or when the duration of the behavior has reached a certain time span. Ratio schedules are used when a trainer wants to obtain a good solid performance of a behavioral event, whereas interval schedules are used to obtain behavioral states or repeated behaviors. If a person wanted to train a dog to lie down, they would use ratio schedules, but if they wanted to reinforce lie down and stay, an interval schedule would probably work best.

When a behavior is reinforced each time it is performed, continuous reinforcement (CRF), the animal's performance increases steadily until they are performing it correctly each time. This is the recommended reinforcement schedule for training new behaviors. Behaviors, learned using a CRF schedule, are receptive to extinction. They may weaken drastically when not reinforced each time.

Once animals learn a behavior well, it is recommended the reinforcement schedule be changed to partial reinforcement (PR) or intermittent reinforcement (IR). These schedules are used to maintain known behaviors by reinforcing them randomly. Animals will then perform the behaviors more rapidly, and the behaviors become resistant to extinction. Variable ratio (VR) reinforcement schedules are included in this category of reinforcement schedules. Although it is a good idea to have wanted behaviors resistant to extinction, many behaviors taught to animals by mistake are reinforced on this schedule as well, making them very difficult to extinguish.

If an animal becomes confused when using a PR schedule, a trainer can use a fixed ratio two (FR2) or three (FR3) reinforcement schedule to get the animal over to the variable schedule using baby steps. This helps the animal understand that they are going to be reinforced for the behavior but not every time they perform it. A behavior should not stay on an fixed reinforcement because the animal will learn this rate and only perform well when they know

Table 6.2 Reinforcement schedules and their effect on behavior.

Reinforcement schedule	Effect on behavior	Common usage
Continuous reinforcement (CR) Fixed ratio 1 (FR1)	Fast acquisition of behavior Easy to extinguish	Teaching new behaviors
Fixed ratio reinforcement: FR2 – reinforce after two behaviors FR3 – reinforce after three behaviors	Behavior weakens after reinforcement is given High rates of behavior worsen this effect Anticipation of reinforcement common	Transitioning an animal from continuous to partial reinforcement
Partial reinforcement (PR) Intermittent reinforcement (IR) Variable ratio (VR)	Steady, strong behavioral response to cue Protects behavior from extinction Reinforcement rate is unknown to animal	Maintenance of a known behavior
Fixed interval 1 reinforcement (FI1)	Fast acquisition of behavior Easy to extinguish	Teaching new repeated behaviors or new behavioral states
Fixed interval reinforcement: FI2 – reinforce after 2 s FI3 – reinforce after 3 s	Behavior weakens after reinforcement is given High intervals of time worsen this effect Anticipation of reinforcement common	Transitioning an animal from continuous to partial reinforcement
Variable interval (VI)	Steady, strong repeated behavior or behavioral state response to cue Protects repeated behavior or behavioral state from extinction Reinforcement interval is unknown to animal	Maintenance of a known repeated behavior or behavioral state

CHAPTER 6

the reinforcer is coming. Animals are able to learn these rates relatively quickly; proceeding to a variable reinforcement schedule as soon as possible will best allow the learned behavior to be strengthened and maintained.

The strength of the reinforcers and punishers used in operant conditioning can be manipulated to some degree by changing the reinforcer or the environment surrounding the reinforcer. There is no need to use deprivation to increase their strength, as animals can be motivated without depriving them of their basic needs. In fact, using food deprivation can inhibit learning by causing the animal to be too focused on obtaining the food or in extreme situations by making the animal weak. Instead of deprivation, opportunistic timing can be used. If food reinforcers are being used, arrange to train just before the animal's regular meal. The animal will be ready for food at that time. If the animal has been alone all day, attention and touch can be used as reinforcers (assuming those things are reinforcing to the animal).

- To create motivation, opportunistic timing of reinforcers is preferred over deprivation.

Designating a treat or toy as special and only using it during training sessions while restricting access to it at other times can be extremely affective. No one wants more food after a feast, and no one wants attention after receiving large quantities of attention. There is no benefit to using a reinforcer after a similar substance sates the animal.

Animals compare reinforcers using negative contrast. In this comparison, one reinforcer loses out to the other. If I give my dog steak as a reinforcer, then switch to dry kibble it is probable that she will not work as hard after the switch. Dry kibble is not as reinforcing for most dogs as steak is for them. Even steak can become common place and boring for animals if it is used too often. Animals can habituate to any reinforcer. It is good practice to vary your reinforcers to allow them to retain their strength. Surprise reinforcers are the best, but it can be difficult to catch animals unaware as their sense of smell is exceptional.

- It is good practice to vary your reinforcers to allow them to retain their strength.

Figure 6.4 A Greyhound, Sancho, showing signs of learned helplessness by not exhibiting any behaviors when approached by a person.

Likewise, punishments can be overused rendering them ineffective through habituation and poor timing. Only the sparing and proper use of punishment can be effective in weakening unwanted behaviors. Inescapable punishments create a condition in animals called *learned helplessness* (Seligman, 1972). When an animal does not know how to avoid or escape punishment, they stop responding to it. But instead of ignoring it as in habituation, they become almost zombie-like. They learn that their behavior does not affect what happens to them (Figure 6.4). They stop trying to learn behaviors, as there is no sense in it any longer. This condition was found through research on human depression, and when an animal exhibits learned helplessness, they appear to be depressed. Overmier and Seligman (1967) found dogs that were exposed to inescapable shock were significantly less likely to try to escape a shock after they were trained how to escape it. Even when they did escape the shock by jumping over a barrier, they were no more likely to try to escape the shock next time it occurred. This suppression of learned behavior is unique to learned helplessness and was contingent on the animal not having control over the occurrence of the punishment. If dogs were able to escape punishment by performing a behavior (negative reinforcement), they did not develop learned helplessness, but if their behavior had no influence on the receipt of the punishment, they were highly predisposed to it.

Another issue related to reinforcement and punishment use is client compliance. Clients would rather use reinforcement when working with their pets. However, people are generally better at noticing undesirable behavior rather than reinforcing desirable behavior.

Table 6.3 Criteria for successful punishment.

Criterion	Comment
Punishment must occur every time the behavior happens	If you cannot be present each time the behavior is performed, you must set up a remote punishment device that punishes every time the behavior is performed
	Only the unwanted behavior can be punished with this remote device
	Indiscriminate punishment causes learned helplessness
	If the punishment does not occur every time the behavior repeats, the animal is likely being reinforced intermittently for the behavior. This makes the behavior resistant to extinction
Punishment must be harsh enough to stop the behavior	Generally, people do not want to use harsh punishments on their animals
	Animals can habituate to different levels of punishment if you start with a weaker one and slowly increase it
Punishment must occur within 2 s of the behavior and before any other behavior has been performed	Associative learning drops off sharply after 2 s following a behavior
	If another behavior is performed before the punishment that is the behavior being punished not the intended one

Punishing behavior (even just a verbal reprimand) can be very reinforcing to the punisher. It is a better use of our time to teach owners how to use positive reinforcement effectively; changing an owner's focus to notice desirable behavior rather than to punish each misstep. Punishment is nearly impossible to administer successfully, see Table 6.3 for the criteria for punishment to be successful.

An animal's attention is a powerful tool during training (Figure 6.5). Without their attention, they are not going to learn the behaviors you want them to learn. Having an appropriate reinforcer goes a long way toward gaining and keeping an animal's attention. Other factors that affect attention are the relationship between the trainer and the animal, the environment within which the training is occurring, the environment in which the animal was socialized, the temperament of the animal (anxiety and fear can inhibit learning), and the animal's genetics. Attention is so vital to learning in animals that it is often the first behavior taught, "look at me."

Once a behavior is taught in one context, it must be taught in other contexts or the animal will only associate that one context with the behavior. It happens frequently that people train an animal to perform a

behavior in one context, yet expect them to perform the behavior in a totally different context. Examples of this phenomenon are seen when dogs trained for obedience trials only heel when on rubber mats. They were taught to heel on these mats in dog obedience classes, and the trials are conducted on them as well. The dogs may not understand that heeling can also occur off of rubber mats. Teaching a behavior on a cue in a variety of situations and environments is called *generalization*. A behavior is not truly learned until the animal will perform it in multiple contexts when given the cue.

Behavior modification using operant conditioning

Behavior can be weakened without using punishment. It is more effective to train an animal to perform the behaviors you want rather than punishing each behavioral mistake they make. One of these behavior modification techniques is called *operant counter conditioning* (Box 6.4). This technique is one in which the animal is taught to perform a wanted behavior in place of the unwanted behavior. When using this technique, the animal should be taught the wanted behavior outside of the situation in which they are deemed to be misbehaving. The behavior must be taught in a relaxed environment for the animal to best be able to learn it. Then, the behavior can be transferred over to the target environment. Notice the cue that elicits the unwanted behavior. Once trained, this cue should elicit the wanted behavior. The animal learns that this new, wanted behavior is reinforcing in this situation, whereas the unwanted behavior is not. A selection of reinforcement rules is used in human

Figure 6.5 A mixed breed dog, Trixie, showing attention toward one of the kennel technicians, Jessica Rice, and a veterinary technology student, Jeanne Rowe.

Table 6.4 Various reinforcement options for operant counter conditioning.

Technique	Full name	Description	Comment
DRO	Differential reinforcement of other behaviors	The trainer reinforces any other behavior besides the unwanted behavior	This is used in circumstances in which an animal does not offer many behaviors. We want to increase any behavior besides the unwanted one
DRA	Differential reinforcement of an alternate behavior	The trainer reinforces a behavior the animal cannot perform at the same time as the unwanted behavior	This is used to substitute a wanted behavior for an unwanted one
DRH	Differential reinforcement of high rates of responding	The trainer reinforces a burst of wanted behaviors	This is used to create quick bursts of a wanted behavior
DRL	Differential reinforcement of low rates of responding	The trainer reinforces the behavior only when the behavior occurs after specific timed pauses	This is used to cause pauses between a series of wanted behaviors

psychology and in animal training when using operant counter conditioning. In these situations, the behavior being reinforced is related to the unwanted behavior in a variety of ways (Table 6.4).

BOX 6.4: BEHAVIOR MODIFICATION USING OPERANT CONDITIONING.

- Operant counter conditioning: different terms used
  - Counter conditioning
  - Response substitution
- Operant extinction: different terms used
  - Extinction
  - Removing the reinforcer for the behavior
  - Can mistakenly be called: ignoring or removing attention

This technique of operant counter conditioning is frequently used in combination with operant extinction. Operant extinction, often called *extinction*, is used to weaken a behavior by removing its reinforcer. It is not a technique in which you only ignore the animal when they perform the behavior because some behaviors are not reinforced by attention. If your dog steals food from a coffee table, you can ignore the behavior forever; however, the dog will never learn to stop stealing the food. This is because obtaining the food is the reinforcer not attention. Sometimes, attention is the reinforcer for the behavior. Attention often reinforces jumping to greet behaviors in dogs. This is why removal of attention when they jump on you and teaching them to sit to greet you instead work so well.

When using extinction, you must first know what is reinforcing the behavior. You can find this out by observing the animal and noting what happens right after they perform the behavior. If you cannot figure out what is reinforcing the behavior or if you cannot remove the reinforcer, then you can still use operant counter conditioning, but you will not be able to use extinction with it. Animals may find performing the behavior reinforcing in itself. This occurs when animals masturbate, and many people believe that it also occurs when dogs bark. If you are able to ascertain the reinforcer and remove it, you can then use extinction.

When the reinforcer is removed first, especially if the behavior has been consistently reinforced at a fixed ratio of one, the animal will exhibit an extinction burst. This affects the behavior by making it more intense and variable. The animal may react by becoming frustrated and even becoming aggressive. To reduce the intensity and length of the extinction burst, operant counter conditioning is used. Using both techniques together, the animal learns the unwanted behavior no longer obtains them any reinforcement, but the wanted behavior is now reinforced instead.

- By using both operant counter conditioning and operant extinction together the animal learns the unwanted behavior no longer obtains them any reinforcement but the wanted behavior is now reinforced instead.

Behaviors that are reinforced on an intermittent or partial reinforcement schedule are difficult to extinguish (Skinner, 1966). The animal has learned they will not be reinforced for each behavior performed, thus will continue to perform the behavior many times reliably without a reinforcer. It may be helpful to put the behavior on a continuous reinforcement schedule before trying to extinguish it. Lerman *et al.*, (1996) found severely mentally challenged children responded more quickly to extinction when behaviors initially intermittently reinforced were switched to a CRF schedule before being extinguished.

Classical conditioning

This type of associative learning is one in which an animal associates a novel stimulus with another stimulus that already causes a reaction (Box 6.5). After repeated pairings, the novel stimulus will also cause this reaction. The paradigm for classical conditioning is the animal associating a conditioned stimulus (CS) with an unconditioned stimulus (US) to elicit an unconditioned response (UR). Again, after many pairings, the CS will elicit a CR, which is often indistinguishable from the UR seen when exposed to the US (Table 6.5).

> **BOX 6.5: DIFFERENT TERMS USED FOR CLASSICAL CONDITIONING.**
>
> - Respondent conditioning
> - Signal learning
> - Pavlovian conditioning
> - Type 1 conditioning
> - Type S conditioning

When thinking about all these stimuli and responses, it may help to remember if a stimulus or response is conditioned, learning had to occur for it to have meaning. If a stimulus is unconditioned, this instead indicates that no learning need occur for it to elicit a response. Therefore, the CS must occur just before a US to elicit the UR as the animal is learning about the CS in this arrangement. The UR occurs naturally after the US, but the CR is learned when the CS repeatedly just precedes the US.

This type of learning was studied by Pavlov in the late 1800s and the early 1900s. His experiments with dogs involved the reflex of salivation. Most of the behaviors related to classical conditioning are involuntary; they include reflexes, emotions, and secretions. Classical conditioning is powerful because the learning takes place within the unconscious mind. Learning of this type cannot be set aside by the conscious brain,

Table 6.5 Classical conditioning schematic.

Cat sees food (US)	Becomes excited (UR)	
Cat hears can opener (CS)	Sees food (US)	Becomes excited (UR)
Cat hears can opener (CS)	Becomes excited (CR)	

although it can be mitigated by experience (Krushinskii, 1960).

Evidence of classical conditioning is seen when a cat learns being put in his carrier signifies he is going to the veterinary hospital. When he is placed in the carrier, he now feels what he feels when at the veterinary hospital. In a real way, the carrier has become the veterinary hospital for this cat. We can use classical conditioning to our advantage by teaching animals to associate the hospital and/or the carrier with stimuli they enjoy. Every piece of equipment at the veterinary hospital can be associated with something that individual animal enjoys, making it easier for us to assess our patients. Procedures and individuals can be associated with desired stimuli as well to facilitate an animal's diagnostics and treatment.

> - Every piece of equipment at the veterinary hospital can be associated with something that individual animal enjoys, making it easier for us to assess our patients.

Not only can animals associate one stimulus with another to elicit a response, they can also associate any number of stimuli with each other, creating a huge chain of associations. Evidence of this is seen in every veterinary hospital. A client comes in and remarks how their dog knows he is coming to the veterinary hospital when the owner turns right on a particular road, as the dog becomes fearful when the client turns the car. The dog has associated the turn with being at the hospital, which he associates with something fear or pain producing. Thus, the fear is elicited by the right turn on a road, which is not fear or pain producing at all. This process is called *higher order conditioning*. Because of this phenomenon, animals can associate an entire string of stimuli with a feared stimulus, creating fear responses when exposed to each individual stimulus.

Animals more readily learn some associations than others. This phenomenon is called *preparedness*. In the work by Seligman (1970, 1971) on prepared-ness, he found that animals exhibited three levels of preparedness to learn specific associations: prepared, unprepared, and contraprepared. When the animal was learning something in the prepared category, they learned it very quickly, often within one trial. Learning something in the unprepared category took many more trials for an animal, and learning something in the contraprepared category took a significant number of trials or it could not be learned. These categories of preparedness seemed tied to the evolution of the animal. Animals seemed to learn some associations easily. For example, the fear of snakes or spiders was learned easily, whereas other associations such as fear of flowers were very difficult if not impossible for them to learn. There are many studies showing this effect. Cook and Mineka (1990) found that primates were more easily trained to associate a snake than a flower with fear after watching videos of monkeys' fearful response to both stimuli.

Overshadowing is present when two CS are conditioned to a US together and one stimulus has a stronger connection to the US than the other. Blocking is similar, but in blocking, only one of the CS is actually conditioned, whereas the other is not. Both of these principles can be illustrated with one example. When conditioning a clicker, the click sound is often paired with a food treat. If the food treat is located within a crinkling bag, that sound may also be conditioned to the food treat at some level. If the crinkle sound and the click sound are conditioned to the food, but one has a stronger connection, then it is an example of overshadowing. If instead only one of the sounds is associated with the food, then that stimulus has blocked the other from forming an association.

Another factor that affects classical conditioning is potentiation. It appears that some pairings of associations create more powerful responses than others. Associations of various sensory stimuli with the gustatory sense are more potent than other pairings. Somehow the animal brain is wired to make stronger associations when taste is involved. This differs from preparedness in that preparedness is related to the ease of learning fear-producing stimuli, whereas potentiation is related to associations of taste and other sensory information with food and eating.

Interestingly, an animal can associate a stimulus with food so strongly that they treat the stimulus as if it were food. This is seen when an animal, after being conditioned to the clicker, licks a clicker when they hear the click sound. They behave as if the clicker is a food treat instead of behaving as if the click sound is

Figure 6.6 A Greyhound, Buck, is showing superstitious behavior by choosing to walk on the dark-colored tiles of the floor. He is afraid of the light-colored tiles.

predicting the presentation of food. This type of association is called *autoshaping*. It can affect the behavior of an animal by changing the response to a conditioned cue in unexpected ways. Autoshaping may be the learning that causes instinctual drift when using operant conditioning in animals (Barker, 2001). Automaintenance is seen when the behavior learned during autoshaping continues despite an apparent lack of reinforcer. In reality, the autoshaped behavior is reinforced through unconditioned and conditioned reinforcers (Barker, 2001).

Animals can learn superstitious behaviors by making associations between stimuli. For example, retired racing Greyhounds are unaccustomed to walking on slick tile floors. The floors at the college where I work have dark-colored tiles along the walls and light-colored tiles in the middle of the floor. When the Greyhounds first come to the building, they walk very close to the walls because they are not confident about walking on the slippery floors. Over time they learn to habituate to walking on the tile flooring, but they also associate the dark-colored tiles close to the wall with safe walking. Thus they learn to walk only on the dark-colored tiles avoiding the light-colored ones (Figure 6.6).

Behavior modification using classical conditioning

Behavior can be modified by changing the associations learned through classical conditioning (Box 6.6). One type of classical conditioning behavior modification technique is called *classical counter conditioning*, whereby the association is changed by changing the US that

Figure 6.7 A Greyhound, Buck, showing signs of learning through classical counter conditioning that the light-colored tiles are fun to walk on.

is being associated with the CS. This will change the conditioned response (Figure 6.7).

BOX 6.6: BEHAVIOR MODIFICATION USING CLASSICAL CONDITIONING.

- Classical extinction
- Classical counter conditioning
- Affective conditioning
- Aversion or avoidance conditioning
- Conditioned taste aversion conditioning

If a dog is afraid of the examination room at a veterinary hospital, they have probably associated some sort of fearful or painful stimulus with their presence in the examination room; otherwise the examination room could be a novel experience that produces fear. Fear can often become generalized and associated with contexts, events, people, and other animals. To change the conditioned response from fear to pleasure, the examination room would need to become associated with something the dog enjoys. This could be play, petting, or a food treat. There must be repeated pairings for the dog to learn the new association (examination room = food treat = happy dog; Table 6.6). The CR does not have to be an emotion. It could be a secretion or a reflex. It is possible to counter condition a blink response or salivation. Amazingly, it is also possible to condition immune suppression and a healthy immune response (Ader and Cohen, 1982 – immunosuppression; Ader and Cohen, 1993 – immune enhancement).

Table 6.6 Classical counter conditioning schematic.

Dog enters examination room (CS)	Nails are quicked (US)	Feels pain and fear (UR)
Dog enters examination room (CS)	Feels fear (CR)	
Dog enters examination room (CS)	Receives treat (new US)	Feels happy and relaxed (new UR)
Dog enters examination room (CS)	Feels happy and relaxed (new CR)	

Although the dog is probably changing its voluntary behaviors at the same time as changing its CR, these voluntary behaviors are not being classically conditioned. They are conditioned through operant conditioning. Operant and classical conditioning are often seen in tandem.

In the aforementioned example, the dog is learning through classical conditioning to be happy in the examination room, but he may also learn to sit instead of pacing. The sitting or pacing behaviors are learned through operant conditioning and are being reinforced by some actions of the owner and/or the veterinary professionals in the room.

CRs can also be changed by removing the association between the CS and the US. Thus, when the CS occurs, the US will no longer follow. This technique uses classical extinction. Extinction within classical conditioning removes the link between the two associated stimuli, which then changes the CR. If the CS no longer predicts the occurrence of the US, then the CR will no longer occur.

If a cat is fed using a can opener, they will learn to associate the sound the can opener makes with obtaining a canned food meal, causing them to be happy. When the can opener no longer opens cans of cat food, the cat then habituates to the sound. They learn the sound no longer predicts they will be fed a canned food meal. Their response changes from happiness to nothing. As with operant extinction, the behavior may go through an extinction burst becoming more variable and intense. The animal may become frustrated and stressed while learning the new paradigm.

Besides learning that one stimulus predicts another, animals can learn that a stimulus means something good or bad for them through classical conditioning. We can manipulate this type of emotional learning by using affective conditioning. To modify an animal's feelings about a stimulus, associations need to be made between the stimulus and something the animal already likes or dislikes. A cat could learn to like getting into her carrier if the cat associated the carrier with other things she likes, such as canned food. Affective conditioning is a type of classical conditioning in which emotions are associated with contexts, objects, or individuals. This technique can be used to create a positive association between an animal and a new baby. The presence of the baby is associated with things the animal likes, whereby the baby consequently elicits a positive emotional response from the animal.

While affective conditioning is a broader type of classical conditioning having to do with the animal's emotions, aversive or avoidance conditioning specifically teaches an animal to avoid a stimulus by making an association between the stimulus and something the animal fears or dislikes. Spray collars triggered by the close proximity of a target use this technique to teach dogs an association between being near an object with a spray in their face. This causes a dog to associate being near that object with being sprayed, thus teaching them the object is bad or to avoid that object. Conditioning of this type can be used to teach a dog to avoid the proximity to a cat's litter box or the garbage can.

Conditioned taste aversion

Classical conditioning contains quite a few specific scenarios for learning, but conditioned taste aversion is so special it has its own category. Taste aversion differs from classical conditioning in that it does not require the two stimuli to be timed closely together. There can be hours separating them. In addition, during taste aversion, the learning can occur even if the animal is not conscious. An animal must experience nausea after eating a substance for taste aversion to occur (Rozin and Kalat, 1971). Taste, color, and odor are all stimuli that can be used by the animal to predict what will happen after they eat a substance. It does not even matter if the nausea is caused by the substance consumed by the animal. The substance could be inert. But if the animal is nauseous because of an illness and they consume a substance, taste aversion can occur. Novel substances are even more likely to be associated with the nausea than recognized substances.

Cats with kidney failure are likely cases for taste aversion because of their medical condition causing nausea. If they are fed a novel diet while experiencing nausea, they will not find that diet palatable because of taste aversion conditioning (Kirk *et al.*, 2000). The cat associates the food with feeling ill.

Augmentation of taste aversion is seen when an animal first learns to avoid a substance through one sensory modality, such as taste, then is presented with that modality (taste) along with another (odor). This second association is even stronger than the first. Augmentation is seen when another stimulus becomes a reliable cue for conditioned taste aversion, strengthening the response through a synergistic effect (Batsell and Batson, 1999). Through augmentation, an animal can learn a stronger response to a CS.

Behavior modification using taste aversion conditioning

Taste aversion conditioning can be used as an effective behavior modification method for weakening predatory behavior in animals (Gustavson *et al.*, 1982 – in coyotes). If an animal learns to associate eating a specific type of animal with nausea, they will stop eating them. Animals can be made to feel nausea and will vomit with the use of apomorphine or lithium chloride. This method can be extremely effective, as it uses classical conditioning that is very powerful.

For taste aversion to work well, the animal must not notice any difference in taste or odor between the treated and the untreated meat. If a predator can assess which meat is treated, they will eat the untreated meat. They will learn an aversion to the emetic not the meat. In addition, the treated meat must be associated with the live animal in the mind of the predator. If this is not the case, the predator will learn not to eat the meat but will still kill and eat the live animal. Evidence for this was found in a study in which penned coyotes were conditioned through taste aversion to avoid laced mutton, but not live sheep (Burns and Connolly, 1980). A similar result was found in huskies in which they became avoidant of the meat, but not the live animal; they also exhibited an increase in interdog aggression when lithium chloride was used to produce taste aversion (Hansen *et al.*, 1997). Another study using 10 adult domestic dogs showed that dogs did form a taste aversion to ground meat from a specific animal (sheep, rabbit, or beef), but this aversion only lasted 24 h (Rathore, 1984).

Social learning

Social learning (Box 6.7) is defined as a type of learning using information received by watching another knowledgeable individual or group (Kubinyi *et al.*, 2009). For evidence of learning to occur, the animal must then produce the learned behavior while no longer in the presence of the individual they watched (Kubinyi *et al.*, 2009). The animal watches another animal's behavior, then they also watch what happens as a consequence of performing the behavior. If an animal performs a behavior and they are reinforced, the watching animal may want to perform the behavior as well. If instead the consequence of the behavior is punishment, the watching animal may learn they do not want to perform that behavior. Social learning should not be confused with social facilitation or social influence, which is a tendency for groups of animals to behave in a similar manner when together (Scott and McCray, 1967). During this phenomenon, no operant learning is occurring in terms of the shared behavior. Of course, there will be classical conditioning going on between the emotional response created by the shared behavior and the accompanying animals.

Mechanisms used to measure social learning include focusing attention on a stimulus, focusing attention on a problem that can be solved, and how the problem can be solved (Kubinyi *et al.*, 2009). When a person or another animal spends time near an object or in a particular place, other animals may also want to spend time there. In this situation, the animals are calling attention to an object or location by proximity. At another level, a person or animal may show through their actions that there is something hidden in a location that can be obtained. This can be shown by the person or animal trying to obtain an object from a location. An animal watching these activities may come to the conclusion that there is an advantage in performing similar actions to obtain a hidden object. The final mechanism used to measure social learning is one in which an animal observes how to solve the problem by watching another animal or person solve it. These mechanisms and the terms describing different forms of social learning are still being defined (Kubinyi *et al.*, 2009), as this is a growing area of interest in behavioral research.

Play is also a form of social learning in animals. Much communication and information about the physical ability of conspecifics are learned by the participants. Playful animals are less aggressive, and groups of animals that play together spend more time together (Beckoff, 1974). Play enhances the ability of animals to learn from each other socially by increasing the time spent together and by making the participants familiar with each other's signals.

Reader (2003), while writing about innovation in primates and bird species, noted social species that were "generalists or opportunists" were likely to exhibit innovation as well as social learning (p. 155). Dogs are generalists and opportunists. They show evidence of social learning from conspecifics as well as from humans, and they often live in groups. The use of animal culture as a way to learn new behaviors is an advantage of living in a group. It is an evidence for behavioral flexibility and cognition in domestic species. Evidence of social learning is seen in both dogs and cats; they found food equally well using a human pointing gesture for orientation (Miklósi *et al.*, 2005) (Figure 6.8).

Behavior modification using social learning

Modeling is a technique of behavior modification in which one animal watches another animal or a human perform a behavior, which helps them to learn how to perform that behavior faster and better (Box 6.8). Evidence of this is found in the study by Slabbert and Rasa (1997) using drug sniffing German shepherd dogs. The dogs were split into four groups: one that stayed with their mothers until 6 weeks of age and the other that stayed with their mothers until 3 months of age. Puppies from each of these groups were further divided according to whether they had trained or untrained narcotic sniffing mothers.

The four groups consist of

1. puppies with mother until 6 weeks and mothers were trained narcotic detection dogs;
2. puppies with mother until 3 months and mothers were trained narcotic detection dogs;

Figure 6.8 Trixie looking where Jeanne Rowe is pointing. This shows dogs look in the direction where humans are pointing.

3. puppies with mother until 6 weeks, untrained mother;
4. puppies with mother until 3 months, untrained mother.

Puppies that stayed until three months with trained mother dogs learned the task of finding narcotics significantly faster than puppies that were either removed at six weeks or stayed with untrained mother dogs. This illustrates that modeling behaviors can reduce training time in dogs.

BOX 6.8: BEHAVIOR MODIFICATION TECHNIQUES USING SOCIAL LEARNING.

• Modeling

Similar evidence was found using humans as the model for the wanted behavior in the studies by Pongrácz *et al.*, (2001). Using a detour task and a desired item, the dogs involved in the study had to learn how to obtain the item by going around the fence shaped in a "V." After viewing a person obtaining the item by walking around the fence, the dogs were easily able to do so themselves.

Gent (2006) found an effect of social familiarity on observational learning in her study using 60 shelter dogs. The dogs learned tasks significantly faster if they were shown how to perform them by familiar people or dogs than if shown by unfamiliar people, unfamiliar dogs, or if they were taught through operant conditioning methods.

Conclusion

Learning is complex. There are many variables that affect the ways in which an animal learns. Their genetic code and their environment will affect how and what they learn.

Animals can learn using nonassociative learning such as habituation and sensitization as well as through associative learning such as operant and classical conditioning and social learning.

Behavior can be modified using a variety of behavior modification techniques. Generally, counter conditioning of operant or classically conditioned behaviors involves changing the consequences or associations between different learning factors. Extinction involves the removal of reinforcement for operant behaviors and of the US for classically conditioned behaviors.

Social learning has recently seen more interest in the animal behavior domain. Animals are now acknowledged to have emotions and perhaps even a rudimentary theory of mind. This allows them to learn through watching others and may even allow them to understand what another animal is thinking or feeling.

A good foundation in how animals learn is vital to working successfully with animals. Animals can be taught to be participants in their medical diagnostics and treatments instead of being forced into them. Learning about how animals learn can foster empathy for them. If you believe an animal is being stubborn, then force seems justified. While if you know the animal is afraid, a plan can be formed to attempt to change the fear to another emotion in order to facilitate humane medical care. Understanding why animals perform certain behaviors can help people work with the animals through the use of learning or behavior modification techniques. Understanding these techniques can help technicians in all aspects of their work with animals throughout their careers.

• A good foundation in how animals learn is vital to working successfully with animals.

References

Ader, R. and Cohen, N. (1982) Behaviorally conditioned immunosuppression and murine systemic lupus erythematosus. *Science*, **214**, 1534–1536.

Ader, R. and Cohen, N. (1993) Psychoneuroimmunology: conditioning and stress. *Annual Review of Psychology*, **44**, 53–85.

Ainsworth, M.D. (1979) Infant–mother attachment. *American Psychologist*, **34** (10), 932–937.

American Veterinary Society of Animal Behavior 2007. The Use of Punishment for Behavior Modification in Animals, http://www.avsabonline.org/avsabonline/images/stories/Position_Statements/Combined_Punishment_Statements.pdf (accessed 25 January 2009).

Barker, L.M. (2001) *Learning and Behavior: Biological, Psychological, and Sociocultural Perspectives*, 3rd edn, Prentice Hall, Upper Saddle River, NJ.

Barry, K.J. and Crowell-Davis, S.L. (1999) Gender differences in the social behavior of neutered indoor only domestic cat. *Applied Animal Behaviour Sciences*, **64**, 193–211.

Batsell, W.R. and Batson, J.D. (1999) Augmentation of taste conditioning by a preconditioned odor. *Journal of Experimental Psychology: Animal Behavior Processes*, **25** (3), 374–388.

Bauer, J.E. (2006) Facilitative and functional fats in diets of cats and dogs. *Journal of the American Veterinary Medical Association*, **229** (5), 680–684.

Beach, F.A., Buehler, M.G. and Dunbar, I.F. (1982) Competitive behavior in male, female, and pseudohemaphiditic female dogs. *Journal of Comparative and Physiological Psychology*, **96** (6), 855–874.

Beckoff, M. (1974) Social play and play-soliciting in infant canids. *American Zoologist*, **14**, 323–340.

Belyaev, D.K. (1979) Destabilizing selection as a factor in domestication. *Journal of Heredity*, **70** (5), 301–307.

Bennett, E.L., Diamond, M.C., Krech, D. and Rosenzweig, M.R. (1964) Chemical and anatomical plasticity of brain: changes in brain through experience, demanded by learning theories, are found in experiments in rats. *Science*, **146** (October), 610–619.

Blake, D.T., Strata, F., Churchland, A.K. and Merzenich, M. (2002) Neural correlates of instrumental learning in primary auditory cortexes. *Proceedings of the National Academy of Sciences*, **99** (15), 10114–10119.

Boissy, A. (1998) Fear and fearfulness in determining behavior, in *Genetics and the Behavior of Domestic Animals*, Academic Press, San Diego, CA, pp. 67–111.

Boitani, L., Francisci, F., Ciucci, P. and Andreoli, G. (1995) Population biology and ecology of feral dogs in central Italy, in *The Domestic Dog: Its Evolution, Behaviour and Interactions with People*, Cambridge University Press, Cambridge, pp. 217–244.

Bourassa, C.M. and Weiden, T.D. (1985) Orienting response and detection of thalamic stimulation: mechanism of perceptual learning in the cat. *Behavioral Neuroscience*, **99** (2), 381–384.

Breland, K. and Breland, M. (1961) The misbehavior of organisms. *American Psychologist*, **16**, 681–684.

Brown, P.L. and Jenkins, H.M. (1968) Auto-shaping of the pigeon's key-peck. *Journal of the Experimental Analysis of Behavior*, **11**, 1–8.

Burns, R.J. and Connolly, G.E. (1980) Lithium chloride bait aversion did not influence prey killing by coyotes, in *Proceedings of the 19th Vertebrate Pest Conference*, DigitalCommons@University of Nebraska, Lincoln, pp. 200–204.

Caulfield, R. (2000) Beneficial effects of tactile stimulation on early development. *Early Childhood Education Journal*, **27** (4), 255–257.

Cheney, D.L. and Seyfarth, R.M. (1992) Dogs that don't bark in the night: how to investigate the lack of a domain of experience? *Proceedings of the Biennial Meeting of the Philosophy of Science Association*, **1992** (2), 92–109.

Cook, M. and Mineka, S. (1990) Selective associations in the observational conditioning of fear in rhesus monkeys. *Journal of Experimental Psychology: Animal Behavioural Processes*, **16** (4), 372–389.

Coppinger, R. and Coppinger, L. (1996) Biologic bases of behavior of domestic dog breeds, in *Readings in companion animal behavior*, Veterinary Learning Systems, Trenton, NJ, pp. 9–18.

Coppinger, R. and Coppinger, L. (1998) Differences in the behavior of dog breeds, in *Genetics and the behavior of domestic animals*, Academic Press, San Diego, CA, pp. 167–202.

Coppinger, R. and Coppinger, L. (2001) *Dogs: A New Understanding of Canine Origin, Behavior, and Evolution*, University of Chicago Press, Chicago.

Cravioto, J. and DeLicarie, E. (1975) Environmental and learning deprivation in children with learning disabilities, in *Perceptual and Learning Disabilities in Children* Vol. 2, Syracuse University Press, Syracuse, New York, pp. 3–102.

Crowell-Davis, S.L., Curtis, T.M. and Knowles, R.J. (2004) Social organization in the cat: a modern understanding. *Journal of Feline Medicine and Surgery*, **6**, 19–28.

D'Andrea, I., Alleva, E. and Branchi, I. (2007) Communal nesting, an early social enrichment, affects social competencies not learning and memory abilities at adulthood. *Behavioral Brain Research*, **123**, 60–66.

Darwin, C. (1859/2004) *On the Origin of Species*, Barnes & Noble, New York Originally published in 1859.

Debner, J.A. and Jacoby, L.L. (1994) Unconscious perception: attention, awareness, and control. *Journal of Experimental Psychology: Learning, Memory, and Cognition*, **20** (2), 304–317.

Ducos, P. (1978) Domestication defined and methodological approaches to its recognition in the faunal assemblages, in *Approaches to Faunal Analysis in the Middle East*, Peabody Museum Bulletin 2, Peabody Museum of Archaeology and Ethnology, Harvard University Publications Department, Cambridge, MA, pp. 53–56.

Estep, D.Q. (1996) The ontogeny of behavior, in *Readings in Companion Animal Behavior*, Veterinary Learning Systems, Trenton, New Jersey, pp. 19–31.

Ferster, C.B. and Skinner, B.F. (1957) *Schedules of reinforcement*, Appleton-Century-Crofts, New York.

Fox, M.W. (1970) Neurobehavioral development and the genotype-environment interaction. *The Quarterly Review of Biology*, **45** (2), 131–147.

Fukuzawa, M., Mills, D.S. and Cooper, J.J. (2005) More than just a word: non-semantic command variables affect obedience in the domestic dog (*Canis familiaris*). *Applied Animal Behaviour Science*, **91**, 129–141.

Fuller, J.L. and Clark, L.D. (1966) Genetic and treatment factors modifying the post-isolation syndrome in dogs. *Journal of Comparative and Physiological Psychology*, **61** (2), 251–257.

Garcia, J., Kimeldorf, D.J. and Koelling, R.A. (1955) Conditioned aversion to saccharin resulting from exposure to gamma radiation. *Science*, **122**, 157–158.

Gent, L.M. 2006 Social familiarity as a predictor of observational learning in the domestic dog (*Canis familiaris*). Unpublished doctoral dissertation, University of Texas at Arlington.

Gibson, J.J. (1958) Visually controlled locomotion and visual orientation in animals. *General Psychology*, **49** (3), 182–194.

Goldstone, R.L. (1998) Perceptual learning. *Annual Reviews in Psychology*, **49**, 585–612.

Goodwin, D., Bradshaw, J.W.S. and Wickens, S.M. (1997) Paedomorphosis affects agonistic visual signals in domestic dogs. *Animal Behaviour*, **53** (2), 297–304.

Grandin, T. and Deesing, M.J. (1998) Behavioral genetics and animal science, in *Genetics and the Behavior of Domestic Animals*, Academic Press, San Diego, CA, pp. 1–30.

Gustavson, C.R., Jowsey, J.R. and Milligan, D.N. (1982) A 3-year evaluation of taste aversion control in Saskatchewan. *Journal of Range Management*, **35** (1), 57–59.

Hall, C.S. (1941) Temperament: a survey of animal studies. *Psychological Bulletin*, **38** (10), 909–943.

Hansen, I., Bakken, M. and Braastad, B.O. (1997) Failure of LiCl-conditioned taste aversion to prevent dogs from attacking sheep. *Applied Animal Behaviour Science*, **54**, 251–256.

Hare, B., Brown, M., Williamson, C. and Tomasello, M. (2002) The domestication of social cognition in dogs. *Science*, **298** (5598), 1634–1637.

Hart, B.L. (1995) Analysing breed and gender differences in behavior, in *The Domestic Dog: Its Evolution, Behaviour and Interactions with People*, Cambridge University Press, Cambridge, pp. 66–77.

Hellemans, K.G.C., Benge, L.C. and Olmstead, M.C. (2004) Adolescent enrichment partially reverses the social isolation syndrome. *Developmental Brain Research*, **150**, 103–115.

Hemmer, H. (1990) *Domestication: The Decline of Environmental Appreciation*, Cambridge University Press, Cambridge.

Horrocks, L.A. and Yeo, Y.K. (1999) Health benefits of docosahexaenoic acid (DHA). *Pharmacological Research*, **40** (3), 211–225.

Hull, C.L. (1943) *Principles of Behavior*, Appleton, New York.

Iso, H., Simoda, S. and Matsuyama, T. (2007) Environmental change during postnatal development alters behaviour, cognition, and neurogenesis of mice. *Behavioural Brain Research*, **179**, 90–98.

Karsh, E.B. (1983) The effects of early handling on the development of social bonds between cats and people, in *New Prospective on our Lives with Companion Animals* (eds A.H. Katcher and A.M. Beck), University of Pennsylvania Press, Philadelphia, pp. 22–28.

Kirk, C.A., Debraekeleer, J. and Jane, A.P. (2000) Normal cats, in *Small Animal Clinical Nutrition*, 4th edn, Mark Morris Institute, Marceline, Missouri, pp. 291–320.

Krushinskii, L.V. (1960) *Animal Behavior: Its Normal and Abnormal Development. The International Behavioral Sciences Series*, Consultants Bureau, New York.

Kubinyi, E., Pongrácz, P. and Miklósi, Á. (2009) Dog as a model for studying conspecifics and heterospecific social learning. *Journal of Veterinary Behavior: Clinical Applications and Research*, **4** (1), 31–41.

Lerman, D.C., Iwata, B.A., Shore, B.A. and Kahng, S.W. (1996) Responding maintained by intermittent reinforcement: implications for the use of extinction in clinical settings. *Journal of Applied Behavior Analysis*, **29**, 153–171.

Li, K.Z.H. and Lindenberger, U. (2003) Relations between aging sensory/sensorimotor and cognitive functions. *Neuroscience and Biobehavioral Reviews*, **26**, 777–783.

Lorenz, K. (1965) *Evolution and modification of behavior*, University of Chicago Press, Chicago.

Macdonald, D.W. and Carr, G.M. (1995) Variation in dog society: between resource dispersion and social flux, in *The Domestic Dog: Its Evolution, Behaviour and Interactions with People*, Cambridge University Press, Cambridge, pp. 199–216.

Mason, G., Clubb, R., Latham, N. and Vickery, S. (2007) Why and how should we use environmental enrichment to tackle stereotypic behaviour? *Applied Animal Behaviour Science*, **102**, 163–188.

McCune, S. (1995) The impact of paternity and early socialization on the development of cat's behaviour to people and novel objects. *Applied Animal Behaviour Science*, **45**, 109–124.

Melzak, R. and Scott, T.H. (1957) The effect of early experience on response to pain. *Journal of Comparative and Physiological Psychology*, **50** (2), 155–161.

Michaels, C.F. and Carello, C. (1981) *Direct Perception*, Prentice Hall, Englewood Cliffs, NJ.

Miklósi, Á., Kubinyi, E., Topál, J. *et al.* (2003) A simple reason for a big difference: wolves do not look back at humans, but dogs do. *Current Biology*, **13**, 763–766.

Miklósi, Á., Pongrácz, P., Lakatos, G. *et al.* (2005) A comparative study of the use of visual communicative signals in interactions between dogs (*Canis familiaris*) and humans and cats (*Felis catus*) and humans. *Journal of Comparative Psychology*, **119** (2), 179–186.

Miller, P.E. 2001 Vision in Animals: What do Dogs and Cats See? Proceedings of the 25th Annual Waltham/OSU Symposium http://www.vin.com/VINDBPub/SearchPB/Proceedings/PR05000/PR00515.htm (accessed 3 March).

Morton, J.R.C. (1968) Effects of early experience "handling and gentling" in laboratory animals, in *Abnormal Behavior in Animals* (Chapter 17) (ed M.W. Fox), MB Sanders, Philadelphia, pp. 261–292.

National Human Genome Research Institute (NHGRI) n.d Allele. Talking glossary. http://www.genome.gov/glossary.cfm?key=allele (accessed 31 January 2009).

Overall, K.L. (1997) *Clinical Behavioral Medicine for Small Animals*, Mosby, St Louis, MO.

Overall, K.L. (2009) Canine behavior: a new synthesis of canine humane care, , North American Veterinary Conference, Proceedings of the, pp. 155–159.

Overall, K.L. and Arnold, S.E. (2007) Olfactory neuron biopsies in dogs: a feasibility pilot study. *Applied Animal Behaviour Science*, **105**, 351–357.

Overmier, J.B. and Seligman, M.E.P. (1967) Effects of inescapable shock upon subsequent escape and avoidance responding. *Journal of Comparative and Physiological Psychology*, **63** (1), 28–33.

Pongrácz, P., Miklósi, Á., Kubinyi, E. *et al.* (2001) Social learning in dogs: the effect of a human demonstrator on the performance of dogs in a detour task. *Animal Behaviour*, **62** (6), 1109–1117.

Pongrácz, P., Miklósi, Á., Vida, V. and Csányi, V. (2005) The pet dogs' ability for learning from a human demonstrator in a detour task is independent from the breed and age. *Animal Behaviour Science*, **90**, 309–323.

Pongrácz, P., Vida, V., Bánhegyi, P., & Miklósi A. (2008) How does dominance rank status affect individual and social learning performance in the dog (*Canis familiaris*)? *Animal Cognition*, **11**, 75–82.

Pongrácz, P., Vida, V., Bánhegyi, P. and Miklósi, Á. (2009) How does dominance rank status affect individual and social learning performances in the dog (*Canis familiaris*)? *Animal Cognition*, **11**, 75–82.

Poppen, R. (1988) *Behavioral Relaxation Training and Assessment*, Penguin, New York.

Premack, D. (1962) Reversibility of reinforcement relation. *Science*, **136** (3512), 255–257.

Price, E.O. (1998) Behavioral genetics and the process of animal domestication, in *Genetics and the Behavior of Domestic Animals*, Academic Press, San Diego, CA, pp. 31–65.

Price, E.O. (1999) Behavioral development in animals undergoing domestication. *Applied Animal Behaviour Science*, **65**, 245–271.

Rathore, A.K. (1984) Evaluation of lithium chloride taste aversion in penned domestic dogs. *Journal of Wildlife Management*, **48** (4), 1424.

Reader, S.M. (2003) Innovation and social learning: individual variation and brain evolution. *Animal Biology*, **53** (2), 147–158.

Rozin, P. and Kalat, J.W. (1971) Specific hungers and poison avoidance as adaptive specializations of learning. *Psychological Review*, **78** (6), 459–486.

Schilder, M.B.H. and van der Borg, J.A.M. (2004) Training dogs with help of the shock collar: short and long term behavioural effects. *Applied Animal Behavioural Science*, **85**, 319–334.

Scott, J.P. and Fuller, J.L. (1965) *Genetics and the Social Behavior of the Dog*, University of Chicago Press, Chicago.

Scott, J.P. and McCray, C. (1967) Allelomimetic behavior in dogs: negative effects of competition on social facilitation. *Journal of Comparative Physiological Psychology*, **63** (2), 316–319.

Seligman, M.E.P. (1970) On the generality of the laws of learning. *Psychological Review*, **77** (5), 406–418.

Seligman, M.E.P. (1971) Phobias and preparedness. *Behavior Therapy*, **2**, 307–321.

Seligman, M.E.P. (1972) Learned helplessness. *Annual Review of Medicine*, **23**, 407–412.

Serpell, J.A. and Hsu, Y. (2001) Development and validation of a novel method for evaluating behavior and temperament in guide dogs. *Applied Animal Behaviour Science*, **72**, 347–364.

Serpell, J.A. and Hsu, Y. (2005) Effects of age, breed and neuter status on trainability in dogs. *Anthrozoös*, **18**, 196–207.

Seyfarth, R.M., Cheney, D.L. and Marler, P. (1980) Monkey responses to three different alarm calls: evidence of predator classification and semantic communication. *Science*, **210** (4417), 801–803.

Skinner, B.F. (1966) *The Behavior of Organisms*, Appleton-Century-Crofts, New York Originally published in 1938.

Slabbert, J.M. and Rasa, O.A.E. (1997) Observational learning of an acquired maternal behaviour pattern by working dog pups: an alternative training method? *Applied Animal Behaviour Science*, **53**, 309–316.

Suomi, S.J. (1997) Early determinants of behavior: evidence from primate studies. *British Medical Bulletin*, **53** (1), 170–184.

Thorne, C. (1995) Feeding behavior of domestic dogs and the role of experience, in *The Domestic Dog: Its Evolution, Behaviour and Interactions With People*, Cambridge University Press, Cambridge, pp. 104–114.

Tolman, E.C. and Honzik, C.H. (1930) Insight in rats. *University of California Publications in Psychology*, **4**, 215–232.

Topál, J., Miklósi, Á. and Csányi, V. (1997) Dog-human relationship affects problem solving behavior in dogs. *Anthrozoös*, **10** (4), 214–224.

Topál, J., Miklósi, Á., Csányi, V. and Dóka, A. (1998) Attachment behavior in dogs (*Canis familiaris*): a new application of Ainsworth's (1969) strange situation test. *Journal of Comparative Psychology*, **112** (3), 219–229.

Topál, J., Gácsi, M., Miklósi, Á. *et al.* (2005) Attachment to humans: a comparative study of hand-reared wolves and differentially socialized dog puppies. *Animal Behaviour*, **70** (6), 1367–1375.

Trut, L.N. (1999) Early canid domestication: the fox farm experiment. *American Scientist*, **87** (March–April), 160–169.

van Oers, H.J.J., de Kloet, E.R., Whelan, T. and Levine, S. (1998) Maternal deprivation effect on the infant's neural stress markers is reversed by tactile stimulation but not by suppressing corticosterone. *Journal of Neuroscience*, **18** (23), 10171–10179.

CHAPTER 6

Virányi, Z., Topál, J., Gácsi, M. *et al.* (2004) Dogs respond appropriately to cues of humans' attentional focus. *Behavioural Processes*, **66**, 161–172.

Weiss, S.J., Wilson, P. and Morrison, D. (2004) Maternal tactile stimulation and the neurodevelopment of low birth weight infants. *Infancy*, **5** (1), 85–107.

Wells, D.L. and Hepper, P.G. (1999) Male and female dogs respond differently to men and women. *Applied Animal Behaviour*, **61** (4), 341–349.

Wells, D.L. and Hepper, P.G. (2006) Prenatal olfactory learning in the domestic dog. *Animal Behaviour*, **72** (3), 681–686.

Wiggins, R.C. and Fuller, G.M. (1978) Early post natal starvation causes lasting brain hypomyelination. *Journal of Neurochemistry*, **30**, 1231–1237.

Williams, R.W., Cavada, C. and Reinoso-Suárez, F. (1993) Rapid evolution of the visual system: a cellular assay of the retina and dorsal lateral geniculate nucleus of the Spanish wild cat and the domestic cat. *Journal of Neuroscience*, **13** (1), 208–228.

Zhang, L.-X., Levine, S., Dent, G. *et al.* (2002) Maternal deprivation increases cell death in the infant rat brain. *Developmental Brain Research*, **133** (1), 1–11.

7 Problem prevention

Debbie Martin[1,2], Linda M. Campbell[3], and Marcia R. Ritchie[4]

[1] TEAM Education in Animal Behavior, LLC, Spicewood, TX, USA
[2] Veterinary Behavior Consultations, LLC, Spicewood, TX, USA
[3] Humane Society of Missouri, St. Louis, MO, USA
[4] The Family Companion, Springville, NY, USA

CHAPTER MENU

Canine and Feline Behavior for Veterinary Technicians and Nurses, First Edition. Edited by Julie K. Shaw and Debbie Martin.
© 2015 John Wiley & Sons, Inc. Published 2015 by John Wiley & Sons, Inc.
Companion Website: www.wiley.com/go/shaw/behavior

Introduction

Benjamin Franklin's adage "An ounce of prevention is worth a pound of cure" is especially appropriate when applied to pets. It is much less work for owners to practice prevention than to correct a problem that has become established. Although this fact alone should make the topic of problem prevention a high priority for anyone working with pets and owners, there are additional benefits to be achieved.

Each year, thousands of dogs and cats are given up by their owners. The majority of these animals are not bad pets but rather victims of unanticipated circumstances or misinformed owners. Reasons cited for relinquishment can often be traced back to poor choices during the pet-selection process, unrealistic owner expectations, and lack of adequate training for the pet. Whatever the cause, the result for many of these animals culminates in the relinquishment of the pet. Programs that focus on prevention, early intervention, and education for owners have the potential to help many of these animals remain in their homes.

The medical community has long recognized the benefits of pet ownership to people. It is an accepted fact that pets enrich lives, improve physical health and offer emotional encouragement to those around them. Studies have demonstrated that the cognitive development of children can be enhanced through pet ownership (Poresky and Hendrix, 1990), as well as a child's level of positive self-esteem (Bergesen, 1989). Pet owners also tend to be less fearful of becoming crime victims when walking with or sharing their residence with a dog (Serpell, 1991).

In a September 1998 presentation at the 8th International Conference on Human–Animal Interactions, P. Raina, PhD, B. Bonnett, PhD, and D. Waltner-Toews, PhD, cited a research project they conducted within a population of senior citizens living in Canada. Results from this study provided evidence that pet ownership serves as an important coping mechanism. This in turn allows the senior owners to deal with stressful life events without the need for healthcare assistance.

The benefits cited above support the importance of a strong bond between owners and their pets. However, this bond cannot develop and grow without ongoing opportunities for positive interactions between pet and owner. Providing education, counseling, and support to owners through all stages of the relationship is one way to ensure that a positive connection between pet and owner continues, thus strengthening the human–animal bond.

Besides the obvious initial financial benefits to clinics, individuals, and businesses that offer training classes and prepurchase services (pet selection counseling), there are additional, often overlooked, advantages. Satisfied owners share information with friends and family. For veterinary practices, this provides a unique opportunity to gain recognition in the community as experts in the care of the total animal. Counseling and animal behavior services can also help create a relationship of trust between the practice and owners spanning the lifetime of the pet, making it possible to market other, equally important, services.

Employees interested in advancing their skills and ultimately their value to employers, often find the field of owner education and counseling on pet behavior to be a perfect venue. Pet counseling programs present an excellent outlet for veterinary clinics that want to reward technicians and experienced staff members with continuing opportunities for professional growth and increased responsibility.

An added advantage of working closely with owners and pets is the ability to build a relationship of trust and improved pet behavior that ultimately results in a cooperative patient.

There are a limitless number of services and programs available that can help owners achieve the goal of problem prevention. A review of common prevention services and topics is covered in this chapter. As discussed in Chapter 1, preventive care "refers to measures taken to prevent the development of behavior problems or disorders rather than treating the symptoms of an existing problem or disorder" whereas intervention care refers to measure taken to improve or alter an existing behavior disorder (psychological or behavioral patterns outside the behavioral norms for the species). Intervention requires a veterinary diagnosis and treatment plan. Chapter 8 will address intervention care.

Preventing fear of the veterinary hospital

Many dogs and cats may accept handling and restraint at the veterinary hospital. However, some patients become so frightened that they fear for their lives, often resulting in aggression. Regardless of whether the patient is accepting or fearful, it is necessary to proactively attempt to make the veterinary hospital experience as pleasant as possible for the patients. This does not necessarily involve a large amount of time. The few seconds or minutes taken initially to allow a patient to relax and become comfortable may save the staff hours in the long run (not to mention decrease risk of injury) but may also save the pet's life. Negative experiences in the veterinary hospital can result in long-lasting aggression issues in handling and routine care from the owner or veterinary staff, as well as fear and aggression toward strangers (Yin, 2009).

> • The few seconds or minutes taken initially to allow a patient to relax and become comfortable may save the staff hours in the long run (not to mention decrease risk of injury) but may also save the pet's life.

Prevention techniques to ensure positive experiences in the veterinary hospital

Time should be taken to build a rapport with new patients and their owners. Assuming the patient is in the preventive stages and is not already fearful, anxious, or aggressive with examination in the veterinary hospital, the following techniques should be employed to prevent negative learning experiences.

The hospital's role of producing a pleasant experience for the pet begins as soon as the patient arrives in the parking lot. The landscaping and approach to the building can even be designed to minimize stress for the patient. Through natural barriers such as bushes or flower beds and wide open walkways, the walk to the front door of the hospital can be a nonthreatening experience for the pet. When possible, provide entrances and exits to the building that minimize congestion. Doorways that provide visualization into and out of the building will allow the pet owner to avoid close encounters with other pets. Safe and secure doors that are easy to manipulate and maneuver reduce the risk of an unpleasant and possibly painful experience. A door that springs shut quickly might start the dog's experience at the hospital with a pinched tail or toes. When possible, have a separate entrance and exit for clients and their pets. This will avert accidental encounters at doorways and avoid crowding because it allows for a smooth flow.

Proper management of the waiting room will also help keep things running smoothly and assure the best experience for the pet. Positive interactions can be initiated by the receptionist offering treats to healthy, nonaggressive patients. (Note that although treats would be used to help treat aggression in the veterinary hospital, only specially trained staff should interact with a patient displaying aggression) (Figure 7.1).

Ideally, patients should be moved to a quiet examination room as soon as possible, especially if there is a large amount of activity in the waiting area. Alternatively, providing visual barriers and cornered off seating areas away from the doors will decrease stimuli and allow pet owners to safely manage their pet. An elevated surface for owners to place their cat or small dog carrier prevents these animals being approached on the floor by passing dogs.

Small, readily consumed treats should be provided to the patients as they are either placed on the scale or walked on to the scale. Providing a nonskid surface on the scale and examination table will help to put canine and feline patients at ease (Figure 7.2).

Scheduling additional time for the first appointment allows the pet to acclimatize to the environment, while

Figure 7.1 A puppy receiving a treat and a pat from the receptionist upon arrival at the veterinary hospital.

Figure 7.2 Puppy on the scale with a nonskid surface while receiving several small treats.

veterinarian? Similarly, the client's questions can be thoroughly answered. Providing a quick questionnaire designed for different life stages of development for the pet owner to complete at each visit will assist the veterinary staff in avoiding overlooking vital information. See Appendices 13–18 Puppy, Adult Dog, Senior Dog, Kitten, Adult Cat, and Senior Cat Questionnaires. Not only will the client leave better educated about their pet but they likely will also become more bonded to the practice.

One of the first items addressed during the initial visit is teaching new pets to become comfortable with the type of handling needed to keep them healthy and well groomed throughout their lives. This will also make procedures run smoothly and save staff time by creating a relaxed and cooperative patient in the clinic. The first puppy/kitten appointment is the ideal time to prepare puppies and kittens for physical exams, venipuncture, teeth cleaning, ear cleaning, and pedicures. It is vital that technicians avoid mishandling patients regardless of their age or behavior. The goal always should be to create a positive association with the examination process that can follow the pet through the rest of its life. Rough or forceful handling methods teach fear and mistrust and often result in a difficult-to-handle adult pet. It also sets a poor example for owners to follow and could be considered malpractice.

- The goal always should be to create a positive association with the examination process that can follow the pet through the rest of its life. Rough or forceful handling methods teach fear and mistrust and often result in a difficult-to-handle adult pet.

- It also sets a poor example for owners to follow and could be considered malpractice.

Dogs and cats should be encouraged to lick peanut butter, canned cheese, canned dog/cat food or meat-based baby food from the table while being examined. Frequently, a complete physical exam including examination of ears, eyes, feet, and teeth can be performed while the patient is licking the treat from the table or from a syringe case held by the owner (Figure 7.3). A treat can be placed in the patient's mouth as the teeth are examined. Peanut butter or squeeze cheese can be smeared on the scale to assist with weighing. A patient that is leery of medical instruments such as the stethoscope or otoscope can be allowed to lick a treat from the instrument's surface. Mild restraint, such as a position

the technician provides guidance regarding preventive medical and behavior care. With new adult patients, the technician should inquire regarding previous experiences at the veterinary hospital. How has their pet responded in the past to being examined by the

Figure 7.3 An adult dog licking canned cheese from a 12-cc syringe case.

that mimics drawing a blood sample, can be practiced while the patient is distracted by the treat. The pet is cooperative because it is focused on the treat but at the same time it develops a positive association with mildly uncomfortable handling. An animal that struggles, growls, or even tries to bite during an examination is not displaying "dominance" but is instead frightened or unsure. Rough handling using "domination techniques" (forcing on the side "until it submits" or grabbing the muzzle) or physically or verbally reprimanding it will only increase fear and can be permanently damaging to the pet. Should a patient show any sign of apprehension or fearfulness, specifically, if it stops taking treats, the process should be slowed or decreased until it begins taking treats again. If the patient wiggles or mildly resists the restraint, the technician should not release the pet until the wiggling stops. Otherwise the pet will learn that wiggling makes people let go. The moment the pet relaxes, restraint should be removed and an exceptional treat should be offered. Continue to practice with the pet, avoiding pushing the animal to the point of reactivity. Again, this is only for mild resistance. If the pet is having an extreme reaction, such as urinating, defecating, or expressing anal sacs, or is more than mildly irritated, do not wait for the pet to calm down or give up. Release the pet to minimize the unpleasant experience. Continuing to restrain a panicked animal until he gives up will not teach the pet to enjoy being restrained and is likely to escalate to aggression in future encounters. A pet that has an extreme reaction to restraint or handling indicates the need for a recommendation for intervention behavior services and treatment with desensitization and counter conditioning (see Chapter 8 for intervention behavior modification techniques).

The veterinarian staff can also change their behavior and approach to a pet to prevent the pet from becoming frightened. Direct eye contact or a direct approach is considered a threat, regardless of our intentions. As humans we often smile, look directly at a pet, and walk straight toward them. As discussed in Chapter 2, all of these behaviors signal confrontation. Although many pets have perhaps learned to understand our inappropriate body language toward them, by simply taking a few easy steps we can put our patients at ease. Polite, nonthreatening communication includes the following: approach the pet on a curve; avoid maintaining direct eye contact (look and then look away); allow the pet to approach you initially (its choice); turn sideways or squat down to appear less menacing; toss treats to the pet rather than reaching toward the pet. By incorporating these techniques, you will quickly put many patients immediately at ease. See Chapter 8 for techniques to approach a fearful dog.

- The veterinarian staff can also change their behavior and approach to a pet to prevent the pet from becoming frightened.

Recognizing the subtle signs of fear as detailed in Chapter 2 (Table 2.2 and Table 2.4, and Figure 2.9 Canine communication in a perfect world) and adapting our interaction with the patient to make the experience more pleasant when possible, allow for two-way communication to occur (Table 7.1).

Ideal characteristics for pet owners

To be a successful "canine or feline parent," there are some simple rules to follow. (i) Be fair. Understand the pet's perspective. Pets are amoral, opportunistic, social (especially dogs), constantly learning, and curious and avid chewers! (ii) Be a good teacher. Control what the pet learns through management and supervision. Guide it to make the right decisions. Rather than focus on what you do not want the pet to do, teach the correct behavior. Set the pet up to succeed. (iii) Clearly communicate to the pet when it is performing the correct behavior. Catch it doing things right and reward it for it. A high occurrence of positive reinforcement will help the pet learn quickly. (iv) Be consistent. Inconsistency and unpredictability cause fear and anxiety, which can be a precursor to behavioral problems. Set the rules of

Table 7.1 Techniques to prevent negative experiences in the veterinary hospital.

Parking lot and approach to building	Open space with natural barriers, if possible provide separate entrance and exit
Waiting room	Seating area away from the door, barriers or partitions to minimize visual exposure, elevated surface to place cat or small dog carriers, escort to a room as soon as possible, receptionist provides treats to healthy, nonaggressive patients
Scale	Treats![a] Nonskid surface
Exam room	In cat-only rooms use a Feliway® diffuser and in the dog-only rooms use an Adaptil™ diffuser. Treats should be given when the patient enters the room, on the exam table, and during the physical exam![a] Place a non-slip surface on exam tables or on floors
Nonthreatening body language	Approach the pet on a curve, avoid maintaining direct eye contact (look and then look away), allow the pet to approach you initially (its choice), turn sideways or squat down to appear less menacing, toss treats to the pet rather than reaching toward the pet
Recognize signs of fear and modify interaction when possible	Allows for two-way communication to occur

[a]Treats should be used whenever possible to promote a positive association. However, ill or fasted patients should not be given treats. Incorporate all other techniques.

the house and make interactions predictable and consistent. (v) Advocate for the pet. Dogs and cats cannot speak up for themselves. It is our responsibility to be their advocate. This includes insuring positive learning experiences and avoiding overwhelming the pet.

The importance of consistency is not always well understood. It has been clarified that the relationship between humans and dogs is not one of submission and domination (Bradshaw *et al.*, 2009). However, we have to control the contingencies of the dog's behavior. That means we need to be consistent in regard to which behaviors are reinforced and which are not. The establishment and enforcement of rules is extremely important. If rules are not consistent, the dog can never figure them out, and cannot function within them to achieve success. This situation would be similar to you visiting with friends who play a card game that you do not know. They ask you to participate and explain the rules to you. You go along with it and after some time think you have the winning hand, put your cards down and claim that you have won. Now of course, your friends add another rule. After two or three times of this, you will become frustrated and likely fairly irritated and not want to participate any longer. Frustration can even lead to aggression. This is how our dogs must feel if we have no rules or constantly change them. They may either compensate for this by developing survival behaviors that yield short-term predictable consequences (such as aggression), or develop learned helplessness (i.e., they learn that their behavior has no effect on what happens around them). Deciding on the "rules of the house" and adhering to them has nothing to do with dominance, but with giving the dog

a chance to operate successfully within the environment and achieve predictable outcomes. Predictability is empowering to an animal. In particular, a highly trainable dog, that is, a dog that is keen on operating in his environment, is in a state of compromised welfare if a consistent rule structure is not maintained. The pet owner is the one who defines the rules of the house. What may be acceptable behavior for my dogs in my house may be unacceptable in someone else's house or vice versa.

- Predictability is empowering to an animal.

- In particular, a highly trainable dog, that is, a dog that is keen on operating in his environment, is in a state of compromised welfare if a consistent rule structure is not maintained.

Desirable behavior should be consistently rewarded (once a behavior is well trained, an intermittent reinforcement schedule can be used). Undesirable behavior should be ignored (a behavior that is not rewarded, that is, not successful, will go into extinction). Of course, a behavior that is self-rewarding such as going through the trash or ripping up a kitchen towel does not go into extinction when ignored. Such behavior needs to be prevented by setting up the environment accordingly, or through supervision and redirection to an alternative, appropriate behavior (such as chewing on a chew toy). In the section titled **Problem Solving Normal Species-specific behavior**, you will learn about other alternatives to address problem behaviors in a positive manner but first we will explore prevention and management techniques.

Canine management and prevention techniques

Prevention of problem behaviors is easier than treatment. Many behavior problems and disorders in dogs can be prevented through early appropriate socialization and training.

Understanding dogs and their characteristics

Understanding what motivates the dog, helps us be better at meeting the dog's needs and preventing issues from arising. In The Culture Clash, Jean Donaldson discusses the characteristics of dogs. Table 7.2 *General Characteristics of Dogs* has been modified from The Culture Clash (Donaldson, 1996).

Always keeping these general canine characteristics in mind allows one to have empathy and to understand why dogs do the things they do. It is not because they are spiteful. Often it is because they are dogs. Those same characteristics that we love about them can also make it challenging to share our homes with them.

Table 7.2 General characteristics of dogs.

Dogs are amoral	They do not know right from wrong. They know safe and unsafe. For example, it is safe to get into the trash when people are absent but unsafe when they are present
Dogs are opportunistic and self-centered	It is about what is in it for them
Dogs are social	This is why they make good companions but is also why it is difficult for dogs to be isolated
Dogs are constantly learning from their actions	Learned behaviors may be appropriate or inappropriate for human counterparts. So even when we are not actively training, they are still learning. Evaluate their behavior from a learning perspective
Dogs are curious and avid chewers	Dogs like to investigate things. They explore their world with their mouths and cannot decipher what items came from the pet store versus the home store

Modified from *The Culture Clash* by Jean Donaldson.

Management of the learning history

Managing and controlling what the dog learns is important to prevent the learning of undesirable behaviors. Puppy and dog owners should puppy-proof the house: use baby gates, an exercise pen, and/or a crate to help manage the dog, especially young dogs. The more opportunity the dog has to practice undesirable behavior (in the eyes of the human), the better he will get at it. Habits begin to form. A preference for chewing on chair legs or pillows can develop quickly without good supervision (Figure 7.4).

Problem prevention includes setting the dog up for success, that is, arranging the environment so the dog can only make the desired choices. If the desired behaviors are successful from the beginning, the dog will repeat those behaviors. The environment should be set up in such a way that unwanted behaviors cannot occur or are much more difficult to perform than the desired behaviors. This includes puppy-proofing the house and utilizing appropriate confinement and supervision.

> • Problem prevention includes setting the dog up for success, that is, arranging the environment so the dog can only make the desired choices.

Although kitchens are a common place for confinement, they also hold several potential dangers. Garbage cans should be kept safely locked away with child-proof latches on the door or be tall enough and fashioned with a lid to prevent access. If a dog gains access to the garbage, it is usually rewarded by some food product,

Figure 7.4 Two adolescent Belgian Malinois left unsupervised chewed a therapeutic pillow.

so it will likely return to it throughout its life if not properly managed. Dangers that lurk in garbage cans include spoiled food, sharp bones, peach and cherry pits, and empty snack bags that can cause suffocation. It is also important to keep all household chemicals safely locked away. Even child-proof caps are no match for a dog's sharp teeth.

Bathrooms provide many temptations for the curious canine. A good rule is to keep bathroom doors closed. Toilet bowl cleaning products, especially the cakes that hang on the inside of the bowl, can be attractive to pets but are highly toxic. Waste basket items such as feminine hygiene products and disposable razor blades can cause serious medical problems if ingested. Medications must be kept out of reach.

Electric cords should be securely taped to the wall using electrical tape. If this is not possible, they should be treated daily with an antichew product. Toxic household plants should be noted and removed from any pet-living areas. Both dogs and cats enjoy ingesting some roughage which may include houseplants. Other potential common household toxins include rodenticides, insecticides, and antifreeze.

Owners should also be educated on responsible pet ownership and keeping their pet safely confined to their property or walked on leash off the property. Just as important as puppy proofing the house, the yard will also need to be made safe. Providing clients with a list of potential plant toxins will allow them to evaluate the safety of plants in their yard and house.

Routine

Maintaining a schedule and routine with puppies and adult dogs makes their lives more consistent and predictable. Ideally, all dogs should be meal-fed twice a day (very young or small puppies may require three meals a day initially), walked off the property twice a day for 10–20 min, and trained using positive reinforcement twice a day for 5–10 min.

- Ideally, all dogs should be meal-fed twice a day (very young or small puppies may require three meals a day initially), walked off the property twice a day for 10–20 min, and trained using positive reinforcement twice a day for 5–10 min.

The importance of walking a puppy or a dog is often misunderstood and is one of the most important problem-prevention tools. Exercise off the property will satisfy the dog's innate motivation to explore

new things, help with exposure and desensitization to stimuli, and facilitate socialization. Walks can also decrease arousal, reactivity, and anxiety. A romp around an enclosed area is no substitute for a relationship-building walk with the owner. The same old yard can also get rather boring where the neighborhood environment is ever changing. The walk should be a combination of a controlled training walk by the owner's side and safe exploration. It is helpful to put walking at the owner's side on cue ("Let's go") and also teach a cue to release the dog to go explore ("Go play"). Walking by the owner's side is not a natural behavior for dogs and will take time to develop. A high rate of reinforcement (a yummy treat every few steps) will be necessary in the beginning. For strong pullers, a head collar or front clip harness may be needed for management initially. These products also help protect the dog from trachea damage due to pulling on a collar. Leashed walks in the neighborhood are an activity that should be a lifelong exercise. They can help prevent behavior disorders such as territorial aggression and fearful and anxious behavior.

An established routine to allow for ample social, physical, and mental stimulation will help set dogs up to be successful in the home environment.

Canine environmental enrichment

Dogs whose exercise and social needs are met are better behaved and more enjoyable pets. Many unruly behaviors that clients are concerned about are a result of a pet being under-stimulated. Exercise and play are important for the pet's mental and physical health and social development. Routine walks that allow for "smell" time are just one way to meet these needs. Toys and games are other ways to provide an enriching environment.

Toys

In the home, a variety of toys should be available to the dog and the toys should be rotated, so it appears that there are always "new" toys. Providing appropriate toys will help generate mental and physical stimulation, an important part of early development. Toys are also great tools to intercept and redirect unwanted behaviors.

Food-dispensing toys are designed to act as puzzles. They can be loaded with a variety of treats or the pet's own diet. When physically manipulated using paws, mouth, or muzzle food is dispensed in a variety of ways. Before domestication, animals used a tremendous amount of mental and physical energy to obtain food. Placing food in a bowl provides little if any challenge for the pet. Food-dispensing toys are ideal for redirecting

Figure 7.5 Variety of food-dispensing toys.

unwanted behaviors including mouthing and destructive chewing. It is best for the client to proactively identify potentially problematic times to occupy the pet with these toys. Many of the more durable varieties can also be used to pacify dogs while adapting to the crate or the owner's absence (Figure 7.5).

Toys designed for chewing purposes are also especially important for puppies that are teething. It is natural for young pets to explore using their mouth. Items such as nylon bones, pressed rawhides, and hard rubber toys can help satisfy these needs and prevent destructive behaviors. There are numerous commercially available chew toys. Despite manufacturer claims, no toy is indestructible. Dogs can destroy and ingest a toy very quickly. Hard rubber toys are more resistant to destruction. When offering a dog a new toy, monitor it closely. Instruct owners to check their dog's toys daily for damage. Toys will become damaged or worn over time and will need to be replaced periodically.

Games

The following are examples of games that can be recommended to clients to help facilitate the human–animal bond. The games are also designed to provide the dog with physical and mental exercise and promote the development of foundation skills such as come, sit, impulse control, take it, and drop it.

Retrieving

Retrieving is an excellent way to combine the use of exercise and foundation training skills. It can be used to teach the cues "take it" and "drop it." Similarly, other cues, such as "sit," "down," and "stay," can be incorporated into retrieving sessions to strengthen those behaviors as well as assist with teaching impulse control to help with over-arousal issues. Even the unmotivated dog owners can exercise their dog while relaxing in

a chair. Although some breeds are natural retrievers, most puppies that do not display such tendencies can be taught the behavior.

Biscuit hunt or find it

Dogs need an outlet for exploratory or searching behavior. If we do not provide them with a human-approved outlet for this behavior, they will likely find one that is less acceptable to us (digging in the garden, stealing items off the counters or out of the laundry, etc.). This is a great game for providing mental stimulation.

When first teaching this game, let the dog see you place the treats about the room. "Hide" the treats in dog-allowed locations (on or near the floor in clear sight initially). Potential locations are on the ledge or the foot of a chair leg or table (not on the table). Avoid locations where human food is placed or any location that you would not want the dog to explore. Place 10 treats about the room while someone holds the dog or it is behind a barrier, watching. Give the cue, "Find it" or "Seek" just before letting it go, explore, and find the treats. Let it find them on its own. It will learn to use its nose! Once the dog understands this game, increase the difficulty level by hiding the treats while the dog is out of sight. Always start the game with your cue word or phrase.

As simple as this activity sounds, the owner is providing the dog with an outlet to explore and use its sense of smell. It is great mental stimulation. This is a wonderful activity for children to be involved in with adult supervision.

Hide and seek

This game is an excellent training game and often a favorite among households with children but should always include adults. As one person gently restrains the dog or while the dog is distracted, the other person finds a hiding place. Once hidden, the dog is called and receives a treat when it discovers the person. Meanwhile the other person has hidden and the sequence can be repeated. Make it easy at first, just going around a piece of furniture or around the corner. As the dog becomes more proficient, the game can be made more challenging. Through play, the owner will also be teaching the dog to come when called.

Round robin

Round robin can be played during family television time. When a commercial comes on, family members take turns calling the dog to them, asking for a sit and rewarding the dog with a treat. When the TV show comes back on, a handful of treats can be scattered on

CHAPTER 7

Figure 7.6 Teaching a dog to chase after a toy can provide an appropriate outlet for a dog's natural desire to chase and mouth and be a fun game to play together.

the floor to end the game on a positive note. This is another activity that will reinforce coming when called and also helps generalize the behavior among all family members.

Chase the toy
Many dogs are highly motivated to chase things. This game can help direct that motivation to an appropriate outlet, a toy. There are commercially available toys or you can make your own by tying a rope to a toy (Figure 7.6). Initially the owner should stand still and make only the toy move. Give a cue, such as "take it" or "get it," just before presenting the toy. Pulling the toy in a direction away from the dog will encourage him to chase it. To prevent injury, over-arousal, or frustration, keep the toy near the ground rather than lifting it up out of reach. Once the dog catches the toy, engage him for a few seconds with a few light tugs on the toy. Then cue "drop it," or do an exchange with a food treat. Other known cues can be added into the game, such as "sit" or "down." This can help slow down the arousal level. As the dog becomes proficient at the game and is focused on grabbing the toy rather than mouthing pants legs or people, the owner can start to move around during the game. Any attempt to catch the owner should cause the person to freeze. The dog should be redirected to the toy. This game helps teach the dog to control his arousal level and also builds on foundation skills such as "take it," "drop it," "sit," and "down." Similarly, it teaches the dog appropriate things to chase and mouth.

Dog parks and dog daycares
Dog parks generally are an uncontrolled situation, which lack supervision from professionals trained in canine body language and behavior. Owners should be aware that potential negative experiences with dogs at a dog park can have a lasting negative effect on their dog.

Dog daycare can be an appropriate option for some dogs and for busy owners. It can provide dogs with an outlet for exercise, companionship, and mental stimulation. Before recommending any daycare, the animal behavior technician should observe the facility and talk to the staff. Centers that combine many dogs of all age groups in play sessions should be avoided. A good daycare will offer small closely supervised play groups with a balance of down time for the dogs. They will also have an evaluation process and be selective regarding dogs that are accepted into daycare. The staff should be knowledgeable on dog behavior, especially body language. Interactions between staff members and the dogs should always be positive-reinforcement based. The veterinary technician should ask the staff how conflicts are managed. Facilities that use squirt bottles and shaker cans to manage dog behavior are not the best options.

Dog parks and dog daycare can be enjoyable for some young and well-socialized adolescent dogs. Even with repetitive exposure, although, it is normal for a socially mature dog to become less accepting of unfamiliar dogs. It is important for the owner to ensure that their dog truly enjoys the experience. The dog should be relaxed, interested in interacting with the people and other dogs, but not overstimulated in the context. Just because a dog comes home tired from daycare, does not necessarily mean he enjoyed it. Dogs that are uncomfortable in the context will be vigilant and unable to relax all day. So for some dogs it can be a great outlet and other dogs may prefer to stay home.

Canine prevention: effects of neutering
There are medical and behavioral benefits and disadvantages of neutering a dog. Behavioral effects of neutering male dogs and the effect of reducing testosterone levels include decreased sexual interest in female dogs, decreased tendency to roam in 90% of dogs, decreased urine marking in 50% of dogs, decreased mounting in 67% of dogs, decreased competitive aggression between males in 60% of dogs (Hopkins *et al.*, 1976), and a slight increased risk of developing senior onset cognitive dysfunction syndrome (senility or dementia).

Spaying the female dog correlates to the following behavioral effects as a result of reduction in sex hormones: eliminates the potential for maternal aggression associated with having a litter of puppies or pseudopregnancy and eliminates the potential for estrus-induced interdog aggression, and a possible increased risk of developing senior onset cognitive dysfunction syndrome (senility or dementia).

Research has also shown a correlation between animals that are neutered being at increased risk of certain behavior issues. One of two studies done by Duffy and Serpell (2006) with approximately 1500 breed club dog owners demonstrated a correlation in the following behavior characteristics:

- Spayed females were more aggressive toward both strangers and owners than intact females.
- Spayed females were more fearful and sensitive to touch than intact females.
- Both males and females that were altered were more likely to beg for food and to engage in excessive licking of people or objects.
- Dog-directed fear/aggression varied quite a bit by breed.
- Neutered males were much less likely to mark their territories.

In the second study by Duffy and Serpell, with a sample of more than 3500 dog owners, the following correlations were identified:

- Neutered dogs of both genders were more likely to show dog-directed aggression/fear.
- Neutered dogs of both genders were more likely to show owner-directed aggression.
- Neutered dogs of both genders were also more likely to have touch sensitivity and nonsocial fear.
- Neutered dogs were also likely to be less energetic/active.

So although differences in behavioral characteristics were associated or correlated with reproductive status, the research does not determine a cause and effect relationship. What is evidenced by this research is that neutering is not an effective treatment for aggression in dogs.

Although neutering has some potential medical and behavior benefits, there are also medical and behavioral disadvantages to altering. The veterinary technician should strive to continue to evaluate research findings regarding the effects of neutering.

Canine prevention: socialization

Dogs experience sensitive periods of development. Of particular importance is the socialization period that occurs between 3 and 12 weeks of age. There is some fluidity of the period but the optimal time for socialization is up to about 12 weeks of age. This period is particularly important because what a puppy learns during this time will have a lifelong effect on its personality and reactions to people, other animals, and environments. This is a well-documented stage of development in which puppies can readily learn to become comfortable with novelty and develop appropriate social skills. Lack of exposure is just as detrimental as a negative experience. Socializing a dog is an active process of positive exposure to novel environments, people, and circumstances and it needs to continue throughout the dog's life. Over the past decades, there has been recognition of the importance of early environmental exposure for puppies. However, all exposure is not the same. Positive, proactive exposure is an active process that takes preparation and planning. When most people think about socialization they think about habituation and exposure; get the puppy out and allow him to habituate to the environment. The problem here is that without positive, proactive socialization, the puppy may actually become sensitized to environmental stimuli. Socialization is not simply about habituation; rather, it is about making exposure fun and positive.

- Socialization is not simply about habituation; rather, it is about making exposure fun and positive.

Rather than just a neutral experience or even worse an overwhelming experience, new experiences should be made positive by utilizing desensitization and classical conditioning or classical counter-conditioning. Undersocialization can cause or exacerbate behavior problems. Enrolling a 7 to 12-week-old puppy into a good puppy class is the single most important thing in the dog's lifetime that a new puppy owner can do for its behavioral well-being. More information about puppy socialization classes is covered in the section titled **Prevention services**.

Canine prevention: crate training

A crate is a valuable tool for house training and management. Teaching a puppy to be comfortable and relaxed in a crate should be done as early as possible. A dog's crate can be a place for him to get away from the complex human world (Figure 7.7).

There are many benefits if a dog is comfortable spending time in a crate. Crates provide for a safe puppy-proof area. They limit access to potential hazards when the dog is unable to be directly supervised. The crate helps control the dog's learning history (limits opportunity to "get into trouble") and assists with elimination training

Figure 7.7 A young puppy taking a break in its crate.

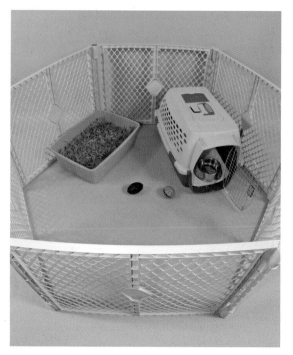

Figure 7.8 An exercise pen, elimination area, crate, and toys provide a safe area for a puppy or dog.

(house training). It can also be a safe way to manage adult and elderly dogs.

An alternative to a crate is an exercise pen. It can prevent destructive behavior while giving the dog a bit more freedom. This is similar to a play pen for toddlers. The crate might be placed within or attached to the exercise pen. Toys and water should be made available in this area. The exercise pen can be used for short periods of time while the owner is home but can also be used if the owner is forced to leave the young puppy (less than 4 months) for an extended period of time (3–4 h). An elimination area may be placed in the exercise pen, to provide an appropriate location for the young puppy to eliminate. This will allow the puppy to relieve itself without soiling the crate. (Figure 7.8).

There are a variety of crates available.

Wire and plastic are the two most common crate types. Fold-up wire crates are easy to transport and allow superior ventilation, but some dogs prefer the closed in, den-like area of plastic crates.

How big should a crate be? That depends. When house training a dog, the crate should be large enough for the dog to get up, stretch, turn around, and lie down. A dog may eliminate in a crate that is too large. Once the dog is house trained, a larger crate is preferred to provide more freedom but still allow for good management.

Initially young dogs should be in the crate or exercise pen whenever they are unable to be supervised. While trying to take care of the children, fixing breakfast, getting school supplies together, or talking on the phone, the young dog might be grabbing food off the table, chewing a pair of socks, and basically learning undesirable behavior. The confinement area should be used to help control the dog's learning history.

The crate can be used throughout a dog's life. The amount of time a dog will spend in the crate will decrease as it grows. Plan to use the crate regularly for at least the first few years.

Although confinement in a dog-proof area is recommended for the safety and learning history of young dogs, overuse of confinement can cause excitability issues. It is important to provide ample mental and physical exercise when the dog is out of the confinement area. This may be accomplished through scheduled training, play, and walks. Alternatively, a dog can learn to be calm in other parts of the house by using the "umbilical cord method": the dog is on leash and goes with the pet owner from room to room. Using a leash teaches the dog in a controlled manner (it cannot wander off) how to acclimate to the human domestic environment. It also allows the pet owner to notice and reward the dog for desirable behavior.

- Although confinement in a dog-proof area is recommended for the safety and learning history of young dogs, overuse of confinement can cause excitability issues.

- SAFETY warning: the collar should be removed before leaving a dog unattended in a confinement area to prevent accidental strangulation!

For instructions on how to teach a dog to love its crate, see Appendix 20: Acclimatizing a pet to a crate. If a dog has already had an aversive reaction to confinement, see Chapter 8 for recreate training.

Canine prevention: elimination training

One of the most common reasons owners relinquish their pet is house soiling (Patronek *et al.*, 1996; Mondelli *et al.*, 2004). Therefore, housetraining should be discussed at the first and every appointment. House training is a term used to describe teaching a dog a "human approved" appropriate elimination area. Usually, this location is outdoors on grass, but dogs can be litter box trained or trained to eliminate on other surfaces such as concrete.

A dog's natural preference is to eliminate on porous surfaces (grass, carpet, bedding, etc.), in a place where elimination has previously occurred, and away from his eating and sleeping areas.

- A dog's natural preference is to eliminate on porous surfaces (grass, carpet, bedding, etc.), in a place where elimination has previously occurred, and away from his eating and sleeping areas.

Successful elimination training depends on the pet owners' ability to effectively communicate where they consider it appropriate for the dog to eliminate. This process will not occur overnight. Punishment, including verbal reprimands, only teaches a dog not to eliminate in front of people, making house training very difficult. The prevention of accidents through management and supervision is the key to successful house training!

- The prevention of accidents through management and supervision is the key to successful house training!

Elimination training can be broken into five key steps.

1. Prevent accidents from occurring: Direct supervision and management, via a confinement area or the umbilical cord technique, are imperative until the desired location has become the dog's preference.

Educate puppy owners on physiological constraints based on the puppy's age. A puppy can hold its urine for one hour and its age in months, when not active. The maximum amount of time a 2-month-old puppy can be expected to have between elimination is 3 h. It may need to eliminate every 30 min when active. Maximum duration of urine retention should not routinely exceed 8 h for any dog older than 7 months of age. Full bladder control may take 4–5 months to develop, but accidents may occasionally occur up to 1 year of age. Once the puppy starts reliably relieving itself outdoors, the intervals between trips outside can gradually be increased.

Water should be available at all times to prevent excessive consumption at one time and subsequent frequent urination. Feeding a highly digestible diet on a set schedule will limit defecation to set times. Most puppies are like clockwork and will need to defecate within 10–20 min after a meal.

2. Reward elimination in appropriate areas: Use a cue phrase, such as, "Let's go outside" or "Outside." Ideally the pet owner should exit from the same door each time and take the dog out on a leash (even if they have a fenced in yard). Many dogs that do not have experience with eliminating while on leash may be hesitant to do so in the future. This can be problematic in settings away from the yard that require a leash. Designate a specific area of the yard for elimination. Once established, it will become saturated with the puppy pheromones, which will help stimulate the puppy to relieve itself. The owner should withhold attention from the puppy until it eliminates. This means basically standing like a pole and not even looking at the puppy. Allow the puppy about 5 min to eliminate; if not successful, take him inside and supervise or confine him and then try again in 10–15 min. *After* elimination is complete, the owner should praise the dog and offer a treat. If the owner begins to praise the puppy while it is still eliminating, it may not complete the void. Wait until just after it has finished. The puppy may be let off the leash for playtime once he eliminates, if in a secure area.

It can be helpful for the owner to add a cue, such as "get busy," when the puppy relieves itself. As the owner predicts the puppy is about to relieve itself by watching its body language, he/she can add the cue just before the puppy begins to eliminate.

3. Anticipate when the puppy needs to eliminate: Set the puppy up to succeed by anticipating when he will need to eliminate. Keeping a journal or log of activity can prove helpful in determining a dog's individual

routine and elimination training patterns. Most commonly, the log will serve as reassurance to the owners that their puppy is having fewer accidents (see Appendix 21: Elimination training log). The log also allows the owner to track when the puppy is full or empty. At first, with a young puppy, it is important to make repeated trips, first thing in the morning, last thing at night, and several times in between. Take a potty break after eating, playing, and sleeping. Puppies are likely to eliminate after finishing one behavior and before beginning another. The idea is that initially the owner will happen to have the puppy outside when he has to eliminate, thus allowing the owner to capture elimination in the desired location.

It is helpful to teach a puppy a signal to go outside. Owners often believe a puppy will clearly signal to them when it needs to eliminate. In reality, puppies usually only show subtle signs of impending elimination such as sniffing the ground, wandering toward the door, circling, or walking slowly. Teaching a puppy to ring a bell to indicate the need to eliminate may be useful, especially in busy households. For instructions on how to teach a puppy to ring a bell to signal the need to eliminate, see Appendix 22: Shaping plan for teaching a puppy to ring a bell to go outside to eliminate.

4. Know what to do when accidents happen: Accidents will happen, so prepare clients on how to react to make it a productive learning experience for the dog. The best course of action if the owner sees the puppy starting to eliminate in the house, is to use the cue, "outside," in a nonthreatening tone to interrupt the behavior. This may momentarily make him stop and give the owner an opportunity to take him outside and reward him for eliminating in the proper location.

Relieving a full bladder is reinforcing. Yelling at or scolding a dog for eliminating in front of you in the house will make him hesitant to go in front of you outside. This makes house training difficult because the owner then is unable to reward appropriate eliminations. Punishment does not teach a puppy where it is appropriate to eliminate, just that it is not safe to do it in front of people. Reprimanding the dog will likely train him to find a quiet place away from people to eliminate. Unfortunately, this might be in the closet, behind the couch, or in the guest room!

5. Clean soiled areas: Because dogs will be drawn to spots where elimination has previously occurred, it is extremely important to thoroughly clean soiled

areas to prevent further accidents. Cleaning products that contain ammonia or vinegar are likely to act as an attractant for pets to eliminate in the same spot and therefore should be avoided. Enzymatic cleaners use natural enzymes to break down the waste, odor, and remove the stain. Because enzymes can be deactivated by harsh chemicals, it is advised to not combine other disinfectants when using an enzymatic product because they are likely to neutralize the desired effects of the enzymes.

To effectively clean an area, first remove as much urine and stool as possible with paper towels. Apply an enzymatic cleaner designed for eliminating pet odors and allow it to dry for 24 h. Then make the area locally aversive to the pet by applying a citrus scent or even more effective, apply the scent of mothballs to the area (wipe the mothball on the fabric or floor). People should not be able to smell the mothballs when they enter the room or sniff the carpet a few feet away, only if they smell the spot where the elimination had occurred. CAUTION: Mothball crystals are toxic to animals and people if consumed. It is unlikely a dog will ingest previously soiled carpet/fabric containing mothball crystals. Do not use mothball crystals on bedding, in areas where the dog is confined, or on objects that may be chewed or ingested (Table 7.3).

Using these techniques, most puppies can be successfully house trained. To be effective, however, all steps must be followed simultaneously and consistently.

Besides the lack of training, there are numerous other reasons for inappropriate elimination. When the dog owner fails to make progress or encounters a regression in house training, the dog should be immediately evaluated by a veterinarian. Excessive urination ($\sim$10+ times a day) can be caused by a variety of medical conditions, including a urinary tract infection or vaginitis. Excessive water consumption and urination can be a sign of

Table 7.3 Five steps to successful elimination training.

1. Prevent accidents	Management and supervision
2. Reward elimination in appropriate locations	Specific location and on leash Cue word, "Outside" Praise and treat after completion
3. Anticipate	Keep a log
4. Know what to do when accidents happen	Interrupt, redirect, reward! Avoid punishment
5. Clean soiled areas	Enzymatic cleaners Locally aversive

a congenital medical disorder (diabetes insipidus). Limiting water intake is generally not advised with house training. In the case of a medical problem causing excessive water consumption, limiting water could be life threatening.

- When the dog owner fails to make progress or encounters a regression in house training, the dog should be immediately evaluated by a veterinarian.

Urine marking is associated with a perceived threat to the territory and is more common in un-neutered male dogs, although neutered males and some females (intact or spayed) might also mark. It is an anxiety-related behavior rather than an issue of elimination training. Neutering and/or treating the underlying anxiety are the key to improving this behavior.

Excitement urination is common in young dogs still developing sphincter control. It is unrelated to house training. Prevention, through low key greetings, is the best solution until the dog develops better muscle control.

Appeasement urination is a normal behavior and can occur in dogs at any age. It is a fear reaction to a perceived threat and unrelated to house training. The dog may squat down, turn slightly to the side, or even roll over while urinating. It is attempting to communicate nonthreat and appeasement. The behavior may be related to underdeveloped urinary sphincter tone in puppies. Positive-based training and using food treats boosts confidence and allows for positive associations with people. Any form of punishment is counterproductive. Avoid threatening body language, including direct eye contact and leaning over or reaching for the dog.

Litter/pad training puppies

Another option many dog owners are considering and hospital personnel should be prepared to counsel on is litter box or puppy pad training. Some reasons for clients to choose this option include small breeds of dogs poorly suited for a harsh outdoor climate and it is an option more conducive to apartment or high-rise living, as well as lifestyles that include traveling with their pet. The type of substrate used can vary from incontinence pad placed in a frame to actual litter box filled with an array of products. There should be close supervision initially due to a puppy's natural desire to shred and perhaps ingest the pads or litter. The techniques of training to

an indoor-approved elimination area are the same as training a puppy to relieve itself outdoors: positive reinforcement for going on the desired surface, supervision, and confinement. As the crate is used for sleeping and eating, the litter box/pad should be located outside of the crate. An exercise pen works quite nicely. Within the exercise pen, a crate area and a separate toileting area provide for a management system that meets all the puppy's needs (Figure 7.8). This system can also be used in the owner's absence.

Canine prevention: independence training

Dogs are social animals; it is not natural for them to be left alone for extended periods of time. Most puppies will show some mild signs of stress when first separated from their mother and littermates. Separation anxiety is a common disorder of dogs manifesting in codependence. Dogs with separation anxiety show signs of distress and may panic when separated from their attachment figure. Often the attachment figure is a person, but occasionally it can be another pet. Distress signs may include barking, whining, howling, pacing, drooling, destructive chewing, urinating, or defecating. When associated with separation anxiety, these signs occur when left alone or confined away from people. The diagnosis and treatment of separation anxiety is an intervention service. However, there are preventive steps that can be taken to minimize the risk of the development of separation anxiety (See Table 7.4: Steps to help prevent the development of canine separation anxiety)

- Separation anxiety is a common disorder of dogs manifesting in codependence. Dogs with separation anxiety show signs of distress and may panic when separated from their attachment figure.

The first 48 h in the client's home can be important for preventing separation issues. The owner should resist the temptation to shower the puppy with attention but instead, simply let the puppy relax in his crate if the puppy has already been introduced to a crate by the breeder. If the breeder has not introduced the puppy to crating, allow the puppy to sleep in a cardboard box or other temporary containment area for the first 48 h before transferring to a crate. The first 48 h will likely be the most stressful and the puppy will not associate the crate with this stress. The transition may also be made easier by installing an Adaptil™ diffuser near the

Table 7.4 Steps to help prevent the development of canine separation anxiety.

Acclimatize the dog to the confinement area	See Appendix 20: Acclimatizing a pet to a crate for steps
Confine when people are home	Dogs should be confined at times when people are home to prevent an association of being locked away only when people leave the home
Confine for variable periods of time	Confinement for short periods of time (5–10 min) periodically throughout the day prevents confinement being associated with long departures
Calm "hellos" and "goodbyes"	Arrivals and departures to and from the dog should be calm and nonchalant
Teaching a relaxed sit or down stay is an exercise of independence	Teach the dog that people leaving the dog can be a good thing
Reward calm behavior	Dogs often get attention for being excited. Teach clients to catch their dogs being calm and reward this behavior
Provide a routine for interactions with the dog	Providing scheduled routine walks, training, and play will help to meet the dog's needs for social interaction and mental and physical exercise
Consider pheromone or music therapy	Adaptil™ is a synthetic form of a pheromone that comes from the mammary tissue of the female dog and is available in a diffuser form that can be used in the confinement area to help decrease stress. Music therapy, such as Through a Dog's Ear™, has also been shown to help calm dogs

puppy's confinement area. After the first couple of days the puppy can be transitioned to the crate.

The puppy should become acclimated to the owner's normal schedule as soon as possible. In the case of clients who do not routinely leave the home, it is important for them to leave the puppy alone for periods of time during their first few days in the household. Other pet owners may find that their current schedule requires they are away from the dog for longer periods of time. It may be necessary to bring in additional support in the form of dog walkers and daycare facilities. However, there should also be opportunity for the dog to learn to be comfortable alone.

When the owners return, they should avoid scolding or reprimanding the dog regardless of what may have transpired while they were away. Reprimands will not lessen the dog's anxiety or teach him not to do the same behavior in the future. Dogs should not be let out of their crate or other enclosed area if they are barking or whining, unless the owner suspects the dog needs to urinate or defecate.

Owners should create departure and arrival routines with no fanfare. They should be unemotional when leaving as well as coming home. Providing a food storage toy in the confinement area can be used to create a positive focus away from the departure of the owner. This should be presented to the dog about 10 min before leaving so it does not become a cue for departure.

Dogs that do not respond to the above preventative strategies or that are showing extreme separation issues should be seen by the veterinarian. Very serious separation anxiety requiring pharmaceutical intervention is

not unheard of, even in puppies as young as 10 weeks of age (Purdue University Animal Behavior Clinic caseload). Often, medication in these cases is only temporary. If left untreated, the anxiety is likely to escalate and the longer the negative learning history, the more difficult it can be to make improvement. Severe cases of separation anxiety can negatively affect the welfare of the dog, damage the developing human–animal bond, and result in relinquishment or even euthanasia.

> - Dogs that do not respond to the above preventative strategies or that are showing extreme separation issues should be seen by the veterinarian. Very serious separation anxiety requiring pharmaceutical intervention is not unheard of, even in puppies as young as 10 weeks of age.

Separation anxiety is the most common behavioral disorder of dogs. It may develop at any age. The condition can sometimes be prevented. However, there can be a genetic or learned component to the disorder. A dog showing signs of separation anxiety is past the preventive stage and indicates a need for a behavior intervention service.

Canine prevention: handling and restraint

Handling refers to manipulating or touching parts of the dog's body, such as its ears, mouth, nose, tail, feet, and so on.

Figure 7.9 Handler touches the ear and clicks with a clicker to mark the event.

Figure 7.10 The hand is removed and a treat is delivered.

To make handling less likely to be an aversive experience, dogs need to learn to associate being touched with earning treats. Although many dogs will tolerate being handled, making it a pleasant experience rather than a neutral or an aversive one is necessary to make future experiences less traumatic for the dog. In short, be proactive! (Figures 7.9 and 7.10).

> • To make handling less likely to be an aversive experience, dogs need to learn to associate being touched with earning treats.

Owners can teach their puppy to enjoy handling by using the puppy's daily food as a training tool. Begin by lightly taking hold of the puppy's collar, then offering a piece of kibble. Touch one ear, then offer kibble, touch the other ear and offer kibble. Touch a paw, and then offer kibble. Continue this with all four feet. Open the puppy's mouth and offer kibble. Touch the puppy on his abdomen, rear end, and private parts and then offer kibble. Repeat this several times a week.

Restraint refers to physically holding a dog still and is often used during routine veterinary procedures. Dogs

learn very quickly that something unpleasant is about to happen when they are restrained. Through experience, they learn that when held still, they may have their nails trimmed, temperature taken, vaccinations given, blood drawn, ears cleaned, or groomed.

Through desensitization and classical and/or counter conditioning, many handling procedures can be performed with little or no restraint. However, there will be times when the veterinary technician or even the pet owner will need the dog to hold completely still. By being proactive, you can teach puppies that being gently restrained is a predictor of good things. Regardless of the age of the pet, it can learn that restraint is nothing to fear. The older the dog, the more likely a negative association with restraint has already developed, unless proactive prevention exercises have previously been implemented.

Clicker or marker training can be very effective in acclimatizing a dog to being handled and restrained. See Appendix 23: Preventive handling and restraint exercises for instructions on how to implement these exercises.

Another alternative is to teach the patient an operant behavior, such as targeting a specific object. A dog can be taught to place his chin in the owner's cupped hand on cue or rest his head on a towel draped across the owners lap. This provides a cued stationary behavior for the animal to perform.

As a veterinary technician, you will encounter patients that are already concerned about being handled or restrained. Signs a dog has become uncomfortable with handling/restraint exercises include stops taking treats, freezes, ears back and/or tail tucked, wants to get away. In this situation, stop and do not escalate any further. Maintain the current level and offer treats until the dog relaxes and begins to take them again. Once the dog is taking treats, release or let go. As discussed earlier, this is for mild fear or resistance. If aggression or extreme fear or anxiety is being displayed, abort the exercise completely and recognize that the dog is not in a preventive stage of learning; behavioral intervention services are indicated.

> • Signs a dog has become uncomfortable with handling/restraint exercises include stops taking treats, freezes, ears back and/or tail tucked, wants to get away.

Canine prevention: safety around the food bowl and relinquishing objects

It is natural for a dog, or person for that matter, in possession of a high-value item to want to keep it. If a dog considers people as a potential threat (often due to previous learning experiences) to a high-value item, serious problems can arise. Educating owners on proper etiquette and implementing prevention exercises in puppyhood will help to prevent future issues with resources. Food, the food bowl, toys, and food-based items (rawhides, pig ears, food storage toys) are considered high-value items for most dogs. "Stolen" items, such as socks, paper towels, or the remote control, can also become high-value items depending on the human's response. To a certain extent, guarding is a normal behavior in dogs. In multiple-pet households, it is imperative to manage resources to prevent competition and consequently, aggression over items between resident animals. It is especially problematic when the guarding of resources becomes a trigger for human-directed aggression.

> • Educating owners on proper etiquette and implementing prevention exercises in puppyhood will help to prevent future issues with resources.

Most dogs guard objects because they are afraid the object will be taken away. The foundation for preventing this behavior is to teach the dog to trust you and that leaving an object is frequently more rewarding than picking up the object. Certain exercises such as "leave it" and "drop it" if taught correctly can prevent a bite from occurring.

As the food bowl is a common area of tension for many dogs, preventive training is imperative. Review Box 7.1 for management recommendations for minimizing tension at feeding time. There are several valuable exercises puppy owners can do with their new puppy while the puppy is eating, to associate people near the food bowl as a welcome thing. The first is to simply walk past the puppy while he is eating a regular meal of kibble and drop a really tasty treat, chicken or cheese, into the bowl. (See Figure 7.11). This will teach puppies to eagerly anticipate the approach of humans while eating. Provided the puppy is comfortable with the approach and there is no body posturing over the bowl, exercises can continue. See Appendix 24 for a detailed process on implementing preventive food bowl training exercises.

> **BOX 7.1: FOOD BOWL RECOMMENDATIONS.**
>
> • Offer food at a set time at least twice a day. Allow up to 20 min for the dog to eat.
> • If any food is left, call the dog away and pick up the bowl when he is out of sight.
> • Place the food bowl in a low-traffic location to avoid the dog being startled. The confinement area or crate is the ideal location.
> • In multiple-pet households, avoid competition over food by having separate bowls and locations for feeding.
> • People should always be the giver of food, not the taker of food. Pulling a food bowl away from a dog while he is eating only teaches him that people are unpredictable and they might try to steal the food bowl.
> • Dogs do not enjoy being touched or petted while eating. (People do not either)

If there is any sign a dog is uncomfortable with the food bowl exercises, such as stiffening, suddenly freezing over the bowl, or eating more quickly, a behavior consultation should be scheduled. It is important to note that aggression toward people over food in puppies is a red flag predicting human-directed aggression later in life. The puppy is not going through a phase and is unlikely to

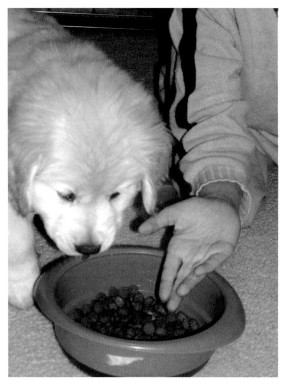

Figure 7.11 A young puppy learning that human hands near the food bowl mean a special treat!

just grow out of the behavior. Immediate behavior counseling should be provided if a puppy or dog is showing aggression toward people over food.

- Aggression toward people over food in puppies is a red flag predicting human-directed aggression later in life.

Because dogs explore the world with their mouths, they are likely to pick up things that for their own safety or due to the nature of the item, their owner will want them to release. In the section titled **Problem solving typical canine behaviors**, strategies for addressing the immediate concern of obtaining an item from the dog will be addressed. However, preventive exercises to teach the dog appropriate items to play with and also relinquishing them to their owner should be implemented.

When the dog is chewing on an appropriate item, the owner approaches and drops a tasty treat; like the food bowl exercise, it teaches the dog to enjoy people approaching. The owner can also do a trade by taking the toy or bone away briefly, giving the puppy a treat, then returning the item to the puppy.

Caution should be given to those fastidious dog owners who want to take everything out of the puppy's mouth. Puppies are exploring with their mouths and if every little thing is taken away from them, there is potential to create a guarding problem. Instead, owners should be instructed to give the puppy a treat for relinquishing the item, examine the item in question but return the object to the puppy if it is determined to be safe. Instructing owners on teaching "take it" and "drop it" with positive reinforcement training can provide a way to communicate effectively with the dog and prevent conflict over items.

The purpose of "drop it" is to teach the dog to drop an object it may have. Again the goal is for the dog to not fear giving a person an object in its possession but to instead look forward to releasing the object. Never punish the dog once he has an object; it is far too late. It will only associate having the object and your presence with "danger." The dog learns it is "unsafe" to have things in its mouth when people are nearby. Some dogs may then try to hide with the object or be placed in a motivational conflict. For example, wanting the object but fearing your response. Instead, if the dog is always rewarded for relinquishing the object, there will be no motivational conflict. If the dog continues to acquire inappropriate objects, the pet owner's management plan for avoiding these situations should be reviewed.

Tug can be an interactive, energetic, and appropriate game to play with a dog. Play fosters a social relationship between people and their dog. Teaching dogs to enjoy playing tug with their owners allows the tug to become a useful tool for motivation and reward. When taught correctly, it allows you to contain and control the dog's arousal (impulse control) and can aid in teaching the dog to enjoy relinquishing a toy (or other item) to the owner.

Teaching a dog to play tug of war will not make him aggressive. Tug can be a physical and mental outlet for energetic dogs. However, it is not recommended to play tug of war with dogs that guard objects and/or display aggression in certain context because previous learning history potentially could make the game unsafe or over-arouse the dog. Caution should be taken with children playing tug of war with any dog and it may be safer to make it an adult only game, because the excitement level may be more difficult to control with children. See Appendix 25 for specific instructions on Teaching tug of war.

There may be certain items some dogs should never have. Really high-value items are animal-based products such as real bones, rawhides, and pig ears. Some dogs just cannot resist the urge to guard these high-value items, almost a primal reaction. In addition, trying to find something of higher value to trade with the dog may be difficult. If a dog only guards a rawhide and truly only guards a rawhide, then simply never offering those objects to the dog is a viable management tool.

Households with small children should be extra aware of guarding issues. A dog with a tendency to guard items in a household with children can be a dangerous situation. No management is 100% effective. Implementation of early prevention exercises is even more vital in households with children to minimize the chance of aggression over resources from developing.

> • A dog with a tendency to guard items in a household with children can be a dangerous situation.

Feline management and prevention techniques

As in dogs, early prevention exercises and training in cats can have a profound impact on the success of their integration into the human household.

Understanding cats and their characteristics

A large part of prevention is educating cat owners about typical behavioral tendencies and characteristics of cats. By developing empathy for the cat's natural tendencies, the cat owner can funnel those desires to appropriate outlets.

As you learned in Chapter 3, friendliness is largely genetic and early experiences play a role in the cat's ability to adapt to changes in the environment. Cats are social animals and they develop a communal smell which identifies members of the group and the territory. One of the cat's most influential forms of communication seems to be olfactory; however, visual and vocal communication also plays an important role.

Feline management recommendations

Feline management recommendations include preventing potentially stress-inducing or dangerous situations and developing a consistent routine.

Special inspection should be given to homes adding a small kitten to the household. A frightened kitten will often seek out a small hiding area. Places such as

behind appliances, sump pumps, and cabinets should be blocked off. Kitten-proofing the house is as important as puppy-proofing it. Kittens are notorious for playing with yarn and string of all sorts. However, if ingested, they can cause potentially fatal intestinal disorders. Just as with puppies, everyday household items have the potential to be dangerous if appropriate management and supervision are not initiated.

Because cats are territorial, threats to the territory by outsiders can cause stress and anxiety. The indoor-only cat that is exposed to the sight, sound, or smell of other cats approaching the house will often display behaviors associated with agitation or stress. Exposure to cats approaching the territory may stimulate urine marking as well as irritation and aggression toward people or other cats in the household. For the comfort of the indoor cat, owners should prevent exposure to outside cats. Some options include blocking visual access out of windows or deterring the outside cats through the use of a motion detection sprinkler.

> • Because cats are territorial, threats to the territory by outsiders can cause stress and anxiety. The indoor-only cat that is exposed to the sight, sound, or smell of other cats approaching the house will often display behaviors associated with agitation or stress.

In regard to territorial ranges, male cats have on average three times more territory than female cats. In the indoor setting, the male cat's average range was 4–5 rooms whereas the female cat's range was 3–3.6 rooms (Liberg et al., 2000; Bernstein and Strack, 2006). In multiple cat households, providing abundant resources/provisions spaced throughout the entire house, minimizes competition between cats over resources. Provisions refer to feeding areas, water stations, resting areas, and litter boxes. By providing access to resources in several locations, resident cats can avoid conflict over the use of the resource at the same time. Similarly, increasing vertical living space through platforms, shelves, and cat trees can avoid confrontation and potential conflict. The increased living space allows for increased territory. Social stress in multiple cat households can be greatly reduced by providing numerous resources in various locations and increasing vertical living space.

Good management in the feline household not only involves setting the environment up to allow for success, it also includes having a consistent routine of interaction with the cat. Set times to train and play each day will ensure the cat's social, mental, and physical needs are met.

Feline environmental enrichment

The majority of cats in the United States are kept as indoor pets, which can cause a severe lack in mental stimulation and exercise. The animal behavior technician can assist cat owners in creating a household setting that provides the cat with an enriched environment, thereby helping to prevent potential behavior problems.

In the United Kingdom, the common belief is cats should have access to the outdoors. Outside access allows for natural outlets for exploration, mental stimulation, exercise, and hunting. Having access to the outdoors can decrease obesity and possibly prevent some behavior disorders in cats.

The accepted position from most pet care professionals in the United States is that cats should be kept as indoor pets. By doing so, owners can prevent injuries such as being hit by a car, poisoning, bite wounds from other cats, and attacks by predators. Indoor cats will be at less risk of contracting diseases such as FIV, FeLV and FIP, or parasites.

Environmental enrichment provides outlets for normal feline behaviors and allows the pet owner to provide for the cat's mental and physical well-being. This is especially important for the indoor-only cat because the human domestic environment is often void of opportunities for normal feline exploratory behavior.

> • Environmental enrichment provides outlets for normal feline behaviors and allows the pet owner to provide for the cat's mental and physical well-being.

Toys and play

Kittens, like puppies, benefit from toys that deliver food and/or treats. Cats are natural grazers and designed to eat small amounts of food at frequent intervals. Food puzzle toys can help to prevent obesity in cats as there is more activity involved in the feeding process and they provide great mental stimulation. Although there are many commercial products available, homemade items such as holes cut out of storage boxes filled with food can be recommended (puzzle feeder). (Figure 7.12).

Hiding food and treats around the house in small dishes or cups will promote exploratory behavior and appease the cat's natural desire to search for food. Although not a toy, some cats enjoy the option of having indoor grass available. Most of them are easily grown indoors and are made up of either wheat or oat

Figure 7.12 A homemade "puzzle feeder" for cats. The round hole is made large enough for the cat to stick his head in the box and the slats allow the cat to paw the food to the large feeding hole.

grasses. Offering fresh grass can prevent them eating house plants while providing roughage to their diet.

Providing exploratory outlets through a variety of interactive toys will help to appease the cat's curiosity. Interactive homemade toys can provide cats with hours of entertainment. A cardboard box with holes for the cat's paws and toys dangling from sisal rope is an easy-to-make homemade toy that most cats will appreciate. Sisal rope is a durable rope made from plant fiber. It is often used for scratching posts for cats. (Figures 7.13 and 7.14). These toys can be inexpensively made to entertain boarding felines and sent home with the owners at pick up.

A set time for play sessions with the owner in the morning and evening is ideal because cats tend to be more active at these times. Cats enjoy playing with toys that encourage pouncing and stalking (predatory sequence). Feather toys on the end of a pole, small stuffed toys, and balls encourage exercise and positive interactions with the owners. Any type of direct play with human hands should be avoided as it can promote inappropriate play and result in potential injury to humans through accidental scratches and bites.

Figure 7.13 The outside of a homemade interactive cat toy. Numerous openings can be cut around the box to allow for multiple exploration ports for the paws.

Figure 7.14 The inside of the same homemade toy. Toys dangling from sisal rope and also a loose ball to bat around.

Vertical space and places to hide

Vertical space is important not only for management but also environmental enrichment. Vertical space creates areas for exploration and additional hiding places. Cat trees, perches, shelves, and elevated hiding places are great options for creating vertical space for cats. Tunnels, boxes, and paper bags can be used at lower levels.

In the veterinary setting, a cardboard box or paper bag placed in a cage with a feline patient can allow the cat a safe place to hide in the novel environment.

Outdoor exposure

Secure outdoor enclosures and fences are available to allow cats to have exposure to the outdoor environment within a confined area. Most are designed to not only keep the pet cat in the yard but also prevent other feline intruders from entering the yard. For safety, supervision by the owner is recommended during controlled outdoor exposure. Acclimatizing a kitten to wearing a cat harness can also allow the owner to manage the cat outside, thus allowing for more exploration. Adult cats that have not had previous exposure to the outside may never be comfortable or enjoy being outside, regardless of the owners' best efforts. Instead, the owner can focus on making indoors as enriching as possible.

Feline prevention: effects of neutering

Neutering the male cat can decrease intermale aggression (testosterone-driven aggression); however, it does not increase amicable behavior or decrease other forms of aggression (nontestosterone driven) (Crowell-Davis et al., 1997; Neville and Remfry, 1984). In female cats, no significant behavioral changes were noted associated with ovariohysterectomy, with the exception of the cessation of behavior patterns associated with estrus (Stubbs et al., 1996). In contrast, neutering of the male and female cat significantly reduces urine marking, 90% in males and 95% in females (Hart and Cooper, 1984).

Feline prevention: socialization

Although the socialization period (2–7 weeks) is usually over by the time the kitten goes to a new home, continued positive exposure to novelty is still important. The cat can be taken on car rides and given a special meal or treat. Treats and play can be utilized while visiting a friend's house or the veterinary hospital to make a positive association with the environment. Friends can be encouraged to come to the house and play with the kitten and give it treats. This may help prevent the fear and hiding often displayed by house cats when a visitor arrives. Kitten classes and fun visits to the veterinary hospital should be encouraged with young cats. Kitten classes will be discussed in more detail in the preventive services section of this chapter.

> • Although the socialization period (2–7 weeks) is usually over by the time the kitten goes to a new home, continued positive exposure to novelty is still important.

Feline prevention: litter box training

Kittens usually enter their new homes ready to use a litter box, unlike puppies which are not always ready to eliminate outdoors. However, as litter box problems are the number one behavior problem seen in cats, it is important to set cat owners up for success.

The rule regarding the number of litter boxes is to provide as many litter boxes as there are cats and one extra box. If the home is multilevel, there should be at least one box on each floor the cat has access to. This is especially important for younger kittens and geriatric cats. In either instance, the need to void may be urgent and youngsters and arthritic seniors may not be able to travel far. The locations should be variable throughout the home as cats tend to prefer to urinate in one location and defecate in another. Litter boxes in numerous locations are particularly important if there are multiple cats as one cat may block the other cat's access to a box. Other pets or small children also may inadvertently block a cat's access to a litter box. All locations should be in low-traffic areas. Many cats have been spooked from using a box in the basement or utility room if the furnace happened to kick on or the washing machine suddenly whirled into spin mode while the cat was in the box. These frightening events can easily be associated with the use of the litter box and many cats will not return to the area, choosing to eliminate elsewhere instead.

Cats generally prefer unscented, clumping litter as the substrate in the litter box (Neilson, 2001). Their ancestors would have been using sand for elimination, so this type of litter may be the closest option to what they seek. Plastic liners are not preferred. Cats prefer larger (1.5 times the length of their body is suggested), uncovered boxes (Neilson, 2008). Most commercial cat litter pans are too small for the average adult cat so it is best to start with a cement mixing pan, an under-the-bed storage Tupperware bin, or a dog litter box. Young kittens should have litter boxes low enough for them to easily step into. Older cats with less mobility may also need lower sided boxes. Being fastidious creatures, cats will be more willing to use a litter box that is kept clean. Scooping at least once daily is recommended.

Prevention of inappropriate elimination is always easier on everyone involved. Kitten classes are a great platform for educating owners regarding litter box preferences. Fielding questions using a pre-exam questionnaire (see Appendices 13–18 for life stage questionnaires) can identify potential problems. Questions should be included regarding litter box habits. For example, how many litter boxes are in the home? Where are they located? What type of litter is used? Unscented or scented? Liners? Covered or uncovered? How often are they scooped? These questions may open the door toward thwarting a potential problem.

The number one reason for inappropriate elimination is due to medical problems. It is imperative that medical reasons for elimination cases be ruled out before a behavioral diagnosis is explored. There are many medical etiologies for both inappropriate urination and defecation, including bladder stones, urinary tract infections, interstitial cystitis, irritable bowel disease, constipation, and hyperthyroidism. If these conditions are allowed to progress, they can be painful for the animal, may cause more serious health issues, and create or exasperate a behavioral problem. Pain from an underlying medical condition can create an aversion to the litter box.

Behavioral reasons for inappropriate elimination generally fall into one of two categories: house training (aversion to the box or preference for another surface) or urine marking (anxiety related). Inappropriate elimination can be a multifaceted issue including medical, house training, and marking components. Cats displaying inappropriate elimination need a thorough medical and behavioral work up to determine an appropriate treatment plan.

- Inappropriate elimination can be a multifaceted issue including medical, house training, and marking components.

- Cats displaying inappropriate elimination need a thorough medical and behavioral work up to determine an appropriate treatment plan.

Feline prevention: crate training

Generally, the carrier comes out in most cat houses for one reason, a trip to the veterinarian. Cats can quickly associate the presence of the carrier with a trip to the doctor, which is not always a pleasant experience for all cats. Cat owners may call to cancel their appointment because they are unable to find the cat or get the cat out from under the bed. Taking some preventive measures early on can alleviate this problem from developing in the first place.

Cat carriers are commonly available in two different materials, plastic or a combination of canvas and mesh. As with puppies, proper introduction is important. Kittens should have the option to go in and out by choice. They will be easily enticed with toys, treats, and comfortable bedding. Clicker training is also an excellent tool for encouraging kittens to enter the crate.

Figure 7.15 Cat cage with multiple levels. A litter box is provided in the lower level and food in the upper level.

Having a cat that is comfortable in a carrier or even a larger cat cage can provide for easy management in multicat households, with introductions to new pets, with convalescence, and also with travel. Commercially available cat cages are large enough to accommodate a litter box, bed, and bowls. They also have several different levels with perches to allow for vertical living space (Figure 7.15).

Feline prevention: handling and restraint

Prevention is very important. Teaching the cat to tolerate restraint and handling at an early age is much easier than treating a cat that is aggressive with handling. Like dogs, cats quickly figure out that being held still or manipulated usually means something unpleasant is about to happen. Canned cat food smeared on the exam room table or delivered on a spoon can be used to facilitate a positive association (classical conditioning) to handling. If the cat becomes frightened and aggressive, avoid punishment. Verbally reprimanding the cat may inhibit its behavior, but it does not make the situation any more pleasant for the cat, or client.

Minimal restraint is generally better tolerated by cats. Towels can be used to aid in the restraint of cats, providing safety and security for the cat and the veterinary staff. Sophia Yin's book, <u>Low Stress Handling, Restraint and Behavior Modification of Dogs & Cats</u>, is a thorough resource for appropriate handling techniques in the veterinary hospital.

> • With cats, the less the restraint that is used, generally, the more the acceptance.

Prevention (canine and feline): introducing a new pet

When bringing a new pet into the household, a few preventive steps should be recommended. Being proactive can sometimes be the difference between successful integration of a new pet versus rejection.

Introductions: dog to dog

Introducing a new puppy or adult dog to resident pets can be of great concern to the owners. Introducing a new puppy to an adult dog that has been well socialized should be relatively smooth. If there is doubt how the interaction will go, neutral territory is best. Adult dogs tend to be less accepting of other adult dogs and the first introduction should be made on neutral territory. It may even be advisable to take the resident dog to the breeder's home or the shelter for the first introduction. Parks and other open areas can also be used. The owner should be relaxed and make all interactions positive ones, using plenty of food treats to reward positive interactions. Sniffing and play bows are good interactions but keep them very brief at first. Any signs of tension should be calmly interrupted and then redirected by cuing a known cue such as come. Once the interactions are going smoothly, they can be moved into the home, repeating the same process.

The resident dog should learn to associate good things with the presence of the new dog. Think of all the activities the resident dog enjoys, such as walks, play, and training. These activities should be performed along with the new dog. Reward appropriate behavior with treats.

It is normal for interactions to include corrections to the puppy from the older dog. This is helping the puppy to learn about dog body language and setting limits on the puppy's interactions. Short of injury, these communications should be allowed between the two dogs. Owners should resist the temptation to interfere as this can complicate relations.

Separate feeding areas should be established for good management. Food bowl guarding is a normal behavior and can be a site of aggression. Chances are they will be on different diets and the separation will prevent them from eating each other's food.

A safe haven should also be established for both the resident dog and the new dog. These areas can be used to give them both a break and allow for alone time. The safe havens should be made as pleasant as possible, using beds and chew toys.

A resident dog that has poor social skills or limited experience with other dogs should be referred for behavior intervention services before the client obtains another dog.

Introductions: cat to cat

The kitten or new cat should be set up in one room. The room should have all necessary resources, including a litter box, scratching station, food, water, bedding, and toys. Although the litter box should be accessible, it should not be in immediate proximity to the rest of the items. It is also a good idea to include a large multilevel cat cage (Figure 7.15).

Introductions to resident cats should be gradual. For the first few days, the new cat should be kept confined in a room. This will give the resident cats the opportunity to become accustomed to the new cat's scent through a closed door. The procedure can be helped along by exchanging bedding between the animals. The scents of the cats can also be mixed by allowing the new cat to explore other parts of the house while confining the resident cats to a room. Another method to mix the scents of the cats is called *artificial allomarking*. A small towel can be rubbed on one cat, then on the other, then again on the first one, then on the second one, and so on. This helps to "mix" the odors and makes a communal scent between the cats.

Ideally, the resident cats and the new cat should become acclimated to their own individual multilevel cat cage. This will aid in the visual introductions of the cats. All cats should be managed in their cage for a special meal time twice a day. Alternatives to the multilevel cat cage are either a travel carrier or a harness and leash. However, all the cats must be comfortable with the confinement method or harness prior to starting the introduction process.

Start at a distance from which the cats can see each other but are not dissuaded from eating their special meal (the furthest distance possible for the layout of the house is best). Each day move the cages a foot closer, until they can be next to each other while eating. Once this has been accomplished, if the resident cats are not

overly interested in the new cat, the owner may consider keeping the new cat in the cat cage for supervised periods of time (if using a travel carrier, place the carrier up on a table or elevated surface) while allowing the resident cats to be loose in the room. This will help to facilitate habituation to the presence of each other. The next step would be to allow the new cat to be loose in the room and the resident cats to be confined to their cat cage. Once it has been determined that amicable interactions are occurring between the cats and they are relaxed in each other's presence, supervised periods of time loose together can be allowed.

If any direct staring, hissing, growling, or other threats are observed, a towel should be placed over the cage to interrupt the threat and the cats should be separated. Aggressive responses should be dealt with by ending the session and waiting 24–48h before attempting again. With the next session, increase the distance between the cats and progress more gradually. Ideally, avoid all negative experiences while introducing the cats. Slower is actually faster because negative experiences will be remembered and will take time to overcome. Pheromone products such as Feliway® may also be useful if the resident cat or the new cat is stressed during the process. It may take 2–6 weeks to accomplish the entire process of new introductions, depending on the individual cats. A quick progression of the same techniques can be used when reintroducing cats after one of the household cats has had a visit to the veterinary clinic. The cat that remained home will often reject the returning cat. Simply mixing their scents and doing a controlled special meal time and gradual introduction over a few hours can be effective in preventing a long-lasting negative reintroduction.

Introductions interspecies

An introduction between a resident dog and a new cat is normally less stressful for both pets than cat-to-cat introductions. The exception to this would be an adult cat that is unfamiliar with dogs or a dog that views the new cat as prey. Before adding a new cat to the household, foundation training is recommended. The dog should be trained to settle on a dog bed or mat so he has an alternative behavior that is not conducive with chasing. In addition, a "look at that" cue (meaning look at an object or animal away from the owner) and a "watch me" cue (look at the owner) should be taught. These opposite cues can allow the owner to make a game of looking at things and looking at the owner, ping ponging back and forth between these two cues. These cues should first be taught in a nondistracting environment with familiar items before incorporating into a session with a new cat in the house. To assess the cat's and dog's reactions to each other, the first interaction should occur with the cat in a multilevel cat cage or elevated travel carrier and the dog on leash. The dog should be rewarded with high-value treats for being able to settle on a mat and play the "look at that–watch me" game. If the dog is intently focused on the cat, the dog should be redirected with a food treat if possible and moved further away from the cat. Once the dog is reliably able to respond to cues and is offering calm behaviors around the cat, gradually allow the cat to have time out of the cat cage with the dog either on leash with the owner or confined to a kennel. The owner continues to reward the dog for calm behavior and response to cues. Eventually, with supervision, the dog can drag the leash (in case redirection is necessary to prevent injury) as the pets become accustomed to each other. If there is any concern about the dog's reaction to the cat, a referral for a behavior consultation should be made and further safety recommendations, such as a basket muzzle, may be necessary. Supervision of both pets is essential during initial introductions.

Care should be taken when introducing a puppy to a household with cats. Many times, this relationship will work out naturally as cats and dogs can be great companions, sometimes better than with their own species. Trouble spots can occur, however, with an overzealous puppy and a fearful cat. Puppies love to chase things but we do not want the cat to be one of them. Attempts can be managed through the use of a leash and redirection to an appropriate toy. Calm behavior while both pets are in the room should be rewarded. Both pets involved need to have safe havens established. For the puppy, this simply means a crate, exercise pen, or a puppy-proofed room. For the cats, this would mean plenty of vertical space and areas they can escape to that are off limits to the puppy. These areas can be set up with cat doors too small for the puppy to get through or areas gated off but off the ground, enough for a cat to slip under.

The cats' food stations, resting areas, and litter boxes should be inaccessible to the puppy and located in the cats' safe area. Establishing these areas will decrease the cats' stress associated with living with a new puppy.

Prevention (canine and feline): children and pets

A pet in a child's life can provide endless hours of companionship and fun. If properly planned, it can be a meaningful and powerful relationship. Pets can be instrumental in teaching a child responsibility, compassion, and empathy.

Some parents may start out thinking they want a dog as a pet for their children but through planning they may discover their life style is more conducive to cat ownership or even a guinea pig. Education can prevent parents from choosing the wrong pet, which may result in relinquishment or, worse yet, injury to the child. Both of these situations can be traumatic for the child and is not a positive learning experience. The experience should be one that promotes responsible pet ownership and the human–animal bond. The pet's well-being should not be solely the child's responsibility. Pet care should always be shared or supervised by all family members to ensure success.

It should be noted that kids and dogs are both egocentric, therefore both do what works best for them. Good kids and good dogs are likely to have misunderstandings every day. Consequently, children and dogs should never be left without adult guidance and direct supervision.

The majority of dog bites involve young children and interactions with a familiar or a family dog. The prevalence of dog bites in children is 2.2% and is double when compared to the general population (Kahn *et al.*, 2004). The majority of children suffer from facial injuries as the result of dog bites (Kahn *et al.*, 2003; Bernardo *et al.*, 2002; Schalomon *et al.*, 2006). The average age of children is 5 years, with boys more commonly bitten than girls. A dog well socialized to children is less likely to bite out of fear. Early appropriate socialization is important for the prevention of future dog bites to adults and children. Predictive factors of aggressive behavior, particularly toward children, include lack of training, little or no socialization with children, aggression over food toys and/or places, being overly sensitive to touch or fearful of people, a history of preying on small animals, or aggression to family members (Lindsay, 2001; Xavier *et al.*, 2008).

Every dog has the potential to bite or show aggression. Even a dog that has been well socialized can still escalate to aggression, depending on the circumstances. Behaviorally normal dogs will get up and walk away in order to avoid confrontation. Children do not always understand the message and parents should be present to intervene and teach their child what is appropriate. It is unrealistic to believe that all dogs should tolerate inappropriate behavior from children. If parents fail to advocate for the dog, unsuccessful attempts to avoid the situation can evolve into aggression. Prevention does not stop with the dog; it also involves teaching children appropriate ways to interact with dogs.

The old adage, "let sleeping dogs lie," is a good rule to follow. Children should be taught to leave dogs alone when the dog is resting, sleeping, eliminating, eating, drinking, hiding, or chewing on a bone or toy. Children should avoid approaching any dog behind a barrier such as a fence, baby gate, or in a kennel. They should be taught to ask for permission to approach and pet an unfamiliar dog. Behaviors from children that have the potential to elicit aggression from a dog include rough play or handling, running after or chasing a dog, hugging, kissing, or crawling on a dog, reaching to pet an unfamiliar or neighborhood dog, teasing, taunting, or barking at a dog, and reprimanding a dog. Children should learn that if a dog is chasing them, they should stop and "be a tree." Movement is often a trigger for the chase and freezing is the safest course of action. Face-to-face interactions between children and all dogs, whether in their own household or elsewhere, should be prevented. Not only may this be perceived as a threat by the dog but the child's face is in a very vulnerable position. Parents should be quick to interrupt and redirect undesirable interactions and reward appropriate ones by the dog or child.

All households with children should include a safe haven for the dog. This area is "off limits" to the children. The dog-only zone can be the crate, an exercise pen, a room that can be closed off, or a combination. Another possibility is circling the dog's mat area with a jump rope and teaching the children they are to stay on their side of the boundary. This dog-only zone should not be a place of punishment but should be made as appealing as possible to the dog. A soft bed and chew toys should be included. The dog's meals can be given here.

The board game Doggone Crazy!™ is intended to introduce the tools children and parents/guardians can use to help reduce the risk of occurrence of a dog bite (Figure 7.16). The board game helps children decide whether a dog is safe or dangerous to approach and teaches children appropriate and inappropriate interactions with a dog. Doggone safe (www.doggonesafe.com) is a nonprofit organization dedicated to dog bite prevention through education and dog bite victim support. They provide educational opportunities for veterinary professionals and the general public.

Cats represent ~10% of bites treated annually in the United States and Canada (dogs 80–85%). The average age of a human for a cat bite is 19–20 years (while for dog bites, the average age is 13) and women are more likely than men to be bitten by a cat. Most cat bites occur on the hands and arms and have a high incident of infection. Often the bites are associated with a person trying to pick up or pet the cat. Bites are more common to be from stray or feral cats (80%) (Barrett *et al.*, 2006). In

Figure 7.16 Doggone Crazy board game. Courtesy of Doggone Crazy. Permission granted by Joan Orr.

the human domestic household, it is usually easy for a cat to evade an approaching child because cats use vertical living space. However, just as with dogs, adults need to teach children appropriate ways to interact with the cat and remain the cat's advocate. Cat-only areas of the house should be designed to allow the cat a safe haven.

Problem solving normal species-specific behavior

We have discussed preventive and management techniques with dogs and cats to set them up for success in the human domestic household. Even with the implementation of these techniques, there are bound to be times that the pet owner will encounter normal behaviors for the species that he/she finds undesirable. This section will explore a general model to help address these behaviors in a positive manner and then apply the model to a variety of normal dog and cat behaviors.

Always, first help the owner decide if the behavior is actually an undesirable behavior. Many owners have read or heard that "Dogs should not be allowed on furniture, sleep in the bed, or eat before you." So they might believe this to be true. What is acceptable behavior for the pet owner will vary from person to person. Some owners enjoy having their cat on the counters, and their dog jump on them, get on furniture, and sleep in the bed; others do not. As long as the behavior is not harmful to the pet, the owner, or other people or animals, it should be the owners who define their expectations for their pet. The animal behavior technician can help owners set realistic expectations and facilitate a harmonious relationship with their pets through consistent and predictable expectations and interactions.

- What is acceptable behavior for the pet owner will vary from person to person. Some owners enjoy having their cat on the counters, and their dog jump on them, get on furniture, and sleep in the bed; others do not. As long as the behavior is not harmful to the pet, the owner, or other people or animals, it should be the owners who define their expectations for their pet.

General problem-solving model

Once you have identified with the owner that this is a behavior that is normal yet undesirable for the owner, it is time to apply the problem-solving model. Although addressing normal undesirable behaviors should be individualized to the particular situation, providing a step-by-step approach can help you keep on track when providing guidance. No two pets or owners are the same and providing a cookbook approach to solving pet owners' concerns should be avoided because it does not necessarily allow for two-way communication to occur. This problem-solving model will allow you to break down behavior and seek positive solutions for addressing everyday canine and feline challenges (it works with people too). This model has been adapted from *Puppy Start Right: Foundation Training for the Companion Dog* by Martin and Martin (2011) (Table 7.5).

The first step is to identify the ABCs. The **A**ntecedent: What is the trigger or stimulus that induces the behavior(s)? The antecedent may be related to a social interaction (human or another animal), a sound, or an inanimate object. Multiple triggers may be identified and the antecedent may be context-specific. Ask yourself, what is the specific situation in which the behavior occurs? At times, the antecedent is not identifiable and may be related to the pet's internal motivation or needs. For example, your dog may be hungry and the temptation of a sandwich just within his reach may be irresistible. The **B**ehavior: Defining the behavior is crucial to solving the problem. What is the problem or undesirable behavior? Looking at the pet's body language and having an understanding of normal and abnormal behavior is helpful. The actual behavior might give insight to the antecedent or trigger, especially when it is related to an internal motivation. The **C**onsequence: The consequence of the behavior should be viewed from the pet's perspective. Initially, ask yourself, what did the pet get out of the situation? Secondarily, especially in social contexts, ask how the consequence of the behavior affects others.

The second step is to determine the motivation. Identifying the ABCs will often give insight into the motivation. Dogs and cats are amoral, opportunistic, and self-centered. They are not spiteful or malicious. In order to simplify motivation, the behavior will be either self-rewarding for the pet or human reinforced. Is the behavior self-rewarding? Self-rewarding behaviors offer an immediate benefit to the pet. For example, a full bladder is emptied and the dog or cat feels better. Is the behavior reinforced by human attention? Human-reinforced behaviors generally relate to behaviors that are socially motivated. For example, a mouthing and jumping puppy is looked at, talked to, and petted. The meowing cat is fed. Some behaviors may be a combination of both: self-rewarding and human reinforced.

Once the ABCs and motivation have been identified, the next step is to explore if the behavior can be prevented or managed. Can the pet owner prevent or manage the behavior in a humane way? For example, can you supervise the dog or cat or confine him so the majority of eliminations are only on a preferred substrate (outside or litter box, respectively)? Can you avoid access to the pantry or shoe closet? Prevention and management controls the learning environment and sets the pet up to succeed. However, it does not address the underlying motivation or change the behavior. Sometimes, managing or avoiding the situation will provide the relief an owner was searching for. No further help is required. Remember though that this has not changed the behavior in any way. So although the trashcan is no longer available to the pet, a desire to search or discover things has not been fulfilled. Providing appropriate outlets for the pet with techniques previously discussed in the enrichment and management sections is imperative.

Table 7.5 Problem-solving model.

Identify the ABCs	Antecedent
	Behavior
	Consequence
Determine motivation	Self-rewarding?
	Human reinforced?
	Both?
Prevention or management	Prevent practicing of the behavior. Proactively reward appropriate behavior
	Provide appropriate outlets
	Prevention/management does not change the behavior; it controls the learning history
Solve it!	Ignore/Avoid reinforcing
	Response substitution

If the behavior cannot be prevented or managed, then there are two options for "solving it." These options depend on whether the pet's motivation is self-rewarding or reinforced by humans. If the motivation and consequence of the behavior is human attention, the behavior should ideally be ignored (not reinforced). Behaviors that are not self-reinforcing or rewarding to the pet will cease to occur if ignored. If the reward for the behavior is social interaction, that is, he jumps on you and you push him away, he nudges you and you pet him, he barks or meows and you let him out of his crate, it is likely that ignoring the pet in these situations will cause the learned behavior to cease. Ignoring means not looking at, talking to, or touching the pet at these times. Initially, the attention-getting behavior will worsen because in the past it has always worked, but if you continue to ignore the behavior, it will disappear.

It is important to realize that pets also need to communicate information to us. So there will be times the pet will be asking for you to meet a specific need through these attention-seeking behaviors. The dog that needs to urinate might come to you and then run to the door. He is trying to tell you he needs to eliminate. Respond to this request. Equally as important to ignoring undesirable behavior is making sure that the mental, social, and physical needs of the pet are being met (prevention). Providing adequate outlets through routine potty breaks, walks, play, and positive training will often drastically decrease the frequency of attention-seeking behaviors.

> • Providing adequate outlets through routine potty breaks, walks, play, and positive training will often drastically decrease the frequency of attention-seeking behaviors.

Behaviors that are self-reinforcing or self-rewarding cannot be ignored. For example, for the teething puppy, chewing on a chair may provide relief. As chewing is self-rewarding, it cannot be ignored. Three steps to follow for response substitution are as follows:

1. Interrupt the behavior by getting the pet's attention. You might call his name in an upbeat tone or softly clap your hands. The interrupter should not be frightening or an indicator of impending punishment. The word "NO" or "Ahh-ahh" should not be used because it has a negative connotation and may cause an aversive emotional response or fear.

2. Cue an alternate appropriate behavior that is incompatible with the undesirable one before the problem behavior begins or after interruption of the behavior. For example, the dog that greets people by jumping on them is cued to "sit" before he jumps. The dog cannot jump and sit at the same time.

3. Reward the pet for the appropriate behavior with a food treat.

Problems with aversive training techniques and equipment

You may have noticed that the problem-solving model focuses on identifying desirable behavior and rewarding the pet. There is no need to communicate to the pet what you do not want or what they did "wrong." Verbal or physical reprimands are often used because the pet owner feels the pet needs to know "he did wrong." Shouting "No" or "Ahh" has a negative association, is positive punishment, or a predictor of positive punishment. A verbal or physical reprimand may suppress behavior, but it does not teach or tell the pet to perform an appropriate behavior in any given situation. Instead teach owners to focus on what they want their pet to do and reward them for those behaviors. Making the pet successful through management and training will enhance the human–animal bond.

Punishment-based training collars such as pinch collars, choke chains, and electric collars are aversive and meant to induce pain/discomfort. The use of these techniques may lead to the development of fear, anxiety, and/or aggressive behavior.

Although aversive techniques often do inhibit behavior, they are riddled with problems and therefore should not be recommended. The effects of coercive or aversive training include the following:
• It damages the human–animal bond.
• Not only does it inhibit the pet at the moment but it also inhibits learning and all behavior. If the pet is worried about being reprimanded it is difficult to try to learn something new. Aversive training can induce learned helplessness.
• It induces anxiety, fear of the handler, or of the environmental situation. One cannot control the pet's perceived association that is going to be made when the aversive is applied. A dog may become aggressive with other dogs because of an association of the correction on a pinch collar and the approach of other dogs. The handler may have intended to correct the dog for pulling to visit the other dogs, but may inadvertently create a serious behavior issue.
• It has been shown to induce aggression toward humans and other animals.

- It does not change the motivation for the behavior. Nor does it teach the pet what is appropriate in the context or appease the pet's desire to perform the behavior. Important warning signs or communication may be inhibited by correction, thus creating a pet that is less likely to give warning and consequently is more dangerous.

> - Although aversive techniques often do inhibit behavior, they are riddled with problems and therefore should not be recommended.

Alternatives to correction-based collars are head halters and front clip harnesses. They can aid an owner who has difficulty controlling the dog. If properly introduced, most dogs tolerate them well. However, some dogs will find them restrictive or perhaps even a little irritating, thus causing frustration. The key is that head collars and harnesses are not designed to inflict pain; instead they provide a leverage perspective which makes it more difficult for the dog to pull forward. They are appropriate and sometimes necessary tools for management with some dogs until the desired behavior has been taught.

Problem solving typical canine behaviors

Even after setting up an ideal environment for learning with appropriate management and a consistent routine, there will still be normal behaviors that a canine will exhibit that may be problematic for the pet owner. Let us apply the problem-solving model to several normal behaviors of dogs such as mouthing/play biting, chewing, taking items, jumping on people, digging, and barking.

Mouthing and play biting

Mouthing is a normal social behavior in dogs. Puppies learn to control the pressure of their bite from playing with other puppies. When one puppy bites too hard, the other puppy yelps and stops playing. This ends the play, teaching the puppy bite inhibition. Although mouthing is normal in canine social circles, it can be problematic when directed at humans. Puppies need to learn that mouthing or biting people is not the way to prompt people to play.

The antecedent is the presence of people and the desire to interact with them. The behavior itself may involve mouthing the hands, grabbing clothes or nipping at the person's legs in a playful manner. The consequence is generally some form of reaction from the person or a

fun game of tug on the person's clothes. The motivation for mouthing is a social one; the dog is seeking a friendly interaction with the person.

Owners can be advised to avoid playing with puppies with their hands, clothes, or shoes. They can also teach their puppy to play with toys or a tug for an appropriate outlet for this behavior. Meeting the social, physical, and mental needs through routine and environmental enrichment will help to minimize mouthing and play biting. When unable to address the problem, the dog should be managed safely in his confinement area to prevent the perpetuation of the undesirable behavior.

Often puppies will exhibit increased mouthing during certain times of the day, which usually correspond with increased level of activity. Many puppy owners report that when the family attempts to settle down for the evening is a common time for increased activity and mouthing. Behaviors such as running laps (zoomies), jumping on people and furniture, along with or without the mouthing are commonly described. This is normal behavior in puppies that is designed to expel excess energy that usually occurs in the evening or another predictable time. Sometimes this behavior can be intercepted by a walk prior to the normal time of onset or by teaching it to settle on a mat with food-dispensing toys.

As it is a solicitation for play and interaction, the owner should immediately withdraw attention to avoid reinforcing the behavior. The instant the puppies teeth touch human skin or clothes, the person should freeze for a second. If the puppy has stopped nipping, an appropriate toy should be offered to provide an outlet for mouthing. The owner should interact with the puppy with the toy instead (Figure 7.17). When

Figure 7.17 Person playing with a puppy with a long tug toy to encourage mouthing of the toy rather than her hands, arms, or legs.

the behavior persists or results in torn clothing or physical injury, it may not be possible to just ignore the behavior. In this case, the puppy owner can redirect and reward an alternate appropriate response (response substitution). The person should calmly and quietly withdraw attention for 2–3 s. Then they can redirect the puppy to sit or perform any alternate behavior other than mouthing and then reward by offering a treat or toy (Table 7.6).

Caution owners to resist the urge to do any type of physical or verbal corrections. Any infliction of pain or discomfort must be avoided. This includes methods such as grabbing the muzzle, pinching the tongue, biting the puppy back, or pushing a fist into the puppy's mouth. Any such methods will serve to make the puppy fearful or defensive, both of which can promote aggression. They do not teach the puppy an acceptable way to play with the owner and can result in a dog that becomes head or hand shy.

Placing the puppy in its crate is helpful when the owner needs a time out. Puppies can become overly tired and overly aroused. If the owners become frustrated with the puppy, they may lose their temper and punish the puppy. At those times it is better to put the puppy in its crate rather than allow it to continue to learn the wrong things.

Table 7.6 Canine mouthing and play biting.

Identify the ABCs	• Antecedent: People present and normal natural social behavior of dogs (especially puppies) • Behavior: Bites or mouths hands/legs or clothes of people • Consequence: Usually some type of social interaction from people
Determine motivation	Generally human attention seeking
Prevention or management	• Avoid play with hands or clothes • Teach the dog to play with toys or tugs • Use confinement if unable to address at the time • Meet the dog's social, physical, and mental needs through routine and enrichment
Solve it!	• Ignore: freeze or remove attention to avoid reinforcing • Redirect to an appropriate toy to mouth when the dog is not mouthing the person • Response substitution when unable to ignore

There are simply times when a puppy becomes overly stimulated and does not have the ability to calm down, similar to an over-tired child. During these times, placing the puppy in the crate or other area of confinement provides the needed opportunity to relax. Confinement can be used to manage the situation but should not be used to punish the behavior. The puppy should be rewarded for going to the confinement area. This technique is not designed to teach the dog appropriate or inappropriate behavior but instead to provide relief to the owner and help calm the dog down. Often, after a few minutes, the puppy will fall asleep.

Chewing

Chewing is a normal exploratory behavior of puppies and adolescent dogs. It is comparable to a human one-year-old child who places objects in its mouth because it is both exploring its environment and teething. Chewing may be associated with teething or a recreational exploration of the world with the mouth. It is important to note that chewing is also an anxiety reliever. Although considered a normal behavior, if it becomes excessive, it could be a symptom of a larger problem. If the chewing is excessive or only associated with the owner's departure, this could be a sign of an underlying anxiety disorder.

The antecedent is the access to items to chew and a normal desire to explore the environment. It could also be associated with the discomfort of teething. The exact behavior will be defined by what items the dog is chewing, although all are nonhuman approved items for chewing. The consequence is the desire to explore and chew has been satisfied. The motivation for chewing is self-rewarding!

Management and supervision are extremely important to prevent dogs from developing undesirable chewing habits. A puppy-proofed confinement area should be utilized when the young dog is unable to be directly supervised. Access to the puppy's favorite inappropriate chew items should be blocked. A lack of stimulation may lead to excessive chewing; ensure all the social, physical, and mental needs are being met through routine enrichment activities. The owner should be encouraged to reward and encourage chewing on appropriate objects; catch the dog getting it right! To prevent a preference for items that have human scent, avoid offering objects to chew that are concentrated with human scent, such as old shoes, socks, or shirts. It will not know the difference between an old or new pair of shoes. Similarly, provide a variety of appropriate chew toys.

Chewing cannot be ignored because the behavior is self-rewarding. The owner will need to use response substitution, call the dog's name in an upbeat tone or clap hands to get its attention, call it to you, and provide an appropriate chew toy. It is best to be proactive. If the owner sees the dog ready to chew on a chair leg, redirect it to an appropriate hard chew toy before it makes the undesirable choice (Table 7.7).

Verbal or physical reprimands will only teach your dog that it is unsafe to chew the chair when you are around. It will instead do it in your absence. Make chewing on appropriate objects more rewarding. It may be necessary to make inappropriate objects aversive through the use of a commercially available taste deterrent. These products need to be applied daily as they do lose their potency and they only seem to work in about 50% of patients. Good chewing habits will be developed through management, supervision, and providing appropriate chewing alternatives.

Stealing objects

Stealing is another common concern of clients and one that is easily reinforced by family members. It should be noted, from the puppy's perspective there is no such thing as "stealing." They are amoral creatures and stealing is a human rationalized statement. Some puppies enjoy being chased and will quickly catch on to the game. Over time the puppy may become anxious when chased and develop guarding issues.

Dogs are opportunistic and they have a great sense of smell. Dogs are also curious and explore their world with their mouth. You can see how a piece of pizza left on the

Table 7.7 Canine chewing.

Identify the ABCs	• Antecedent: Access to items to chew and a natural desire to explore • Behavior: Chewing of nonhuman approved items • Consequence: Desire for exploration and chewing has been fulfilled
Determine motivation	Self-rewarding!
Prevention or management	• Manage access • Supervision • Provide a variety of appropriate chew toys • Reward appropriate chewing • Meet the dog's social, physical, and mental needs through routine and enrichment
Solve it!	• Response substitution; interrupt, redirect, reward

counter might go missing. Dogs are likely to check out the kitchen counter, trash cans, or coffee table at some point. What they learn when this happens will set the course for future behavior.

The antecedent is items within reach and normal exploratory behavior. The behavior itself may involve taking food or nonfood based items found in the house and ingesting or chewing them. From the dog's perspective the consequence can be ingestion of yummy food, exploration with a novel chew item, or a fun game of chase while the owners try to retrieve the item.

The motivation can be exploratory or appetitive. It can also develop into an attention-getting behavior. If the dog learns that taking an object in front of people gets a reaction, it is likely to repeat it. On the other hand, many dogs will check the counters, trash can, and tables because they smell food. If this behavior pays off on occasion, this will make for a very strong behavior resistant to extinction. It is just like playing the slot machine: sometimes you hit the jackpot. Typical consequences that perpetuate counter surfing and object stealing may include finding food, a game of chase, a verbal reprimand (this is attention), physical contact, or any combination of the above.

Preventing this behavior involves good management by all family members. Keeping items picked up and floors free of socks and other temptations will allow the dog to be successful. It may be necessary to block access to the problem areas through the use of baby gates or an exercise pen. Keep the counters clean and place the trash can in a cupboard or closet. Many covered trash cans designed to make it difficult for a dog to access the contents are commercially available. Proactively, teach the dog to settle on a dog bed located outside of the kitchen or away from the table. Resting on his bed is the place to be when people are in the kitchen or sitting at the table (Figure 7.18). While the process of "settle on a bed" behavior is being taught, the dog should be crated or confined to an area during meal times to prevent the practicing of undesirable behavior. A frozen food storage device (toy) will help occupy the dog on his bed or in his confinement area. Advise owners to only offer treats and food outside of the kitchen so the area is not associated with obtaining food. It is important that the dog is provided appropriate opportunities to appease his exploratory motivation through games suggested in the section titled **Canine environmental enrichment**.

There are a variety of possible scenarios with this behavior and the response will vary depending on the circumstances.

Scenario 1: Dog checks out the counter or coffee table but there is nothing it can get. It is best to just ignore

Figure 7.18 Dog settling on a mat just outside the kitchen while the owner prepares food.

this behavior. Exploration is normal and if it does not pay off (with food or human attention) it will decrease in frequency.

Scenario 2: The dog is checking the counters and there are items in reach but it has not obtained it yet. The best course of action is to use response substitution; gently interrupt/distract by clapping your hands to get your dog's attention, give him a cue you have previously taught ("Leave it," "Place," "Sit," "Come"), and reward him for the alternate behavior.

Scenario 3: The dog has an item. It is important that owners avoid chasing the dog because this just makes for a fun game of "keep away" and increases the dog's perceived value of the object. It can also lead to guarding of objects.

- If it is a low value object (i.e., a paper towel, tissue) that will not harm the dog, it is best for owners to ignore the situation. They should not look at or say anything to the dog; instead they can leave the room. The dog may follow. Any reaction from the owner will increase the value of the item and risks reinforcing the behavior as a way to get the owner's attention. The dog likely will grow bored of the item on his own and walk away. Owners should reevaluate their prevention and management system, to avoid continued opportunities for the behavior.
- If the dog obtains a high-value object (i.e., cell phone, wallet, candy bar) or one that may cause him harm, the owner has three options:

1. Response substitution: If the dog knows a release cue, the owner can prompt the release and reward for complying.

2. Distraction: If the dog does not yet know a release cue, the owner can create a distraction by such means as ringing the door bell, crinkling cellophane or giving another pet or person a hug or acting silly and running out of the room with the dog's favorite toy. This diversion will likely cause the dog to drop the item to investigate. The item can be picked up while the dog's focus is elsewhere.

3. Exchange: If the dog is not dissuaded by the distraction, then the owner can use a special treat such as a piece of cheese, hotdog, or sandwich meat, to prompt the dog to release the item. The dog can be led away from the object by giving it several treats. Once he is in another room or outside, the owner can return to pick up the object without having the dog underfoot.

The distraction and exchange should not substitute for appropriate management and teaching the dog to willingly relinquish objects (Table 7.8).

Owners should be advised when a dog retreats under a bed or table and hunkers down over a stolen item, the dog should NOT BE CONFRONTED. Safely distract the dog out of hiding using a toy or special treat in exchange for the object. Guarding as a young puppy can be the first sign that the puppy is not comfortable or is in conflict and should be investigated more fully.

Verbal or physical reprimands are not advised as they will only teach a dog to explore and take items when people are not around and ultimately can lead to a serious guarding issue.

Commercial pet deterrents are available to punish this exploratory behavior, but they should not be used as a

Table 7.8 Stealing objects.

Identify the ABCs	• Antecedent: Access to items and a desire to explore/chew
	• Behavior: Takes or investigates nonhuman approved items.
	• Consequence: Game of chase and/or desire to explore and chew has been met
Determine motivation	Self-rewarding but can also be attention seeking
Prevention or management	• Block access, keep items out of reach
	• Teach to settle on a mat
	• Meet the dogs social, physical, and mental needs through routine and enrichment
Solve it!	• Ignore
	• Response substitution
	• Distract
	• Exchange

first option strategy. Gadgets and gizmos are never a substitute for teaching an appropriate response and they can have unpleasant side effects, eliciting fear and anxiety in dogs.

Jumping on people

Jumping is a normal and friendly greeting behavior of dogs. Puppies learn to solicit attention and feeding through jumping and licking the commissure of their mother's lips and muzzle. Dogs jump on people in an attempt to show affection and it is usually intended as a friendly gesture. If the pet owners do not want their dog to jump when greeting them or others, then it will be necessary to teach the dog an alternate greeting behavior.

The antecedent for jumping is the presence of people and a natural greeting behavior of dogs. The behavior can be defined as jumping on a person in friendly greeting. The context (arrival home after a long or short departure) and the target of the jumping (familiar versus unfamiliar people) may vary from case to case. The consequence generally involves some type of social interaction from people.

The motivation for the behavior is excitement and social interaction. Because dogs are social, typical human responses that perpetuate jumping may include an eye glance, a verbal reprimand, physical contact, such as pushing the dog off, or any combination of the above.

Prevention and management techniques should be geared toward rewarding an alternate behavior and managing the learning history to set the dog up to be successful from the beginning. Owners should initially make their social interactions and greetings very calm. The higher the excitement level, the more likely the dog will jump. To prevent the escalation of jumping, owners should avoid encouraging the puppy to jump on them. However, because many owners actually enjoy it when their dog jumps on them, an alternative is to teach the dog to jump when cued. To help prevent others from reinforcing the dog for jumping, a leash can be utilized to prevent the behavior. Expecting a sit may be too much at first with young puppies or over-exuberant greeters. Owners should be encouraged to catch their dog with four feet on the floor and reward the dog for not jumping.

Alternatively, telling the dog what to do before it makes the undesirable choice of jumping will help it learn faster. The owner should also reward the dog often for sitting. The dog will learn that sitting, rather than jumping, results in people turning, looking at, talking

Figure 7.19 A puppy being rewarded with treats and attention for a calm greeting.

to, and petting it. Thus, the act of sitting becomes an appropriate greeting behavior. (See Figure 7.19).

A release cue, such as "make a friend," can teach the dog when it is time to visit and greet guests. Combined with "settle on a mat," the dog is rewarded for going to his mat while the guest enters the home and then calmly released to "make a friend" if appropriate in the context.

Regardless of how well a preventive system is implemented, there are likely to be times that jumping will still occur. Counseling owners on how to respond to jumping should promote a positive learning experience for the dog. Remember, we are teaching them a human-approved appropriate greeting that is not a natural greeting behavior in their repertoire. If the dog jumps, the owner should avoid reinforcing it with any form of attention (eye contact, talking, or even reprimanding). The best response is no response at all. It might be necessary for the person to step back or away to avoid the initial contact and protect himself/herself. If the person is sitting, he/she can calmly and quietly stand up and look away. When the dog is not jumping, it can then be rewarded with calm attention and even better, a treat placed on the ground or close to the ground.

Table 7.9 Jumping on people.

Identify the ABCs	• Antecedent: Presence of people and natural greeting behavior • Behavior: Jumps on person • Consequence: Tactile contact and attention
Determine motivation	Human attention seeking
Prevention or management	• Calm greetings • Reward 4 feet on the floor • Use a leash if needed • Reward sitting often • Teach "settle on mat" and "make a friend" cues • Meet the dog's social, physical, and mental needs through routine and enrichment
Solve it!	• Ignore/avoid reinforcing • Response substitution if necessary

There are times when trying to ignore the behavior of an over-exuberant dog is not possible because it hurts or the dog simply continues to jump. Likely just making any contact with the person can act to reinforce the behavior. If the behavior cannot be ignored, response substitution can be used:

1. Calmly and quietly withdraw attention for 2–3 s.
2. Redirect the dog to sit, down, or any behavior incompatible with jumping.
3. Reward the alternate behavior with a treat and calm attention. Over-exuberant praise is likely to result in more jumping (Table 7.9).

It is important to emphasize to owners that verbal and physical reprimands should be avoided. Shouting "NO," swatting, pushing, or kneeing the dog in the chest, may inhibit the jumping, but they are counterproductive techniques that can often result in fearful or shy dogs. It would be analogous to introducing yourself to a person by reaching to shake his/her hand and the person yells at you or slaps you. Punishment for jumping does not teach a dog how to interact appropriately and may cause or directly contribute to the development of serious aggression toward the owners or others.

Digging

Some breeds of dogs are more likely to dig than others. Terriers are notorious for being diggers. Terrier comes from the Latin word, "Terra" meaning "of the earth." Many terrier and some hound breeds have been selectively bred to dig and chase vermin underground. Regardless of the dog's breeding, all dogs have the potential to dig.

Antecedents for digging can include access to digging areas, normal exploratory behavior, and potentially escape behavior. Sometimes the behavior will involve digging holes in flower beds or in the middle of the yard. If the digging occurs along a fence line it could be an attempt to escape the confinement. Digging can have a variety of consequences such as finding things, a cool/warm spot to rest, or escape.

The motivation for digging is self-rewarding. Digging can occur for a multitude of reasons. The motivation can include the following:

1. Thermoregulation: To keep warm or cool when outside for prolonged periods of time.
2. Hunting: Insects or other animals. Dogs can smell and hear animals in the ground.
3. Burying: Hiding a treasured item to be recovered later.
4. Escape or anxiety: This usually involves digging along a fence line. For example, a dog may become panicked by a thunderstorm or an intact male dog may be motivated to roam the neighborhood.

Supervision will play a role in preventing this behavior from starting in the first place. If a dog that enjoys digging is left unattended in a suitable digging location, it will do what is natural for it. Blocking access to these areas can remove the temptation for the dog. Lack of stimulation may lead to excessive digging. Routine scheduled walks, play time, and training are important. Time in the backyard alone should not be a substitute for human initiated exercise and interactions.

To provide the dog with an appropriate place to dig, owners may decide to give the dog a digging box. Similar to a sand box for a child, a digging box for the dog can provide it with hours of appropriate digging entertainment (Figure 7.20). The digging box can be made enticing to the dog by hiding treats in the substrate and rewarding it for showing interest in the digging spot.

Figure 7.20 Example of providing a digging box for the dog to provide an appropriate outlet for this exploratory behavior.

So what should the owners do if they catch their dog digging in an inappropriate location? Verbal or physical reprimands will teach the dog it is unsafe to do in front of people, so it will learn to do it when it is safe; no people around. Digging cannot be ignored because the behavior is self-rewarding. The owner will need to use response substitution.

1. In an upbeat tone, call the dog's name or clap your hands to get his attention.
2. Call him to you.
3. Redirect him to an appropriate digging area, a short game of play, or other incompatible behavior, and reward (Table 7.10).

Advise owners to be proactive. If they see their dog getting ready to dig, redirect it before it makes the undesirable choice.

Placing the dog's feces in the unwanted digging spot will make that area unattractive. However, without supervision, management, and appropriate alternatives, the dog may find a new location to dig.

Barking

Some breeds of dogs are genetically predisposed to barking. The ability to vocalize was an important feature required for some dogs to do a job. Classic examples are some of the herding breeds, such as shelties and corgis, which depended on barking to move livestock on a farm. Barking is also a method for dogs to communicate within their own species and with humans. Different pitches in barking can mean different things. There can be multiple antecedents and consequences for barking, therefore identifying the ABCs of this behavior will be important.

Table 7.10 Digging.

Identify the ABCs	• Antecedent: access to digging areas, exploration, escape, anxiety
	• Behavior: Digs in yard or flower beds
	• Consequence: finds things, makes a comfortable resting spot, escapes
Determine motivation	Self-rewarding!
Prevention or management	• Direct supervision
	• Block access
	• Provide digging location
	• If applicable, address underlying anxiety
	• Meet the dog's social, physical, and mental needs through routine and enrichment
Solve it!	• Response substitution

Possible triggers or antecedents for barking include desire for human attention, physical and mental needs (hunger, elimination, social contact), a sound (car door, doorbell), or presentation of a feared stimulus. The behavior will vary in the pitch of the barking and the accompanying body language of the dog depending on the trigger/antecedent that started it. High-pitched barking is generally a distance-decreasing signal (come closer), while low-pitched barking is a distance-increasing signal (go away). The consequence of the behavior will also be variable. Consequences that typically perpetuate barking include human responses in the case of barking triggered by social or physical needs and cessation of the sound or stimulus in the latter example.

The motivation for the behavior will vary. It can be self-rewarding and it also can be human attention seeking. The antecedents and consequences will make the distinction in motivation.

Prevention of excessive barking often relies on the owners being able to meet the physical, mental, and social needs of their companion. Some dogs have more needs than others. Early and continued proper socialization can help curb the development of stimuli or sound-induced barking.

Blocking visual or auditory access to the dog's triggers will inhibit the practicing of the barking behavior. This can be accomplished by blocking access out of the front windows or gates with window film, blinds, or screens. A white noise machine or classical music can be utilized to minimize outside sounds. Classical music has been shown to have a calming effect on dogs in the shelter setting (Wells *et al.*, 2002).

The important foundation skill of settling on a mat should be trained early and incorporated with times that might induce high arousal and consequently barking. The owner can proactively redirect the dog to settle in his kennel or mat when the owner is preparing food or answering the door. It is much easier to ignore a quiet dog than it is to ignore a barking one. Counseling owners to recognize and reward their dogs when they are quiet and calm can also be helpful in preventing unwanted barking.

Depending on the circumstances barking can either be ignored or response substitution can be applied. Attention and communication barking, if undesirable to the owner, should be ignored. However, it is important to educate owners that frequent attention barking is usually a sign that the dog's mental, physical, and social needs are not being met. Ignoring the barking will prevent owner reinforcement of the behavior but does not address the underlying issue. If the dog is barking at a stimulus, response substitution (interrupt, cue an alternate behavior, reward) can alleviate the situation at the moment (Table 7.11).

Dogs bark; this is normal. However, excessive barking or reactivity can be a sign of underlying fear and/or anxiety. Behavioral intervention services may be warranted.

Problem solving typical feline behaviors

Feline behavior concerns that are normal behaviors for cats include play biting and/or scratching and scratching which causes damage to property. The same problem-solving model can be used to analyze and create positive solutions for these natural behaviors.

Play biting and scratching

Play biting and scratching is a normal behavior of cats. Cats will bite and scratch in other contexts not associated with play but here we are specifically addressing a play behavior. They interact and explore their world with their feet and mouth. Cat bites and scratches have the potential to cause severe infections so should not be taken lightly. On average, 80% of cat bites caused by punctures will become infected. It is important to address feline play biting and scratching of humans because it can become a dangerous problem in the human household. The antecedent for this particular behavior is the presence of people and the cat's desire to play. The behavior itself may involve the cat stocking the owner and ambushing them as they walk down a hallway. It is often displayed when owners play with the

cat with their hands. The consequence of the behavior is generally some kind of reaction from the human. The motivation for this particular type of biting and scratching is human attention.

To prevent this behavior, owners should be advised to only play with their cat with toys. Playing with the cat with their hands can create a problem that can be very damaging to the human–animal bond. Providing environmental enrichment and a set routine for play time and training can funnel this desire to appropriate outlets. Although not recommended with puppies, obtaining two kittens at the same time is advantageous, especially in regard to providing an interactive playmate.

Recommended treatment for play biting and scratching involves a combination of ignoring and response substitution. When preventive measures have failed, owners should be instructed to immediately freeze and withdraw any attention, the moment the cat begins to mouth or scratch them. If the cat knows a stationing cue (go to a perch or cat tree) or a sit cue, the owner can cue that after withdrawing attention for a few seconds. If no cues are known, then the cat should simply be ignored for a few seconds while the owner remains still. In both scenarios the cat should be redirected to an appropriate toy (wand type chase toys) to play with the owner (Table 7.12).

As with dogs, positive punishment (squirt bottles, verbal reprimands) should be avoided because it creates fear

Table 7.11 Barking.

Identify the ABCs	• Antecedent: social interaction, physical or mental needs, response to a sound or other stimuli • Behavior: Variety of forms of barking depending on the trigger • Consequence: Attention, needs met, stimuli goes away
Determine motivation	Can be human attention seeking or self-rewarding
Prevention or management	• Meet the dog's social, physical, and mental needs through routine and enrichment • Proper early and continued socialization • Block access to stimuli • Reward quiet and calm behavior • Teach "settle on a mat"
Solve it!	• Ignore or • Response substitution

Table 7.12 Feline play biting and scratching.

Identify the ABCs	• Antecedent: People present and normal, natural social behavior of cats (especially kittens) • Behavior: Bites or scratches hands/legs of people • Consequence: Usually some type of social interaction from people
Determine motivation	Generally human attention seeking
Prevention or management	• Avoid play with hands • Play with cat with appropriate toys • Obtain two kittens at the same time • Meet the cat's social, physical, and mental needs through routine and enrichment
Solve it!	• Ignore: Freeze or remove attention to avoid reinforcing • Redirect to an appropriate toy to mouth when the cat is not biting or scratching the person • Response substitution if the cat knows a stationing or sit cue

and distrust and can lead to more serious aggression. Positive punishment does not appease the cat's motivation for friendly play nor does it teach the cat an appropriate way to interact with people.

Destructive scratching

Scratching is a normal behavior of cats. Approximately 60% of house cats will scratch furniture without the presence of any underlying behavioral problem (Morgan and Houpt, 1990). The potential problem of scratching should be considered before obtaining a cat. Because the behavior is normal, it is not realistic to eliminate the behavior completely. Scratching objects serves to remove dead cells from their nails. Scratching is also used as a form of territorial communication or marking. It leaves both a visual and chemical scent on the object. Pheromones secreted from the scent glands between the pads of the feet are left on the surface. The antecedent for scratching items is access to items that stimulate the behavior in the cat as well as an innate desire to scratch. The behavior is more common in multicat households where there is social tension among cats. In solitary cat households, the presence of other cats outside the home may be a trigger. While some cats seem to prefer to scratch on vertical surfaces, other cats will choose to scratch horizontal ones. The behavior will vary depending on the individual cat's preferences. The motivation for this behavior is self-rewarding and consequently, it will not go away if ignored.

Owners should attempt to prevent the undesirable scratching by providing an appropriate outlet. Keeping the cat's nails trimmed may also decrease the need to scratch. The cat's preferred location and surface attributes (position-vertical/horizontal, height, type of material) should be noted. A scratching post or board that mimics the preferred attributes should be provided near the object the cat is likely to scratch. This provides a human-approved alternative. All cat owners should provide their cat with multiple scratching posts/boards. Most commercially available scratching posts/boards will be covered with sisal, fabric, carpet, or corrugated cardboard. Favored locations for scratching seem to be near sleeping areas and in other prominent areas of the home which the cat chooses to frequent. Encourage owners to reward the cat for interest in the scratching post. Catnip and the dispersion of toys near or on the scratching post/board may make it more intriguing. Blocking access to certain items and supervision will be necessary while funneling scratching to a preferred location. If unable to block access, making the location unattractive, via the use of double sided sticky tape or plastic, is an option. Feliway® spray (www.feliway.com)

is a commercial product that can be applied to scratched objects to induce cheek gland marking of objects, which is preferable to scratching. Plastic coated sheaths may also be routinely applied to the cat's nails to prevent damage to furniture.

If the cat is scratching an inappropriate object, the owner should use response substitution; gently interrupt the behavior, call the cat away, reward, and redirect to an appropriate scratching area (Table 7.13).

Excessive scratching can be a sign of anxiety and may warrant behavioral intervention services to address the underlying anxiety issue.

Prevention services

The behavior technician should take the lead to provide prevention services within the hospital. Because prevention services do not require a diagnosis and treatment plan from a veterinarian, this is an amenity the technician can provide without the need for direct supervision by the veterinarian. Not only will vital experiences and information be shared but also the high achieving technician can manage and supervise these services, adding to job satisfaction.

This section explores several prevention services, including pet selection counseling, puppy and kitten classes, juvenile, adolescent, and adult dog classes, private training lessons, and special topic seminars or classes.

Pet selection counseling

Pet selection counseling is one of the most valuable, yet under-utilized, services available to owners. Also

Table 7.13 Feline destructive scratching.

Identify the ABCs	• Antecedent: Innate behavior of cats • Behavior: Scratches nonhuman approved objects causing destruction • Consequence: Pacifies innate desire
Determine motivation	Self-rewarding
Prevention or management	• Avoid access to objects or make them less attractive • Feliway® to promote cheek marking • Reward appropriate scratching • Plastic sheaths applied to nails • Meet the cat's social, physical, and mental needs through routine and provide appropriate scratching areas
Solve it!	• Response substitution and redirect to appropriate scratching location

referred to as *pre-adoption* or *pre-purchase counseling*, this type of service provides guidance prior to the acquisition of a pet. It can decrease the possibility of mismatches by ensuring that owners have the information necessary to make educated decisions before bringing a new pet into the home.

> • Pet selection counseling is one of the most valuable, yet under-utilized, services available to owners.

A well-planned program encourages clients to consider whether this is the appropriate time to acquire a new pet and whether the pet they are interested in is suited to their lifestyle. This is also an opportunity to assess expectations of the entire household toward a new pet and instill realistic expectations about the responsibility associated with pet ownership.

There are several components present in every successful selection service. They are keys to having a program that achieves the desired results.

Although knowledgeable counselors can advise and guide clients in their selection of an appropriate pet, they should not be expected to choose the specific breed, age, or sex of the pet for the owner. Counselors should possess and demonstrate a working knowledge of the breed or species-specific traits for many of the animals commonly considered as household pets. This includes the normal growth and developmental stages. Species-specific and breed-specific behavior refers to those behaviors commonly engaged in by members of a species or breed within a species.

A good example of species-specific behavior is the inherent desire felines have to scratch. This trait serves multiple purposes. Scratching allows cats to expend excess energy, stretch their bodies, flex their feet, and tone muscles, mark their territory both visually and with scent, and remove the dead sheaths from their claws. All domestic cats, including those that are declawed, exhibit this behavior in some form or another. A knowledgeable counselor, aware that this behavior is not something owners can prevent, will instead educate owners on a variety of ways to redirect scratching toward appropriate objects.

Breed-specific behavior is often readily observed. For instance, while scent hounds, like Beagles, tend to pursue their prey with their noses to the ground, sight hounds such as Greyhounds generally run with their head up, looking toward the object of their pursuit.

Singing canaries have no distinguishing physical characteristics, but they do have their own behavior traits.

Roller Canaries sing with their beaks closed and have lower, softer, more rolling melodies to their songs. Chopper Canaries sing with fully open beaks and produce louder, vibrant, choppier musical notes that some people might consider too shrill.

It is important that counselors learn about behavior traits and the reasons they exist. This enables them to direct owners toward a pet with traits they are seeking. Counselors who understand the importance of species and breed specific behavior can provide accurate explanations of why one pet may be better suited to a home than another animal that the client may be considering.

Although a veterinary degree is not necessary, pet selection counselors should be familiar with common genetic disorders within a breed. This allows them to make valuable recommendations of pets that would fit into a specific home.

The English Bulldog breed serves as a good example. This dog was listed number 10 in the 2008 American Kennel Club list of most popular breeds. It tends to be a favored sports mascot and is one of the most recognized breed of dogs in the United States. Many people consider English Bulldogs to be tolerant, family-friendly pets. They are also predisposed to several genetic disorders, including hip dysplasia, brachycephalic airway obstruction syndrome (BAOS), keratoconjunctivitis sicca (KCS), and pulmonic stenosis. An English Bulldog would not be the best choice for an active individual seeking a dog to accompany him/her in rigorous outdoor activities or for people living in hot, humid climates.

Families also benefit from information about the care and maintenance requirement for various types and breeds of pets. This topic is often the first thing potential owners think of. They want to know how much and what type of food a pet eats, its housing and space requirements, whether an animal sheds excessively, needs frequent professional grooming, and yearly vaccinations. The counselor must be prepared to provide answers to these and other similar questions.

In situations where clients are interested in pets that counselors are unfamiliar with, it is beneficial to research and gather information about the animal prior to making any recommendations. Counselors can use the opportunity to collect information and develop a comprehensive library listing common physical and behavioral traits, normal developmental stages, care and husbandry. Creating a list with the pros and cons of ownership on each animal being researched and links to reliable web sites that provide additional detailed information will increase the client's confidence in a counselor's ability.

Knowledge about animals alone does not guarantee a successful counseling session. An equally important trait that counselors should possess is the ability to communicate meaningfully with clients. This entails the skill of listening to, processing, and correctly interpreting what the client is saying and the aptitude to clearly and concisely communicate suggestions back in a manner that is conducive to reaching the best decision possible. Tactfulness and diplomacy are the standard trademarks of good counselors. Additionally, counselors should strive to be nonjudgmental and avoid interjecting their own personal feelings into the session.

Counseling sessions

Preadoption counseling can be provided in several different formats. Each one has its own set of positive and negative points. Several of the most popular designs are discussed here.

Counselors who work privately with people during one-on-one sessions can establish themselves as important mentors. This personalized relationship has the potential to increase client receptivity and compliance with alternative suggestions. Individualized sessions are usually scheduled as appointments. This allows them to fit into the daily routine of the clinic or business while still meeting the needs of each client. Counselors are able to tailor the information presented to the individual situation. In some cases counselors can arrange to accompany the clients and evaluate the pet prior to the owner making a final decision. Additionally, preselection counseling offers an opportunity to schedule a follow-up visit once a new pet is decided upon and opens the door to a lasting relationship with the clients.

In-home counseling offers the same advantages as individual sessions done in the office. However, there are additional benefits associated with home visits. Technicians can schedule visits for evenings or weekends when the clinic may be closed, but the client is available. As a bonus, technicians are provided with an inside view to the home environment. This information is handy when educating clients on setting up the home for a new arrival.

There are several possible disadvantages to doing private counseling sessions. They can be extremely time intensive in the preparation work. Private preselection appointments may require a time commitment or initial cost that some clients are not willing to make. In-home visits involve travel time to and from the client's home, in addition to the time spent during the sessions.

Besides private sessions, another option is group sessions. One obvious benefit of group counseling class is the ability to schedule the session months in advance. This provides opportunities for marketing the service throughout the community, which can attract a large group of participants. Additionally, people not actively seeking a pet one month, may decide to later, and these classes will be available for them at that time. Group classes allow people to share stories, ask questions, and learn from each other, with the counselor serving the role of both facilitator and educator. Group sessions are generally less costly than private counseling, something that may encourage otherwise reluctant clients.

Drawbacks to group pet selection classes include the obvious inability to provide the same amount of personalized attention to the needs of individuals as private counseling. Some of the information covered may not be pertinent to all of those in attendance. Additionally, there is no guarantee the group in attendance would be large enough to justify the time and energy involved in preparing for the session. People may be reluctant to fully participate or ask questions in a group setting and would benefit more from private sessions.

There are additional considerations when developing pre-selection counseling sessions. For instance, who will attend the sessions. One excellent predictor of how successful counseling will be is the number of family members involved in the process. Ideally, everyone in the family will participate in the counseling session. This includes all adults and children old enough to understand and express themselves. Doing this allows everyone to have input into the decision and will assist the counselor in making suggestions. Although not everyone will experience the same amount of attachment to a new pet, involvement of the entire household can help ensure that all family members are comfortable living with the pet.

Counseling forms

Pet selection forms are meant to provide the counselor with insight into the client's preconceived expectations of a pet. They can also identify potential areas in which the client may require further education. There are a variety of forms and handouts available, which can be personalized or adapted to meet the needs of each individual user, or counselors can develop their own form from scratch. See Appendix 19 for a sample of a pet selection form to be completed by the client. Regardless of the origin of the form selected, there are essential pieces of information that should be included in every counseling session.

• Pet selection forms are meant to provide the counselor with insight into the client's preconceived expectations of a pet. They can also identify potential areas in which the client may require further education.

Household composition

The personal information section allows clients to provide basic data about family members, such as the number of adults and children residing in the home and whether anyone suffers from allergies or other medical conditions that could be affected by a pet. If there are small children, individuals with allergies, or elders in the residence, the counselor can help to direct clients toward pets that may be more appropriate for the entire family. As an example, a bird that produces large amounts of feather dust (Cockatoo, African Grey, and Cockatiel) is not the best choice for a home where a family member has asthma or allergies.

Previous pets

Counselors often also ask for the history of the family's current and past pets. Some animals do not necessarily make good first-time pets. It is useful to examine why any former pets are no longer owned by the individuals. If the reasons were related to anything other than illness or old age, the counselor should inquire further about what has changed in the household to make owning a pet successful this time. Clients who have not owned a pet in a number of years may also need to be brought up to date with new training techniques and philosophies.

Household logistics and dynamics

Other considerations are the size, location, and type of home, whether there is a yard, the size of the yard, and, if the yard is fenced, the type of fence. The size and location of the home do not directly preclude owning a pet but it can influence the final selection. Families living in apartments or homes where residences are bunched close together would have a better chance of success with a small bird, like a budgie, cockatiel, finch, or canary, rather than larger parrots such as a cockatoo, macaw, or conure. The latter birds are capable of ear-piercing screams and can result in complaints from nearby neighbors. When there is no yard, or a small, unfenced yard, clients need to carefully evaluate the exercise needs of the pet that they decide upon. High-energy dogs like Border Collies are not usually good candidates for apartment living, unless owners are able to provide adequate daily mental and physical

exercise, perhaps in the form of agility, herding or fly ball.

As today's families are busier than ever, it is important that any new pet fits into the household's daily routine. Counselors should inquire about how many vacations, business trips, and other types of travel the family takes regularly. If owners are frequently on the road, what type of accommodations are they prepared to make for the pet's care during their absence? One option can be family and friends who enjoy pets and are willing to perform pet-sitting duty in their home or the owner's home during trips. Dogs and cats may not be the best pet if the owners anticipate frequent use of boarding kennels.

In many households, family members are engaged in nonstop activities every day. This can include lengthy commutes back and forth to work, accompanied by long days spent on the job. Children may spend all day in school with evenings and weekends devoted to extracurricular activities. It then becomes important to determine how much time will realistically be available for pet care and interaction. While there is not a set amount of time owners must spend with their pets on a daily basis, puppies and kittens will always require more time than adult dogs and cats. Will someone be available to provide the dog with opportunities to exercise and relieve itself during the day? The amount of time each pet needs will vary according to the individual animal.

Visitors to the home add another dimension in the area of lifestyle. Active households where there are a variety of people frequently coming and going each day may prefer a pet that is friendly and outgoing. An animal that is quiet and reserved may adapt better to a calmer, more sedate environment. Pets often react differently to adult visitors than to teenagers or toddlers.

Are there any major changes on the horizon for the household, or have there been any major changes within the past 6 months? This includes, but is not limited to, marriage, an adjustment in living arrangements, relocation, pregnancy, or a new baby, children moving away or moving back home, or a change in work status or hours. If the answer to any of these questions is yes, careful consideration should be given to the timing of bringing in a new pet.

One related question involves why the decision was made to acquire a new pet at this time. The answer to this question can provide much insight for counselors. Did they watch a new movie or read a book starring a specific animal? Did they just purchase a new home? Do they feel that their children are now old enough to care for a pet?

Anticipated responsibilities

Families often make erroneous assumptions about who will assume responsibility for various pet-related duties. Therefore, this topic is one that should be discussed with everyone in the family. There should be a clear idea about who in the family will feed, walk, train, and cleanup after the pet. Parents who bring a pet into their home as a way to teach children responsibility should understand that, in most cases, children cannot be reliably expected to perform these duties. This means that parents must be prepared to assume animal-care duties when necessary.

Living arrangements

Is the pet expected to spend life outside, inside, or a combination? If indoors, will the pet have free access to the entire house, including being allowed on furniture, or restricted to a specific area? What arrangements are owners willing to make in order to safeguard the pet and the home when the pet is left alone? How much time will the pet spend alone each day? These topics can easily cause dissension in a household. One family member may have an entirely different view of what is acceptable and anticipated from another family member.

Financial considerations

The first connection most people make when financial investments of pet ownership are mentioned involves the initial purchase price of the pet. Breeders may charge hundreds or thousands of dollars for a purebred dog or cat. Shelter adoption fees are generally less and many pets are advertised as "free to a good home" in local papers. However, even a free pet has associated costs. All counseling forms should contain questions asking owners about their understanding of expenses related to regular and emergency medical treatment, spaying or neutering, food, treats, toys, and training. This is where veterinary clinics can provide realistic guidance about yearly medical procedures and costs for food.

Husbandry considerations

Some pets require regular grooming sessions where they are bathed and their coat is clipped. Frequent brushing is important for longhaired pets to prevent matted hair from developing. Almost all dogs and cats shed, which is something to remind families about during counseling. Birds shed feathers regularly, and some produce a very fine powder-like feather dust that can leave residue on furniture and cause respiratory problems for some people. Clients should be counseled on the potential husbandry needs of pets they are considering.

Management and training considerations

Not every owner has the willingness or ability to deal with challenging behaviors new pets may demonstrate. First-time owners and people who have not lived with a pet for an extended period of time may be unaware of, or have forgotten, the realities of owning a pet. In this connection, the counselor can list behaviors commonly reported as troubling for owners and discuss whether the clients feel confident about dealing with them. Behaviors cited for dogs and cats should include vocalization (barking/meowing), destructive chewing, house training issues, scratching furniture, exploratory behavior, mouthing or nipping, and other similar issues. When talking with individuals interested in birds and exotics, it is important to counsel about screaming, biting, aggression, and the impact diet and husbandry can have on behavior.

Adopting multiple pets at the same time

People sometimes believe it is best to acquire two pets at the same time. There are some advantages to this situation. Working owners may find multiple animals provide each other with companionship and entertainment during the owner's absence. Caring for two pets may or may not require a significant amount of extra work. As an example, the additional time spent on the care and maintenance of two kittens may be almost negligible. However, if the two pets are puppies, it often takes considerable more time and effort.

Bringing two new animals into a house together presents additional challenges. Training two animals at the same time can be a difficult task. When raised together, animals may bond more closely to each other than their human companions. Anxiety and separation issues can become apparent if the two animals must be separated later in life. Undesirable behaviors can easily be transferred from one pet to the other.

If the client is insistent about owning two pets, the technician could recommend acquiring only one pet. Once that pet is trained and understands the household rules, then bring in another one. The resident pet can then serve as a model for the new one.

Personal preferences

An area of the session where all members of the family can have a great deal of input is the section where they discuss their personal preferences for a new pet. One exercise that promotes participation and feedback from everyone is to provide a separate sheet of paper to all family members and ask them each to write down three activities they visualize themselves doing with a new pet. Possible answers may include hunting, lap warmer, companion for themselves, their children or other family pets, competition prospect, jogging partner, and protection. In some cases, the variety of answers from members of the same family can be an eye-opening experience. This often opens the door to further discussion and a better understanding among family members.

Other areas where there can be differences of opinion involve the size, weight, age, and coat length of the pet. Where one family member prefers a puppy or kitten, adult dog or cat, others may look forward to a bird that talks, sings, or does tricks. Still others in the family may dream of living with an unusual or exotic pet, such as a reptile or amphibian.

The last section of a pet selection form can request that clients create a list with the top three to five types or breeds of animals they are considering, as well as any questions or concerns that were not mentioned on the form.

Pet-selection reports

Although counselors may have handouts and information available during the session, clients may find it even more helpful to receive a list of magazines, videos, DVDs and books they can use for additional referencing during their search. Counselors are positioned to direct owners to materials that provide reliable, scientifically accurate information in an easy-to-follow format. This will prevent owners accessing information of questionable quality.

After everyone has had an opportunity to review all the information provided, there are several possible outcomes. The counselor may recommend one or more of the pets that initially interested the client. Sometimes the animals suggested are not part of the owner's original list of candidates. However, if the counselor has carefully guided clients through the selection process, the recommended animals will not be unexpected. If the clients have indicated a specific breed or species in their consultation, it is important those animals be incorporated into the pet selection report. The counselor may indicate potential issues with those choices but should not exclude them from the report. Completely excluding or negating those possibilities could alienate the client. See Appendix 28 for an example of a pet-selection report.

So that there is time to research unusual or unfamiliar types of pets, the counselor may set up another meeting, via an in-person appointment, phone call, or email report, in order to provide the client with more specific suggestions.

A client may decide, based upon solid, logical advice from the counselor, that this is not the right time or circumstances for a new pet to join the family. Even though it may cause initial disappointment, tactful counselors can turn the experience into a positive experience by helping owners understand how changes in lifestyle could make pet ownership possible in the future. Counselors can also offer to assist these clients when they are more prepared to select a pet.

Finding a source for obtaining the pet

Often families will take the information provided and begin to search for a pet on their own. The counselor can assist by providing various resources to aid in the search. A good suggestion can be to visit a dog or cat show and talk to competitors that have the breeds they are interested in. Counselors can format a list of breeders known to produce healthy problem-free litters. This client should interview the breeder, asking specific questions and be knowledgeable of acceptable answers. Speaking to breeders can be intimidating to a client. Instructing and empowering clients with a list of questions will help them be more confident during breeder interviews. (see Appendix 26 for a Breeder Interview Questions form). Kennel clubs and feline associations often publish registries of breed rescues and breed associations. Specialty organizations for support and therapy dogs may have animals unsuitable for their purposes, but that would otherwise make an excellent pet.

Animal shelters and breed rescue can also be a source for the public. Adopting a pet can help save a life and provide owners with a feeling of self-satisfaction. However, there are some cautions for clients. Avoid facilities where there are obvious signs of overcrowding or lack of adequate medical treatment. Many shelters observe and assess adult dogs and cats for health, sociability, fear, and level of activity. This may help people to identify a pet that will be well-suited to their lifestyle and needs.

Rescues often specialize in one type of purebred dog or cat, but there are rescues for special needs animals such as senior dogs and cats or small-size dogs. Many of these groups lack a physical shelter, and instead rely upon a network of trained members to "foster" animals in their homes. The pet receives individual attention and training while in the home. Additionally, information on how the animal interacts with children and other animals can be easily observed and relayed to the adopter. Potential adopters should anticipate both written and in-person interviews, and several meetings with the pet before the rescue will approve placement. Many rescues also require an in-home visit before finalizing any adoption paperwork. Groups that attempt to talk people into adopting a pet, lack up-to-date medical records, or refuse

CHAPTER 7

to allow a potential adopter into the facility, should be avoided.

Clients should be advised to avoid pet shops, puppy mills, and breeding farms. Animals from these locations are usually the by-product of mass breeding, poor husbandry practices, and inadequate management techniques.

> • Clients should be advised to avoid pet shops, puppy mills, and breeding farms. Animals from these locations are usually the by-product of mass breeding, poor husbandry practices, and inadequate management techniques.

Other services can be included as part of the pet selection sessions. Counselors may offer to accompany clients who have located a potential new pet and assist in evaluating interactions with the animal. Veterinary clinics may offer a short post-purchase office visit where owners receive behavior counseling and set up follow-up medical care for their new pet.

Pet selection counseling is the first step in problem prevention and encourages creation of a strong human-animal bond. Pet selection counseling results in the selection of a more suitable pet, better educated owners, and establishment of a positive ongoing relationship between the client and the veterinary clinic that will carry through for the life of the pet and beyond.

> • Pet selection counseling results in the selection of a more suitable pet, better educated owners, and establishment of a positive ongoing relationship between the client and the veterinary clinic that will carry through for the life of the pet and beyond.

Puppy socialization classes

For many years, little attention was given to any type of classes targeting puppies. Most training was reserved for dogs 6 months of age or older and concentrated on skills for people interested in obedience competition. This attitude has changed as studies have increased our understanding of the impact early socialization and training can have on behavior.

In 1998, the National Council on Pet Population Study and Policy conducted a study exploring factors leading to behavior-related surrenders of dogs and cats. The owners of 1984 dogs that were surrendered to 12 shelters across the United States were asked to list up to five

reasons that they were relinquishing their pets. Not surprisingly, behavior problems were listed as a reason for canine relinquishment more than any other single category.

Additionally, approximately 96% of all the dog owners reported that their dogs lacked any type of training. Owners who taught their canine companions at least some basic training skills were less likely to surrender them due to behavior problems.

Although this study was not directed at training, it helped provide some insight into the importance of training by suggesting that owners who work with their dogs to teach them even a few basic foundation skills and cues are less likely to give them up due to (mis)behavior.

In the July 2003 issue of the Journal of American Veterinary Medical Association, a study was published that evaluated the association between retention of dogs in their adoptive homes, attendance at puppy socialization classes, and several other factors. The study involved 248 adult dogs that were adopted as puppies from a humane society. Owners were asked to complete a questionnaire regarding demographics, retention of the dogs in the homes, and the dogs' early learning events.

Dogs that participated in puppy socialization classes, wore head collars as puppies, responded to their owners' cues, and lived in homes without young children had higher retention rates. Analysis of the answers suggested several practices that veterinarians may recommend to enhance the likelihood that puppies will remain in their first homes. First on the list was enrolling 7–12-week-old puppies in early learning and socialization classes. Additionally, the lower retention rate of dogs in homes with children further emphasized the vital role technicians can play by helping owners develop realistic expectations and effective tools necessary to manage daily interactions between their children and dogs.

> • Dogs that participated in puppy socialization classes, wore head collars as puppies, responded to their owners' cues, and lived in homes without young children had higher retention rates.

These studies highlight the significance of a well-run puppy class in providing multiple opportunities to educate owners on problem prevention, behavior management and, if necessary, modification techniques.

Experts in canine behavior now recommend that owners take advantage of the optimum periods of learning and enroll puppies in classes as early as 8 weeks of age.

Puppy classes can provide benefits to the veterinary practice by promoting a successful union between clients and their pets early in the relationship. Handling and socialization skills introduced in puppy classes may help create a more cooperative patient for examinations. When classes are held inside the veterinary clinic, they can become an excellent practice builder, and provide opportunities to recommend additional products and services beneficial both to the pet and the clinic. Similarly, puppy classes that are held in the veterinary practice can help develop a symbiotic relationship between the clinic and the instructor, regardless of whether that person is an employee of the clinic or teaches classes independently.

All animals that attend class must be healthy and remain current on all vaccinations, which results in pet owners returning to the practice for updated exams and preventative medical treatments. Conversely, the clinic provides a constant source of referrals for the instructor. Not only can puppy classes provide veterinary technicians with a supplementary source of income, they can also provide a much needed stress relief from the life and death situations encountered everyday in the veterinary hospital. The veterinary technicians involved in puppy socialization classes will experience a boost in their own morale. Puppy class is about enhancing the bond between a puppy and its owners at a time when the owners are usually still excited with the new puppy.

Logistics

There are multiple key components involved in developing and implementing a puppy class, including the logistics of a puppy class. The logistics of puppy class involve deciding on a location for class, identifying competent instructors, selecting criteria for canine and human participants, deciding on a class style, and implementing strategies to minimize health risks.

Location

The ideal location should be climate controlled, easy to sanitize, puppy- and escape-proof, easily dividable, and free of interruptions.

An indoor, climate-controlled facility is preferred because outdoor locations will cause delays in class sessions due to weather. As the goal is for the class to be completed during a short window of time (the socialization period), delays in class would be problematic.

Similarly, outdoor locations can be difficult to sanitize properly. Porous surfaces such as grass, dirt, mulch, or carpet cannot be effectively sanitized, whereas nonporous surfaces are easily disinfected. If other dogs have been in the facility, then the puppy class location should be disinfected prior to class. Accidents (urine or stool) during class should be cleaned with disposable towels and a parvocidal disinfectant to minimize contamination.

In a puppy socialization class there will be one or two short off-leash play sessions. Classes need to be held in a facility or room that can be secured so as to prevent accidental escapes. Either the doors to the facility should be locked or the room should be secured with sturdy gates (Figure 7.21).

With large classes (more than six puppies) the ability to divide the room provides the instructor the ability to maintain an appropriate setting for puppy class. Barriers and divisions reduce the risk of overstimulation of the puppies. Gates, exercise pens, and other barriers can be used to divide the room and group the puppies appropriately.

Instructors should be able to see the clients and puppies easily. The space should provide enough seating for all human participants. There will need to be enough room for exploration areas, a play area, and an exercise pen.

The novelty of the environment, people, and other puppies will prove to be highly distracting to the puppies and their human counterparts as well. All other distractions should be minimized. A location that is free of disruptions during the class time is imperative. In a training facility, other classes should not be held in the same area simultaneously. In a veterinary hospital, puppy classes can be offered after hours or in a nonactive area of the hospital.

Instructor characteristics

Competent, knowledgeable instructors are one of the most important requirements for class. Instructors should have a strong understanding of learning theory, canine body language, and puppy growth and development. They must also possess excellent communication skills.

Instructors should demonstrate a well-versed understanding of learning theory. Although it may not be important for clients to have an extensive vocabulary of official terminology, instructors must be able to explain the basic concepts in an easy to understand format. This means it is imperative for technicians to be well-informed on the differences between Classical Conditioning (learning by association) and

Figure 7.21 Secure area that is able to be divided for puppy socialization class.

Operant Conditioning (learning by consequences) (see Chapter 6).

Dogs communicate with each other predominantly through movement and body postures. Primates (including humans) rely primarily on vocalization as a way of communication. This difference in styles is one reason for the misunderstanding that commonly occurs in owner/pet interactions. A puppy class instructor should be knowledgeable about canine body language and be able to teach pet owners how to interpret dog communication. An instructor who is familiar with basic canine body postures is able to help owners recognize emotional signs of stress and fear.

Understanding the growth and developmental stages of puppies allows instructors to structure classes that make the greatest impact in the shortest amount of time. Science has recognized that there are multiple sensitive periods that puppies pass through as they mature. The most significant of these periods occurs between 3 and 12 weeks of age. During this period, puppies learn behaviors that allow them to communicate as adult dogs and are developmentally ready to meet and interact with other species, including people. Puppies exposed to increasingly complex enrichment during this period tend to adapt better to changes as they mature.

An appropriate instructor to puppy ratio should also be considered. Ideally, puppy classes should have one instructor or assistant per three or four puppies. This allows for individual guidance during exploration and exposure activities in class.

Owners, as a group, have very diverse needs that dictate what they are willing and able to do when training their dogs. Each has different physical abilities and learning styles that must be taken into account.

Physical factors that affect an owner's ability to perform training exercises include age, health and physical limitations. Classes should be structured to meet the needs of all students. This may entail using an elevated platform to teach "sits" and "downs" for owners who are in wheelchairs or unable to get down on the floor with their dogs.

Individuals tend to rely upon specific approaches when learning. Visual learners retain information best by observation. Auditory learners rely upon hearing what is said. Tactile/kinesthetic learners learn through moving, doing, and touching. The best classes incorporate all the above methods in each session.

It is important to adopt teaching methods that provide owners with a variety of opportunities to learn, practice, and perfect their skills. As a rule of thumb, a well-structured class is one where individuals are encouraged to use their preferred learning styles, instructional activities are designed to appeal to a variety of different learning styles, and evaluation of successful owner education takes into account the different learning styles.

Participant characteristics

When developing a puppy socialization class, guidelines for the participants, canine and human, are necessary to provide an environment conducive to socialization.

What puppies will be accepted into classes? What is the minimum and maximum age for a class? What vaccinations will be required for each puppy prior to starting class? What safeguards will be implemented to verify the health of new puppies entering classes and protect the health of puppies currently attending classes?

There is much discussion about the safest age for a puppy to begin class. However, in an open letter, R. K. Anderson DVM, Diplomate ACVB and ACVPM, Professor and Director Emeritus, Animal Behavior Clinic and Center to Study Human/Animal Relationships and Environments University of Minnesota, encourages veterinarians and puppy owners to make socialization in class a first priority, beginning about 8 weeks of age and continuing through 12 weeks. See Appendix 29 and 30 for letters from Purdue University and Dr. R. K Anderson regarding the recommendations for early puppy socialization classes.

Both letters noted above address concerns about health issues. Dr. Anderson's letter states, "Experience and epidemiologic data support the relative safety and lack of transmission of disease in these puppy socialization classes over the past 10 years in many parts of the United States." He further states that the risk of a puppy dying from distemper or parvovirus disease is much less than the risk of euthanasia due to a behavior problem.

- Dr. Anderson's letter states, "Experience and epidemiologic data support the relative safety and lack of transmission of disease in these puppy socialization classes over the past 10 years in many parts of the United States." He further states that the risk of a puppy dying from distemper or parvovirus disease is much less than the risk of euthanasia due to a behavior problem.

Based upon current available information, many classes use the following guidelines for accepting puppies into class: Puppies are required to be at least 8 weeks of age and have had a minimum set of Distemper-Adenovirus 2-Parvo and Bordatella vaccinations prior to attending class. Furthermore, owners must provide proof of ongoing preventative veterinary care throughout the class.

Puppies who attend class should be in their socialization period (between 7 and 12 weeks when starting class). The puppies need to have recently been examined by a veterinarian, in an active vaccine protocol, and considered healthy for puppy class. Ideally the puppy should have been in its current home for a minimum of 10 days prior to starting class. Ten days is the incubation period for many viruses. If the puppy had exposure before being obtained by their current owners, signs of illness should be evident within 10 days.

Puppy classes focus on the socialization of young puppies and the education of new puppy parents. Consequently, there are some limitations associated with a puppy socialization class. The tendency to allow older puppies (older than 12 weeks when starting the class) into a socialization class can negatively affect the older puppy and other participants. However, the information provided in a puppy socialization class can be valuable for all dog owners, regardless of the dog's age. The instructor may consider allowing the owners to audit the class (attend without the puppy). Another option would be to have them attend with the puppy (should be under 4.5 months old), but during off-leash play time the puppy is managed in another area. This option would depend on the individual puppy and whether the owners are able to successfully manage the puppy in class.

Puppy classes are not designed to address abnormal behaviors, including profound fears, phobias, aggression, or excessive reactivity. A puppy showing signs of a behavior disorder can still benefit from attendance in a puppy socialization class, as long as the puppy can be managed in a way that is not disruptive to the class and does not negatively affect the experience of the other puppies in the class. "Problem puppies" should also be enjoying the class and have positive experiences. If a puppy is in its socialization period and is showing profound signs of fear, failing to acclimate to the situation, excessively reactive or disruptive, then the puppy is not in an appropriate setting for learning nor is it enjoying the class. A referral for intervention services would be indicated.

In regard to the human participants in puppy class, the entire family should be encouraged to attend. It is recommended that anyone under 18 years old be accompanied by an adult and children under 8 should have two adults present (one to supervise the children and one to supervise the puppy).

Class style

Although some basic cues are taught during puppy classes, the emphasis at this point is not on training skills, but on the all-crucial skills of socialization and problem prevention.

Conventional series-style puppy classes are the most common and easiest to manage. They have a definite beginning and ending date. However, owners who miss the start of a session must wait until the next one begins, which may result in loss of important socialization time. Additionally, puppies are generally in class with the same puppies throughout the entire session and do not have the advantage of socializing with new puppies entering the class.

A rotational style of class has become increasingly popular in recent years. Open enrollment classes offer flexibility as puppies can enter the classes at any time, but require excellent organizational skills to keep track of student progress. As puppies can begin at any time, new puppies are constantly being introduced to the group, which provides the greatest impact.

Disease prevention

Minimizing the risk of infection is crucial for the safety of the puppies. Besides the health and vaccine requirements previously recommended, as each puppy arrives for class, the instructors should take a brief moment to greet the puppy and owner. While interacting with the puppy, the instructor should note the following:

- Mental state: Bright, alert, responsive, and active.
- Mucous membranes: gums and tongue are pink.
- Eyes, ears, nose, throat (airway): Free from mucopurulent eye or nasal discharge and not sneezing or coughing.
- Tail and rear end: Coat free of fecal staining (possibly from diarrhea).
- Skin and coat: No evidence of hair loss, free of crusty skin lesions, or external parasites (fleas/ticks).

In addition to a brief examination of each puppy upon arrival, the following guidelines will minimize the risk of contamination:

- Veterinary staff who have been working with healthy or ill animals all day should change clothes and shoes before class.
- Disinfect surface areas before and after each class with 30 parts water: 1 part bleach mixture or a Parvocidal product. This is especially important if other dog activities occur in the facility or it is a veterinary hospital.

- Wash any food storage items after each use (dishwasher-safe items should be run through a dishwasher cycle if possible). Better yet, use disposable food storage toys (such as yogurt cups, cottage cheese containers, or empty syringe casings) and throw them away after use.
- Properly clean up puppy accidents (stool or urine).
- Remove solid waste and spray with disinfectant and wipe up with disposable or washable towels.

By following the above guidelines, the risk of spreading infectious diseases is minimized.

Puppy socialization class format

A high-quality puppy socialization class will have many components, including a people-only orientation class, short play sessions, positive exposure to sights, sounds, and novelty, preventive exercises, puppy parenting tips, and introduction to positive reinforcement training.

> - A high-quality puppy socialization class will have many components, including a people-only orientation class, short play sessions, positive exposure to sights, sounds, and novelty, preventive exercises, puppy parenting tips, and introduction to positive reinforcement training.

Orientation

Providing a mandatory orientation prior to attendance in socialization classes will minimize any surprises for the owner as well as the instructor. Orientation prepares the puppy parent for class and should be a prerequisite to attending socialization classes. It allows for the human participants to learn about what to expect in puppy class. Because orientation is a human only class (puppies stay home), puppy parents can learn without the distraction of their puppy (Figure 7.22).

Puppy play sessions

Controlled, off-leash short play sessions (5 min or less) with other puppies in a secure environment allow young puppies to familiarize themselves with a variety of different breeds of dogs. Well-organized group play is the benchmark of a good puppy class. It provides a situation where puppies learn how to properly interact with other puppies and begin to learn the vital skill of bite inhibition. In some instances it is possible to observe giant-size puppies, toy breeds, and many sizes in between playfully interacting together. Instructors take advantage of the play time to help owners understand how to interpret what the puppies body postures signify.

Figure 7.22 Weekly puppy class orientation.

- High pitched yips or screams are a sign of pain or fear and can be normal communication.
- Look at the body language of the puppy.
  - Is the body relaxed or tense?
  - Are all participants having fun?
- Self-regulated.
  - Puppies are able to adjust the play on their own.
  - Ebb and flow of activity level.
    - Some running/chasing or wrestling.
    - Followed by a short break and a role reversal.

From the course Puppy Start Right for Instructors with permission from Kenneth Martin, DVM, and Debbie Martin, RVT, VTS (Behavior).

Puppies teach each other about bite inhibition and the value of appropriate play behavior. Owners often call their puppies away from play to give them a treat and then release them back to play. In this way the puppy learns that play does not always end when called by the owner.

Play sessions are not intended to be a free-for-all. First-time puppies often hang back during play sessions and some may even attempt to hide. Instructors should strive to help new puppies become comfortable. Small, reluctant, or fearful puppies may be placed in a separate play group where they acclimate to the environment slowly. An alternate suggestion is to partition off a small area using dividers or exercise pens. The shy puppy can then observe and interact with the group more slowly (Box 7.2).

BOX 7.2: COMPONENTS OF NORMAL PLAY.

- Role reversal.
  - Puppies take turns being chased or chasing, being on the bottom and being on top.
  - It is not just one puppy "winning" all the time.
- Asking for more.
  - When there is a break in the play, the puppy that was on the bottom or being chased asks for more by trying to re-engage the other puppy.
- Play can be rough and vocal.
  - They might tumble around and bite at each other's legs or neck.
  - Some puppies are vocal while playing and will bark and growl.

Occasionally you will encounter puppies in the socialization period that lack appropriate communication skills or the ability to self-regulate play. This could be due to lack of play during primary socialization, early removal from the litter, genetic predisposition, or learning.

With puppies in their socialization period, it is best to let them learn how to communicate with each other on their own. Exposure to a variety of play styles and breeds of dogs during the socialization period is important for puppies to learn that not all puppies play the same. Allowing a puppy to appropriately communicate (with conflict/calming signals or even a little reprimand–i.e., show of teeth, yip, grumble) to another puppy that its play style is not appropriate is a life skill that should be developed during this time. Ideally, puppy class instructors should try to let the puppies handle it on their own and should avoid frequent interventions.

However, there will be times the instructor should intervene. According to Puppy Start Right for Instructors (Martin and Martin, 2012), puppy play should be interrupted when the following conditions occur:
- The target puppy is fearful, does not recover and begin to solicit play, or keeps trying to escape or hide.
- The instigator of play does not reciprocate the message from the target puppy.
- Other puppies are showing signs of fear even when not involved in the play. Perhaps the play is vocal or involves chase and the observer puppies are concerned and not recovering.
- The instructor is unsure if all the puppies are enjoying the play because role reversal has not happened for a while and the "underdog" might or might not be having fun.

• Puppies are having trouble self-regulating; they are having fun but there is no slow-down period.

Just as important, or even more important, is how play is interrupted. The goal with an interruption in play is to promote learning and decrease tension. The recommended technique is using distraction. A treat or squeaky toy can be placed in front of the instigators nose to get its attention. It can then be lured away from the other puppy and rewarded with a food treat. The puppy should be allowed to return to play. The goal is to distract the puppies in a non-confrontational manner in order to calm down the play session.

• The goal with an interruption in play is to promote learning and decrease tension.

Interruption techniques that should be avoided include verbal reprimands, grabbing the puppy's collar or picking it up. These techniques do not provide a positive learning experience for the puppies.

Verbal reprimands such as an "Ahh" or "No" will only add tension to the situation and can cause a negative association with play. All the puppies (even the ones not involved) learn, "When I interact with other puppies, humans fuss. Therefore, other dogs are not fun."

Grabbing the puppy by the collar will increase tension and frustration, and should be avoided even if the collar grab is followed with a treat. This method could work if the puppy had a long learning history (several months) outside of the play context that collar grabs are great. This will not be the case in a puppy class because the puppies are only 2–3 months old.

Picking the puppy up to interrupt play should be discouraged because when it is used repetitively to interrupt play, this can be a negative learning experience associated with people. Puppies may learn to avoid people in order to avoid being picked up. Picking the puppy up is likely to increase tension and frustration and could potentially reinforce an unwanted emotional response, such as fear or aggression. People providing "back up" will not teach the puppy how to interact appropriately in these contexts. The exception to this rule is if there is truly abnormal behavior occurring and there is concern about injury to a puppy.

If after attempting to interrupt the play between two puppies, the puppies return to inappropriate play again right away, it will be necessary to implement some management. Using an exercise pen for the instigator of the play will allow the target (other) puppy to engage in play with the other puppies in class. To make the exercise pen a positive experience for the puppy, the owner or an assistant should stand next to the pen and hand the puppy a small treat every few seconds (especially when other puppies come near).

Exploration and exposure

A large part of puppy class should be devoted to teaching owners how to provide exposure to a variety of novel environments, people, objects, surfaces, and sounds in a fun and positive manner.

Instructors should teach clients to utilize desensitization by gradually exposing their puppy to novelty in combination with classical conditioning or classical counter-conditioning through the liberal use of treats. The puppy should be acclimated to a new environment by staying clear of the "action" when first arriving. Owners need to be proactive; they should assume the puppy could be afraid of a new person, object, or environment and use treats liberally to prevent a fear response and make a positive association from the start. Similarly, the owner should control what the puppy learns and keep experiences positive. This is accomplished by teaching owners how to read their puppy's body language and be the puppy's advocate.

Setting up exploration and exposure stations in puppy class allows the instructor to coach the client in developing these skills (Figure 7.23).

Preventive exercises

The importance of preventive exercises has already been discussed in detail in an earlier section of this chapter. Preventive exercises to be taught and practiced in a puppy socialization class should include crate training and independence exercises, food bowl prevention,

Figure 7.23 Exploration stations set up for a puppy socialization class.

Figure 7.24 A puppy receiving treats from its owner while the instructor demonstrates gently holding the puppies collar.

how to play with people, and handling and restraint exercises, including the collar grab (Figure 7.24).

Puppy parenting tips

Puppy class should help to educate owners on normal canine body language, learning, and positive problem solving. Typical topics to be covered would include play biting and mouthing, elimination training, digging, stealing items, chewing, and jumping.

Introduction to positive reinforcement training

Although not a training class, puppy socialization class should introduce owners to positive reinforcement training techniques. Beginning to teach attention (eye contact), targeting, sit, come when called, and leash manners with clicker training gets puppies and owners prepped for developing these skills further with additional classes.

For an example of a curriculum for a 5-week puppy socialization class see Appendix 31: Sample puppy socialization class curriculum.

Kitten classes

Veterinarians and owners have long recognized the many advantages of attending classes with puppies. However, in the past few years it has become equally accepted that there is a similar benefit for kittens enrolled in classes.

Kittens that are handled by humans early in life tend to become easier to handle as adults. When kittens also receive ongoing socialization to people, dogs, and other animals (including other cats), they are able to grow into well-adjusted felines and may become very social family members. Kitten classes provide many of the same benefits as puppy classes. Owners learn important

aspects of how to raise a healthy kitten, including how to prevent behavior problems, understanding what is normal behavior, and how to redirect unwanted behaviors in an acceptable direction. Single kittens or kittens that are hand-raised have an opportunity to interact with other kittens of their own age. Classes also help kittens learn that travel in the cat carrier is not always a bad thing. The ultimate goal of all these classes is to strengthen the human–animal bond through education and training. Additionally, socialization classes help promote a positive relationship between the veterinary clinic and the cat, which results in a more relaxed and compliant patient during future visits.

The time period during which kittens most benefit from socialization and learning is shorter than that of puppies. In his article "Developmental behaviour in kittens and puppies; puppy and kitten classes for problem prevention", Peter F. Neville DHc BSc(Hons), states "With a kitten, the time available for providing adequate psychological development in terms of producing a friendly pet is even shorter. Though evolved to be a solitary predator, a home bred kitten is destined to transfer the social bond it has with its mother to form a lifelong strong social tie with its new owners. If kittens aren't handled by at least four people in their maternal home before they reach the age of eight weeks, the chances of being able to transfer that bond reduce almost with every day. The critical difference for kitten owners is that if their kitten has not been raised in the right environment, it may be too late by the time they take on their pet at 12 weeks of age, while the puppy owner will still have a chance up to about twenty weeks to make up for any shortfalls in the early environment."

Studies have demonstrated that kittens held and lightly stroked during the first few weeks of life experience greater behavior and physical development than littermates not handled. Attending a kitten class during the early part of their lives takes advantage of their adaptability.

Classes for kittens are not structured in the same way as puppy classes. Kitten classes generally only last 2 or 3 weeks and most experts agree that the kittens in class should never be older than 14 weeks of age. After kittens reach 14 weeks of age, they are more likely to fight than play. It is advisable to encourage owners with kittens older than 14 weeks of age to attend the class, but without bringing their kitten.

Based upon current available information, many classes use the following guidelines for accepting kittens into class: kittens are required to be at least 8 weeks of age, have lived in the home for a minimum of 7 days and have written proof of Distemper-respiratory vaccine,

Rabies vaccine, if old enough, negative feline leukemia (FeLV) and immunodeficiency virus (FIV) blood tests. They must also be free of all internal and external parasites and have no signs of upper respiratory infection.

Just as with puppies, kitten owners must provide proof of ongoing preventative veterinary care throughout the class. Although there is no way to give a 100% guarantee of health, these requirements provide the best possibility of ensuring only healthy kittens attend class. Additionally, most experts agree that pets are more likely to lose their homes due to behavior problems, than become ill at a kitten class.

Other considerations include where will kitten classes be held? Many classes are held in the veterinary clinic so that kittens can associate a visit to the doctor as a positive experience. However, classes can be held in any secure area. Rooms should be large enough to place equipment and comfortably seat owners, yet small enough so instructors are able to restrict the kittens' movements. The classroom area must be easily cleaned and disinfected between sessions. A variety of small easy-to-transport supplies are essential for classes. Many can be bought ready to use, or with a little imagination can be created from everyday items around the house. They include the following:

- scratching posts – vertical and horizontal,
- empy cardboard boxes stacked so that kittens can hide inside or jump onto during play,
- a variety of toys (PVC piping or other tubing that can be used as a tunnel, readymade cat tunnels, etc.),
- pin-pong balls inside a shallow tub,
- fishing pole-type toys,
- interactive toys such as Cat Tracks, food-stuffed Kong toys,
- cat baskets or kennels (various types and sizes),
- litter boxes with a variety of different litter.

Additionally, it is wise for instructors to provide synthetic pheromone spray or diffuser in the room.

Classes usually accommodate three to five kittens per session so there are adequate opportunities for instructors to observe and manage the kittens. The size can be increased if there are additional assistants, but should still be limited to no more than 10.

Although some basic skills are taught, the main emphasis of this class is to teach owners. Actual training should be limited to short, two to four minute increments with rest and play in between each session. Patience and consistency are the elements to successful learning as each kitten has its own individual rate of learning new skills.

During the weekly kitten classes, instructors typically include play sessions, body handling, name recognition, introduction to other pets, introduction to a harness and leash, clicker training basic behaviors, walking on leash, and teaching owners how to play with the kitten. Discussions about the importance of environmental enrichment at home, basic behavior, and problem solving can be incorporated into the class, but if owners report out-of-the-ordinary or severe challenges, it is important to refer them to a qualified behavior specialist for a consultation. For a sample of a 2-week kitten class curriculum see Appendix 32.

Juvenile/Adolescent/Adult canine classes

Socialization and exposure is an active and lifelong process. If a puppy parent were to stop socializing a puppy at 3 months of age, the puppy would be more likely to become fearful as an adolescent dog. It is much more difficult to socialize a puppy after 3 months of age without early positive foundation memories. As the puppy developmentally becomes more suspicious of novelty, positive exposure is probably equally important as during the socialization period. Even the well-socialized young puppy might regress if positive exposure does not continue into adolescence. After completion of a puppy socialization class, young dogs should enroll into a class designed for juvenile and adolescent dogs.

The juvenile stage in a dog's development is from about 3–6 months of age. The adolescent stage is from approximately 6 months–2 years of age. This timing can vary with individual dogs. The adolescent period is the most trying time behaviorally for dog owners. It is also an important time to offer clients additional support to keep these dogs mentally and physically stimulated. Offering adolescent dog training classes is a vital service that can prevent owners from relinquishing their pet during this difficult stage. Veterinary behavior technicians can play an important part in designing and teaching adolescent dog training classes.

Technicians and other staff members who are interested in teaching classes will want to acquire the proper knowledge, skills, and experience from reputable organizations (see Chapter 1).

Clinics offering classes will need to have ample space with secure flooring. Some may have an appropriate area on the premises. If a room is not available, renting space elsewhere in the community should be considered. Church halls, community recreation halls, and picnic shelters are a few options that could be considered. The clinic will need to provide a certificate of insurance when offering classes outside the facility.

When designing a program the family pet and average owner should be kept in mind. The class format should be loaded with practical and easy-to-accomplish exercises. Real-life role playing is valuable to help owners visualize what they should be doing at home. The juvenile/adolescent/adult dog classes should continue to provide exploration and exposure opportunities to novelty, incorporate problem prevention and problem solving exercises, and build on the foundation training skills that have been started in puppy socialization class. The following foundation skills are important for a young dog to learn to help owners communicate effectively with the adolescent canine:

- Attention (look at the owner): A high rate of reinforcement for paying attention to the owner will make this a favorite activity for the dog. Building in the ability to focus on the handler even in the face of distractions requires a detailed training plan designed to gradually introduce distraction while keeping the dog successful.
- Look (look at something in the environment but no need to explore it): It is unrealistic to think that dogs can tune out every little distraction. People are unable to do this. We hear a sound or see someone coming into the training class and it is natural for us to attend to it. Dogs are no different. The more the owners try to make their dog ignore everything, the more likely that conflict and frustration between the owner and dog will develop. By creating a cue that is the opposite of attention, the owner is able to flip-flop back and forth from attention and look, thus, in the end, making for a more attentive dog and a less frustrated owner.
- Settle on a mat: This foundation behavior has many uses. Once the behavior has been taught, the dog can be cued to settle on its mat while the owner is cooking, eating, or watching TV and when visitors arrive at the door: any time the owners need the dog to be at a distance from them. This cue provides an alternative to jumping on people, bolting out the door, begging, or stealing food off the counter.
- Target: Teaching the dog to touch its nose to the owner's hand when cued provides for a way to quickly teach a "come when called." By providing a specific target behavior (touch the owner's hand), the dog is clear about what is expected. This behavior is first taught up close and gradually the owner cues the behavior from further away. A nose touch to hand target behavior can also be used to refocus or direct the dog in the face of distractions. Targeting can be a quick way to jump start a new behavior such as teaching a spin, over or under an object, or even to walk by the owner's side.
- Loose leash walking (LLW): This is a valuable skill that does not come naturally to dogs. The importance of routine walks for mental and physical stimulation has been discussed earlier in this chapter. If walking the dog is unbearable because it pulls, the owner is less likely to take it for routine walks. Juvenile and adolescent classes should focus on making this a fun and enjoyable behavior for the dog and the owner. A management tool, such as a front clip harness or head collar, may be necessary initially for some dogs while the owner works on making the loose leash walking more reliable.
- Greeting behaviors and door manners: As discussed in the problem prevention section, dogs naturally want to greet people by jumping up toward their face. This is an innate behavior that is often reinforced. Juvenile and adolescent dog classes should help provide owners with the skills to teach appropriate alternatives to jumping. Skills that could be taught include teaching the dog that the sound of a door bell or knock is the cue to settle on its bed and training the dog that sitting (instead of jumping) is reinforced. Exercises to practice these skills with a variety of people in the class allows for further socialization at the same time.

The clicker is the ideal training tool when teaching new behaviors or improving an existing behavior. Many dogs are simply confused by their owner's erratic way of communicating. People use their voices for many things, where the clicker is reserved only for the dog. The precision of the clicker to mark a behavior allows for clear communication between the dog and the owner. Clicker training is discussed in more detail in Chapter 8.

The class format could be either a traditional linear series with clients signing up for a set of classes that has a start and end date, or a modular format with an open enrollment that provides for more flexibility.

For the linear series, specific exercises are introduced and practiced each week. Each consecutive class builds on the exercises from the previous week. The same students and dogs complete the class together, usually over a 6 to 8-week period.

Modular classes take more planning and organization but they allow for client convenience and flexibility. The client prepays for a set number of classes; the more they buy the cheaper the per-class cost. Weekly classes are designed around skills (coming when called, loose leash walking, manners at the door, etc.) and the clients can choose which classes they take. Some trainers will have a beginner, intermediate, and advanced level for each skill (i.e., beginner level "come when called" is on Monday at 7 pm, intermediate level "come when called" is on Monday at 8 pm). However, to maximize class size, offering the skill and combining all levels in one class has some advantages for the client as well. The beginner students see the advanced dogs working and

Figure 7.25 Separate training station and barriers to help minimize distraction in a group class.

it inspires them to train their own dog. The advanced dogs are provided with the distraction of the more unruly beginner dogs. With this type of modular class, stations are set up with specific exercises including beginner, intermediate, and advanced instructions. The clients work at their dog's level and the instructor provides guidance and feedback. During the class they rotate through the various stations to work on several different exercises associated with the skill.

Instructor to student ratio is very important in adolescent and adult dog training. The dogs tend to be more excitable and easily distracted. Many dogs also experience a social regression during adolescence, which can pose some difficulties. Instructors and assistants must be prepared to provide some individual attention if a student is having difficulty mastering the exercises. Having barriers and dividers provides an environment that is conducive to learning because distractions can be minimized (Figure 7.25). Three students per instructor/assistant is ideal.

Whether teaching modular classes or linear classes, the first session should be an orientation without the dogs. This prerequisite may have been met with attending a puppy socialization orientation and completing a socialization series. New clients will need to be provided with general instructions and learn their own training skill basics without the distraction of the dogs being present.

Class dynamics need to be carefully managed in adolescent and adult dog classes. Dogs may range from well-socialized alumnus of a puppy program to dogs who are in the group environment for the first time. Both situations pose different challenges.

Geriatric canine classes

The aging dog can benefit from group classes as well. A class full of young active dogs learning foundation skills is less likely to meet the needs of a geriatric dog and its owner. The behavior technician can be instrumental in designing and providing classes that take into consideration the difference in activity level of the geriatric dog. Many dogs develop arthritis as they age and engaging in a training class that requires frequent sitting or mobile activities could be uncomfortable for the geriatric dog. However, mental stimulation and moderate physical activity are important to prevent cognitive and physical decline in older dogs. A geriatric class can be centered around teaching clients how to massage their dogs, provide puzzle type toys for mental stimulation, teaching the dogs to "stretch" on cue, and also educate owners regarding clinical signs for canine cognitive dysfunction syndrome (DISHA: **D**isorientation, **I**nteraction changes, **S**leep–wake cycle changes, **H**ouse soiling, **A**ctivity changes).

Private in-home or in-clinic prevention/training appointments

The private in-home instruction option is becoming increasingly more popular among both dog owners and instructors. This is another area in which veterinary technicians can play a role while adding to their income.

There are many advantages to such a program. Training the dog in a low-stress environment will speed up the learning process. Adolescent dogs are highly distractible and they are likely to be better focused in their own home. Owners are most concerned about their dog's behaviors at home during the daily routine. Specific behaviors can be identified and modified where they are most problematic. When designing an in-home program, the instructor can also take into consideration the household dynamics such as behavior of family members.

In-home private training should be a customized program that is initiated with an interview session. In addition to contact information, other areas of information should include household members, their ages, and schedules. The family's history of previous dog ownership, details of why and where the dog was acquired, as well as early environmental history can be beneficial. During the interview process, the technician can observe the dog and inquire about any learning history, including past training experience. Together the client and technician can develop clear training goals for the dog and owner.

Problem behaviors may be identified. With training issues, these can be addressed in the training program. The technician may determine an issue is no longer in the preventive stage and therefore needs to be attended by a veterinarian. Owners may request assistance with a dog barking when guests come to the door but the veterinary technicians may determine the dog is in a high level of arousal with the potential to bite. Owners may not realize when a situation is no longer simply a lack of training but has become a behavior disorder.

In-clinic private training appointments with the behavior technician can be utilized for teaching owners how to fit a head collar or front clip harness. These private lessons could also be used to work on one specific skill such as walking on a loose leash.

Special prevention topic seminars or classes

The behavior technician can be assigned to develop public interest seminars on a variety of prevention topics for the hospital staff, clientele, and general public. For example, a technician with exceptional knowledge of avian or exotic pets may design a seminar for pet owners regarding handling, husbandry, environmental enrichment, and nutrition for the particular species. Other ideal prevention topics include pets and children, such as preparing for a newborn in a house with pets or managing a house with a toddler and pets.

Prevention seminars provide clients with a deeper understanding of their pets, can prevent the development of serious problems, and consequently decrease relinquishment rates.

Integrating behavior wellness into the veterinary hospital

A behavior wellness exam is an opportunity to check up on a pet's behavioral health and answer any related questions a client may have. Behavior wellness exams can be offered in conjunction with a routine physical exam or as a separate service.

Owners may be embarrassed to bring up behavior concerns to their veterinarian, because they often feel they are the cause of their pet's problems. Staff members can set the client at ease by bringing up the subject and providing them with a form to complete that will identify potential medical and behavioral concerns. Behavioral wellness visits are another ideal niche for the veterinary behavior technician.

A behavior check list/questionnaire should be used to obtain a general behavioral and physical health overview. In Appendices 13–18 there are samples of questionnaires for cats and dogs at different life stages. The adult form can be used with adolescent and adult examinations. This check list should become part of the pet's permanent file.

Puppy and kitten visits

The entire hospital staff should play a role in the counseling of new puppy and kitten owners. The staff can make the biggest impact when the new pet is novel and endearing as a puppy or kitten. This makes it the ideal time to educate clients on being successful pet owners. How clients and their new puppies and kittens are handled and counseled in the clinic on their first visit can help guarantee a satisfied client and development of a strong human–animal bond.

The entire clinic staff should be knowledgeable in what will be discussed with clients. The veterinary behavior technician can be the ideal person to educate clinic staff on behavior and coordinate the roles of each team member who interacts with owners. Regular staff meetings or seminars provide an excellent opportunity to educate the staff, answer questions, share concerns, and offer suggestions. This process ensures the consistency of information given out and promotes a team-oriented approach to behavior education.

The behavior team, including a veterinarian, should decide on appropriate literature to be included in the puppy and kitten packets. Most packets will include information on preventive medicine, such as recommended vaccine protocols, heartworm and other parasite preventives, as well as resources on the prevention of problems and handouts for positive solutions to normal puppy and kitten behaviors. Other pet care professionals in the community recommended by the hospital may also be invited to provide brochures and business cards to be included in the packet.

The best way to organize behavior resources for new puppy and kitten owners is in a 3-ring binder. The handouts can have holes punched in them and be included in the binder along with vaccination records and other veterinary informational handouts. The binder with a clear sleeve on the front cover will accommodate a page with the hospital logo and other contact information.

Utilizing a questionnaire, such as the New Puppy (less than 4 months) Questionnaire or the New Kitten (less than 3 months) Questionnaire in Appendices 13–18, ensures all vital information is obtained during the first puppy and kitten appointments. The questionnaire could be e-mailed to the client prior to the appointment or provided at check-in.

As discussed earlier in the chapter, techniques for preventing fear of the veterinary clinic should be implemented with all appointments, but is of particular importance with the new puppy or kitten.

Fearful puppies and kittens

Fearful puppies and kittens should be identified and treated as soon as possible. Although fear is genetically influenced, early experiences also play a role. The best chance of modifying fearful behaviors is when the pets are still within their sensitive socialization period. If the behavior is dismissed, it is sure to escalate as they mature and could lead to aggression. It is the veterinarian's and the veterinary behavior technician's responsibility to emphasize the importance of early intervention.

In the case of a new puppy or kitten that is still in its socialization period and showing mild fear, a technician can be of great assistance. Owners left on their own can cause further damage by overwhelming their pet. Through the appropriate implementation of classical counter-conditioning and desensitization, mild fears can usually be addressed quickly.

A young pet with severe fear and/or anxiety should be referred to a Veterinary Behaviorist. It has been hypothesized that anxiolytic medication used early may assist in extending the socialization period (direct communication with Dr. Andrew Luescher, Purdue University's Animal Behavior Clinic).

High-risk puppies

Research has shown (Guy *et al.*, 2001) certain factors may predispose a puppy to developing conflict-related aggression (aggression toward family members) (Table 7.14). These puppies may seem more fearful and anxious in general and may demonstrate handling issues or may show guarding behaviors around the food bowl or toys. Conflict behaviors may be observed in these and other situations (see Chapter 2 for a description of conflict behaviors). Puppies that have suffered a serious illness before 4 months of age are at a higher risk then puppies that have not had a serious physical illness. High-risk puppies are often hyperexcitable and have difficulty calming and may lack impulse control. The research also showed a correlation between canine aggression toward owners with first-time owners and owners interacting with a high level of anthropomorphism. The risk increases if there is a lack of training or if harsh training techniques are used (including the use of training tools such as choke, pinch or shock collars). Confrontational "domination" techniques are also likely to increase anxiety and aggression. High-risk puppies often form negative associations quickly, even after only one event. Puppies at high risk or that are demonstrating early signs of conflict-related aggression

Table 7.14 High risk factors for puppies to develop conflict-related aggression (aggression toward family members).

Increased fear and anxiety	Including early handling and/or guarding issues
Had a serious illness under 4 months of age	Including parasite infestation, skin disorders and other serious physical stressors
Hyperexcitable	May show an inability to calm and lack impulse control
Not walked off the property routinely	That is, lack of mental stimulation, which also contributes to hyperexcitability
Anthropomorphic owners	Increases inconsistency and unpredictability in the environment
Lack of training or harsh, aversive training	Punishment is rarely administered appropriately but rather inconsistently and unpredictably, causing an increase in anxiety

(Guy *et al.*, 2001)

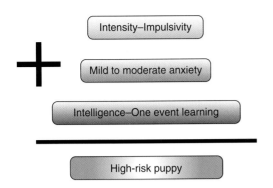

Figure 7.26 High-risk puppy paradigm.

should be diagnosed and treated by a veterinarian or veterinary behaviorist as early as possible (Figure 7.26).

The adolescent behavior wellness examination

Consideration should be given toward scheduling a specific behavior wellness exam for every adolescent dog and cat between 9 and 12 months of age. Scheduling the session for 30–60 min is ideal.

Adolescence is the most trying time in pet ownership. Although dogs and cats may appear fully grown physically, they are not yet socially mature. During this difficult time, there is often no physical reason for a veterinary visit. Pets have been neutered and vaccination protocols completed by 6 months of age, just as they are entering adolescence. This is the age that most dogs and cats are relinquished. By scheduling a behavior wellness exam, technicians can provide an opportunity for the client to learn about this difficult stage and assist clients with positive solutions for normal behavior.

Offering products related to behavior health such as head halters, front clip harnesses, and food storage toys will increase revenue. It also provides staff members with the opportunity to educate clients on proper use and fitting of these items. When offered as a separate service, the behavior wellness exam also provides an opportunity to review other recommendations such as flea and heartworm prevention.

A behavior wellness exam may also identify actions that can potentially lead to a severe behavior problem if left untreated. Many owners are unaware of the warning signs that veterinary behavior technicians see as potential red flags for developing issues. Pet owners may not see the dog that hides behind the owner or barks at incoming guests as potential signs of aggression. It is unfortunate that many do not recognize the warning signs as being problematic until a bite has

occurred. By that time the prognosis is much worse. By identifying signs early, bites may be prevented, the human–animal bond maintained, and the animal's life saved. The best way to identify these signs is with a behavior wellness exam.

Another goal of the adolescent behavior wellness exam is to educate clients when they are given poor or outdated advice. The media and internet are filled with unproven, unscientific, and potentially dangerous recommendations. Neighbors and friends are quick to give advice in all areas of pet care but are largely uneducated. Dog trainers may present themselves as experts in behavior. This is a highly unregulated field and although some advice may be beneficial, there are many unknowing dog trainers who can contribute to or even create behavior problems. A behavior wellness exam can help provide clients with appropriate recommendations and resources.

The canine and feline management and enrichment previously discussed in this chapter will be crucial information for the veterinary technician to be fluent with and communicate to the client.

Discussions on training should be included in a behavior wellness exam. All pets benefit from mental stimulation. Training is a great way to enrich the lives of pets and can create a set of positive behaviors in place of less desirable behaviors. It is likely the most troublesome dogs are also the most intelligent. Veterinary staff members need to quickly identify training issues and come up with positive solutions that will fit into the life style of the client and meet the pet's needs.

Training recommendations may be made, including qualified trainers (see Chapter 1 for recommendations of choosing a trainer and Appendix 5 Trainer assessment form) and whether group, private or in-home classes would be the most beneficial.

Some behavioral issues pertaining to lack of stimulation are not evident in kittens but can become increasingly important in adulthood. A noted weight gain is another important reason to stress more mental and physical stimulation in the adult cat.

Pointed questions on changes in the environment should be included. As cats are influenced greatly by their surroundings, any changes should be as stress free as possible. It is also important that the client understands how cats show signs of stress. The average cat owner would likely place an anthropomorphic label such as "spite" or "getting back at them" when a cat eliminates outside of a litter box or sprays. Making them aware of the motivating factor behind a behavior will help them become more proactive with solutions for problem behavior.

The adult behavior wellness examination

Feline and canine adult behavior wellness exams can be incorporated into the annual or semi-annual exams. Obtaining an updated questionnaire at each visit will allow the staff to recognize any changes in the physical and behavioral health from previous visits. If we do not ask, the client many not ask for help until they are at their "wits end." When the bond between the owner and pet has been damaged to this point, it can be much more difficult to reconcile (see Chapters 4 and 5). Early intervention is always best. Routine questions designed to uncover potential problems early are key.

The senior behavior wellness examination

An important time for practices to include a behavioral exam is when a pet becomes a senior. This timing is going to vary greatly between species as well as individual breeds of dogs. Many giant breed dogs can be considered geriatric as early as 6 or 7 years of age. Smaller breed dogs and cats tend to have a longer life span and therefore my not show signs of aging until 11 or 12 years of age. Other effects on the aging process may include long-standing health problems, the environment, and general care received throughout their lives. When the veterinary staff see signs of a pet becoming aged, they should always question the owners about behavioral changes. This can be a topic owners fail to bring up on their own as they feel it is normal or it is an area they do not realize veterinary staff are well-versed in. It is extra important in this stage of a pet's life to ask about behavioral changes as there is no other time when physical and behavioral problems are more closely linked together. It can also be a time when an owner's bond is the greatest with the pet.

Any behavioral changes in geriatric pets should be followed up with a full medical work up. A physical examination should be performed along with a complete blood count (CBC), blood chemistries, thyroid levels, urinalysis and a neurological exam. In many cases, the first sign of disease in pets is changes in their personality and activity level. You can also have a physically healthy pet showing signs of cognitive loss through changes in behavior. This is where being well-versed in management, nutrition, pharmacology, and behavior modification is important. By offering support to the client in these areas you may be prolonging the pet's life span as well as improving the quality of life.

Common behavioral changes seen in geriatric pets center around house soiling, anxiety, and aggression. Because medical factors are often the causative factor, a combination approach to treatment (medical and behavioral) will be necessary.

Cognitive dysfunction can occur in both dogs and cats. It is by definition an impairment of memory and learning. The DISHA signs are often used as a screening tool.

Disorientation

Interaction changes

Sleep-wake cycle changes

House soiling

Activity level changes

Common symptoms of cognitive dysfunction syndrome include loss of house training, excess vocalization, abnormal sleep–wake cycles, failure to recognize familiar people, standing in corners or going to the hinged side of the door, and abnormal motility such as circling and pacing. Although no cure is available, the progression of the disease can be slowed through pharmaceutical and behavior modification.

Behavior wellness conclusion

If behavior wellness is not a top priority of veterinary practices, valuable information on behavior problem prevention, along with potential medical problems, may go undetected. It is the responsibility of the veterinary staff to meet the needs of their client's pets both physically and behaviorally.

Conclusion

A behavior problem is a behavior that is a problem for the pet owner, which can be due to lack of training or conditioned unwanted behaviors. The goal is to prevent "behavior problems" and to certainly prevent them from becoming a "behavioral disorder," which usually has an emotional foundation. Most behavior problems are much easier to prevent than they are to treat. The veterinary clinic is the ideal location to educate owners before problem behaviors become well established. This is a valuable role for the behavior technician to fill in veterinary practice. Prevention and enrichment from puppy and kitten to the geriatric dog and cat is a position in which the veterinary technician can excel and make an impact on the welfare of numerous pets and their owners.

References

Barrett J., Frey R., Thomson G. Animal Bite Infections. Gale Encyclopedia of Children's Health, 2006. http://www.healthline.com/galecontent/animal-bite-infections (accessed 15 May 2014).

Bergesen, F.J. (1989). The Effects of Pet Facilitated Therapy on the Self-Esteem and Socialization of Primary School Children. Paper presented at Monaco'89, the 5th International Conference on the Relationship Between Humans and Animals.

Bernardo L, Gardner M, Rosenfield R, Cohen B, Pitetti R. A comparision of dog bite injuries in younger and older children treated in a pediatric emergency department. *Pediatric Emergency Care* 2002 Jun; **18** (3): 247-249.

Bernstein, P.L. and Strack, M. (1996) A game of cat and house: spatial patterns and behavior of 14 cats (*Felis catus*) in the home. *Anthrozoos*, **9**, 25–39.

Bradshaw, J. W. S., E. J. Blackwell and R. A. Casey (2009). "Dominance in domestic dogs–useful construct or bad habit?" *Journal of Veterinary Behavior: Clinical Applications and Research* **4** (3): 135-144.

Crowell-Davis, S.L., Barry, K. and Wolfe, R. (1997) Social behavior and aggression problems of cats. *Veterinary Clinics of North America: Small Animal Practice*, **27** (3), 549–568.

Donaldson, J. (1996) *The Culture Clash*, James and Kenneth Publishers, Berkeley, California, USA.

Duffy, D.L. and Serpell, J.A. (2006) Non-reproductive effects of spaying and neutering on behavior in dogs, in *Proceedings of the Third International Symposium on Non-Surgical Contraceptive Methods for Pet Population Control*, Center for the Interaction of Animals and Society, School of Veterinary Medicine, University of Pennsylvania, Alexandria, Virginia, USA.

Guy, N.C., Luescher, U.A., Dohoo, S.E. *et al.* (2001) Demographic and aggressive characteristics of dogs in a general veterinary caseload. *Applied Animal Behaviour Science*, **74** (1), 15–28.

Hart, B.L. and Cooper, L. (1984) Factors relating to urine spraying and fighting in prepubertally gonadectomized cats. *Journal of the American Veterinary Medical Association*, **184** (10), 1255–1258.

Hopkins, S.G., Schubert, T.A. and Hart, B.L. (1976) Castration of adult male dogs: effects on roaming, aggression, urine marking, and mounting. *Journal of the American Veterinary Medical Association*, **168**, 1108–1110.

Kahn, A., Bauche, P., Lamoureux, J. and the Members of the Dog Bites Research Team (2003) Child victims of dog bites treated in emergency departments. *European Journal of Pediatrics*, **162**, 254–258.

Kahn, A., Robert, E., Piette, D. *et al.* (2004) Prevalence of dog bites in children. A telephone survey. *European Journal of Pediatrics*, **163**, 424.

Liberg, O., Sandell, M., Pontier, D. *et al.* (2000) Density, spatial organization and reproducive tactics in the domestic cat and other felids, in *The domestic cat: the biology of its behavior*, 2nd edn (eds D.V. Turner and P. Bateson), Cambridge University Press, Cambridge, England, pp. 119–147.

Lindsay, S.R. (2001) *Handbook of Applied Dog Behavior and Training* Vol. 2, Iowa State University Press, Ames.

Martin, K. and Martin, D. (2011) *Puppy Start Right: Foundation Training for the Companion Dog*, Sunshine Books, Waltham, MA.

Martin K., and Martin D. Puppy Start Right for Instructors. Online course http://www.karenpryoracademy.com (accessed 15 May 2014). 2012.

Mondelli, F., Prato Previde, E., Verga, M. *et al.* (2004) The bond that never developed: adoption and relinquishment of dogs in a rescue shelter. *Journal of Applied Animal Welfare Science*, **7** (4), 253–266.

Morgan, M. and Houpt, K.A. (1990) Feline behaviour problems: the influence of declawing. *Antrozöos*, **3**, 50–53.

Neilson JC. Pearl vs. clumping: litter preference in a population of shelter cats, in *Proceedings. American Veterinary Society of Animal Behavior* 2001; pp. 14.

Neilson, J.C. (2008) Is bigger better? Litterbox size preference test, in *Proceedings. American College of Veterinary Behavior/American Veterinary Society of Animal Behavior 2008 Scientific Paper and Poster Session*, pp. 46–49.

Neville, P.F. and Remfry, J. (1984) Effect of neutering on two groups of feral cats. *Veterinary Record*, **114** (5), 447–450 May.

Patronek, G.J., Glickman, L.T., Beck, A.M. *et al.* (1996) Risk factors for relinquishment of dogs to an animal shelter. *Journal of the American Veterinary Medical Association*, **209** (3), 572–581.

Poresky, R.H. and Hendrix, C. (1990) Differential effects of pet presence and pet-bonding on young children. *Psychological Reports*, **67**, 51–54.

Schalomon J, Ainoedhofer H, Singer G, Petnehazy T, Mayr J, Kiss K, Hollwarth M. Analysis of dog bites in children who are younger than 17 years. *Journal of Pediatrics* 2006 Mar; **117** (3) 374-379.

Serpell J: Beneficial effects of pet ownership on some aspects of human health & behaviour, *Journal of Royal Science of Medicine* 84, December 1991

Stubbs, W.P., Bloomberg, M.S., Scruggs, S.L. *et al* (1996) Effects of perpubertal gonadectomy on physical and behavioral development of cats. *Journal of American Veterinary Medical Association*, **209** (11), 1864–1871.

Wells, D.L., Graham, L. and Hepper, P.G. (2002) The influence of auditory stimulation on the behaviour of dogs housed in a rescue shelter. *Animal Welfare*, **11**, 385–393.

Xavier M., J. Fatjó, M. Amat and V. Mariotti 2008. Preventing Canine Aggression: What Works and What Doesn't. Proceeding of the SEVC Southern European Veterinary Conference. Oct. 17–19, 2008 – Barcelona, Spain.

Yin, S. (2009) *Low Stress Handling Restraint and Behavior Modification of Dogs & Cats*, Cattle Dog Publishing, Davis, California, USA.

8

Specific behavior modification techniques and practical applications for behavior disorders

Julie K. Shaw

TEAM Education in Animal Behavior, LLC, Spicewood, TX, USA

CHAPTER MENU

The focus of this chapter is to standardize, through terminology and description, commonly prescribed treatments, including management, training styles, specific training exercises, training tools, and commonly prescribed behavior modification techniques.

As described in detail in Chapter 1, it is the veterinarian's responsibility to diagnose behavior disorders and prescribe the treatment plan. The veterinary technician is the "case manager" triaging and coordinating the communication cycle between the pet owner, veterinarian, and qualified trainer. The technician also teaches the pet owner why aspects of the treatment plan were chosen, how each aspect of the treatment plan will improve the problem, and how to apply them.

The veterinary technician must be a fluent communicator, teacher, and trainer to successfully instruct the pet owner on understanding and applying the prescribed treatment plan. A canine behavior plan of care form has been included in the appendix to expedite treatment plans from the veterinarian to the technician/trainer (see Appendix 7). This text will follow the plan of care form in its organization.

As the case manager, the veterinary technician will advocate for both the client and patient, making sure the treatment plan is functional and productive, while also teaching and being the support system for the pet owner. The veterinary technician must fully understand the science behind the techniques, translate the techniques into language the client can relate to, and instruct the pet owner on how to place treatment techniques into their daily routine. A complete and confident understanding of the techniques will give the technician the ability to modify techniques to best fit the individual client's lifestyle.

> • The veterinary technician must fully understand the science behind the techniques, translate the techniques into language the client can relate to, and instruct the pet owner on how to place treatment techniques into their daily routine.

Common veterinary behavior disorder diagnosis and descriptions

A "diagnosis" refers to the categorization of clinical signs into diagnostic categories that provide the veterinarian with information. The clinical information suggests an underlying cause and specific treatments for the disorder. The diagnosis is not meant to label the animal but to describe a set of clinical signs and to expedite communication between professionals. For example, a dog that has been diagnosed with fear aggression toward unfamiliar people indicates the animal has displayed a set of behaviors indicating fear-motivated distance-increasing behaviors. This is comparable to diagnosing an animal that cannot process sugars appropriately due to insulin production insufficiency of the pancreas as having diabetes. Just as with any medical disorder, behavior disorder diagnoses are used to describe a set of past or present conditions that may need to be treated or managed to prevent relapses.

As with any medical diagnosis, the veterinary technician must understand the general meaning of each behavioral disorder diagnoses, the specific aspects of treatment, and the effects on the human–animal bond. The following are common behavioral diagnoses with their descriptions (Table 8.1).

Aggression

Aggression is the most common reason dogs are presented to referral behavior practices. In general, aggression refers to threatening or harmful behavior directed toward another individual or group. Often an animal is presented with multiple types of aggression with multiple causations.

Aggression is a normal communication tool and is not necessarily a pathological or abnormal behavior. Normal aggression is demonstrated in situations that warrant aggression. The intensity of the aggression by the animal is modified, depending on the situation and the relative level of the threat. For example, a normal aggressive display would be if a stranger broke into the home unannounced and was bitten. Abnormal aggression occurs when the animal perceives threat where it does not exist and has difficulty modulating its aggressive response as the perceived threat changes.

> • Aggression is a normal communication tool and is not necessarily a pathological or abnormal behavior.

The context of the situation will determine whether the aggression is normal or abnormal and may be influenced by a combination of genetics and experience.

Often high arousal or frustration is a complicating factor to aggression. High arousal tends to cause the animal to react rather than respond to a situation, making it difficult for it to respond consciously.

Many types of aggression can be thwarted or prevented if the veterinary technician is able to detect early warning signs in puppy and kitten classes (see Chapter 7).

There remains some controversy with regard to aggressive behavior classification among veterinary behaviorists. In this chapter, diagnosis will be defined according to motivation or trigger, behavior, and target.

Conflict-induced aggression

Conflict-induced aggression is a conflict-resolution strategy, resulting from an approach-withdrawal conflict or the inability to predict the environment. Conflict-induced aggression is usually directed toward family members. It differs from fear-based aggression in that the dog or cat does not usually attempt to leave the situation, unless the motivation to withdrawal becomes greater than to remain in the situation. Many dogs that have conflict-induced aggression also show fear-based aggression in other contexts. Conflict-induced aggression is also not limited to owner-initiated interactions. The pet may be social and solicit owner interaction and attention at times.

Fear aggression typically occurs when a person approaches the pet and tries to interact; the pet shows appeasement or displacement behaviors (curves body, sniffs ground) and aggresses if unable to avoid the interaction.

> • Fear aggression typically occurs when a person approaches the pet and tries to interact; the pet shows appeasement or displacement behaviors (curves body, sniffs ground) and aggresses if unable to avoid the interaction.

Conflict-induced aggression typically occurs when the pet seeks out the pet-owner, perhaps even solicits attention, then shows conflict behaviors (freezes, shifts eyes) and aggresses. The pet could leave the situation but chooses not to because of conflicting motivations (desire to be with the pet-owner and uncertainty of what will happen next.)

Table 8.1 Common behavioral diagnoses.

Behavior	Description or motivation	Species	Target
Aggression	Conflict-induced	C,F	FP, UFP[a]
	Possessive	C	FP, UFP
	Petting-induced	F	FP, UFP
	Disease or pain-induced	C,F	A
	Fear/Defensive-induced	C,F	A
	Idiopathic	C,F	A
	Inter-dog (IDA) + motivation	C	UFA
	Inter-cat (ICA) + motivation	F	UFA
	Inter-cat – household (ICA-H) + motivation	F	FA
	Inter-dog – Household (IDA-H) + motivation	C	FA
	Alliance-induced	C	FA
	Status-induced	C	FA
	Learned	C,F	A
	Maternal/hormonal-induced	C	A
	Play-induced	C,F	FP, UFP
	Redirected	C,F	A
	Territorial	C,F	UFP, UFA
Ingestive	Coprophagia	C	
	Pica	C,F	
	Predatory Behavior	C,F	
Eliminative	Housesoiling	C,F	
	Urine marking	C,F	
	Excitement urination	C	
	Extreme fear/appeasement urination	C	
Anxiety Disorders	Generalized anxiety	C, F	
	Global fear	C, F	
	Separation anxiety	C, F	
	Sound / Thunderstorm phobia	C, F	
	Specific fear or phobia	C, F	
	Acute conflict behaviors / stereotypy	C, F	
	Compulsive disorder	C, F	
Other	Cognitive dysfunction	C, F	
	Hyper-excitability	C, F	
	Conditioned-unwanted behavior	C, F	

[a]Conflict-induced aggression is most commonly associated with aggression toward family members and more rarely toward unfamiliar people.
C, canine; F, feline; FP, familiar people; UFP, unfamiliar people; FA, familiar animal; UFA, unfamiliar animal; A, all.

- Conflict-induced aggression typically occurs when the pet seeks out the pet-owner, perhaps even solicits attention, then shows conflict behaviors (freezes, shifts eyes) and aggresses. The pet could leave the situation but chooses not to because of conflicting motivations (desire to be with the pet-owner and uncertainty of what will happen next.)

The pet is in a motivational approach-withdrawal conflict. The pet wants to interact with the person, but at some point it becomes uncomfortable with the social interaction because of unpredictability or uncertainty. It anticipates that something unpleasant or undesirable (from the pet's point of view) is about to happen. The conflict is likely similar to the feeling a human gets when a person remains in your personal space too long, or a person hugs you and holds you a little longer than you would like. A hallmark with conflict-induced aggression is the display of conflict behaviors before the aggression. Unfortunately, most pet owners are unaware of what the pet is communicating and it escalates to growling, snapping, or biting.

Conflict-induced (and other forms of) aggression is often rewarded through removal of the threat (stimulus backs off negatively reinforcing the aggression) and the conflict/fear is resolved; the animal consequently will be more likely to continue to use aggression in these contexts and may become more offensive in its behavior as the outcome becomes more predictable. Over time, the animal may stop showing fear and/or conflict behaviors or the conflict behaviors are minimized. Therefore, when working with an animal with a long history of aggression, the technician should proceed with caution and be fully aware of past bite history, as warning signs may not be displayed.

Conflict-induced aggression is most frequently owner directed and often includes a comorbid diagnosis of possessive aggression or the guarding of resources.

> • Conflict-induced aggression is most frequently owner directed.

Conflict-induced aggression is seen in dogs and cats but is diagnosed less frequently in cats, likely because fewer direct human–cat interactions occur and therefore there are fewer opportunities for conflict. Most cases of aggression in cats is fear-induced, with the exception of petting intolerance where the cat may be in a motivational conflict of "I want to sit on your lap, but I do not want to be petted."

Conflict-induced aggression may first be seen in puppyhood as inappropriate play, fear-based aggression, and guarding of the food bowl or other resources (Guy et al., 2001). It frequently begins when a puppy is sociable (mouthing, play biting, jumping on familiar people, or displaying some form of attention-getting behavior) and the behavior is then punished by the owner. The puppy still wants to interact with the owner, but is afraid and in a motivation conflict. The motivational conflict occurs because the pet owner's behavior is inconsistent and unpredictable from the puppy's point of view. Some puppies may get more aroused and interact with rougher play biting rather than leaving or avoiding the pet owner. Eventually the motivation changes from play to fear, to frustration, and conflict, resulting in the development of conflict-induced aggression (Figure 8.1).

> • Conflict-induced aggression may first be seen in puppyhood as inappropriate play, fear-based aggression, and guarding of the food bowl or other resources.

Treatment includes addressing how the dog is managed, addressing basic temperament issues (fearfulness or anxiety) and the cause of the conflict (owner's inconsistency). One of the most important components of treatment is structuring consistent, predictable, and positive human–pet interactions in order to reduce fear and conflict. Social interactions, in the form of cue-response-reward, add predictability and facilitate classical CC resulting in a positive emotional state.

Consistent rules provide the dog with the possibility to predict events in the environment and thus increase confidence.

Possessive aggression
Possessive aggression is described as guarding of an item from people. Aggression over a possession, food, or handling may be subcategories of conflict-induced aggression.

> • Aggression over a possession, food, or handling may be subcategories of conflict-induced aggression.

Possessive aggression often begins with a puppy possessing a "valued" or stolen item, is then chased by the pet owner (which may initially be "fun") followed by the unknowing pet owner attempting to take the object away, sometimes in an antagonistic fashion. The puppy may become fearfully aggressive and when the pet owner backs off, the aggressive behavior becomes negatively reinforced, creating a strong learning component.

In the case of aggression over the food bowl, guarding food is a somewhat normal behavior of dogs, especially when directed toward other animals in the home. When excessive and directed toward animals or humans near the food bowl, it may be a subcategory of possessive aggression.

Petting-induced aggression
Petting-induced aggression in the cat can be either offensive or defensive. It is believed to be a subtype of conflict-induced aggression. The cat seems to enjoy the

CHAPTER 8

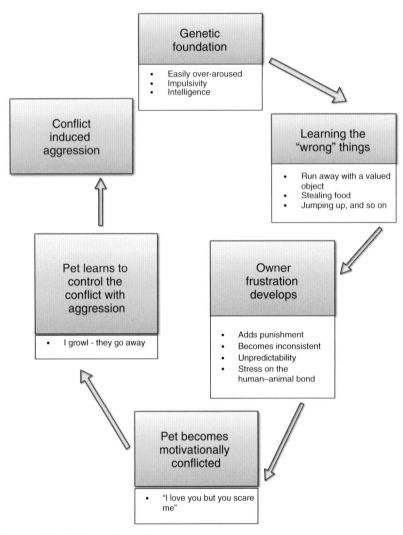

Figure 8.1 The development of conflict-induced aggression.

petting and then suddenly attacks the person petting it, jumps down, runs a short distance, sits, and grooms itself. Often the cat's pupils are dilated. In all likelihood, the cat was placed in a motivational conflict, wanting to remain on the lap but no longer desiring to be touched.

Disease-induced or pain-induced aggression

Disease-induced or pain-induced aggression occurs either primarily or secondarily from a gross medical condition. The aggression may occur primarily because the animal is more irritable because of the disease process or in the attempt to avoid or remove pain.

Aggression may occur secondarily long after the disease or pain is resolved because the animal has learned through classical conditioning (i.e., being restrained = pain, the veterinary hospital = fear.)

Decreasing pain and fear during all veterinary visits and teaching handling exercises during puppy and kitten classes may help prevent pain-induced aggression and a later veterinary hospital aversion or phobia from developing.

Fear/defensive aggression

Fear aggression is sometimes referred to as *defensive aggression* and occurs when the animal perceives a situation as threatening. Initial descriptions of the aggression may include a dog demonstrating defensive postures including head down, approach withdrawal, ears back, tail down, looking away, and lip licking. Cats attempt to use physical contact as a last resort in a fearful situation and prefer active avoidance or withdrawal.

Aggressive responses may be followed by withdrawal and distance-increasing responses. Fear aggression occurs when the animal chooses "fight" over freezing or flight. This "choice" may occur because of not being able to leave the situation or by being in a motivational conflict about leaving the situation (i.e., "I want the stranger to leave my safe area and I do not want to leave my safe area".) Animals that are fearful frequently learn to control the fear-provoking stimulus using aggression and may later become more offensive in their aggressive displays as they learn that aggression results in removal of the threat. The predictability of the consequence from previous learning experiences can result in more offensive rather than defensive aggression. However, even though there may be less outward signs of fear in the animal's body language, the motivation for the aggression is still fear.

"Control" in this context refers to an animal's ability to predict its own outcomes. Research conducted over decades suggests that control is an unconditional (primary) reinforcer and is especially reinforcing to animals that suffer from anxiety.

- "Control" in this context refers to an animal's ability to predict its own outcomes.

It is critical that all fear-eliciting stimuli are identified before modification can occur. The pet's emotion to the fear-provoking stimuli is modified and then a new response is taught.

Idiopathic aggression

Idiopathic aggression refers to an unexplained and intense aggression and is reserved for animals that have had a complete medical and behavioral investigation in which no identifiable aggression-provoking stimuli can be determined. The aggression has been described as explosive, out of context in its severity, and unpredictable. Idiopathic aggression is usually only diagnosed by a veterinary behaviorist who has acquired an in-depth medical and behavioral history.

Inter-dog aggression (IDA)

Inter-dog aggression (IDA) is described as aggression between dogs unknown to each other. "IDA" does not define the motivation behind the behavior and therefore usually includes a motivation description (i.e., territorial, fear, and conflict). Common motivations may include fear/defensive, status (usually between intact males), territoriality, conflict or poor canine communication skills (under socialized or communication skills were not learned in early puppyhood).

Underlying fear or anxiety often contributes to IDA along with learning. Some dogs that have been attacked in the past assume an offensively defensive position – "I'll attack you before you can attack me."

Inter-cat aggression (ICA)

Inter-cat aggression (ICA) refers to interactions between known and unknown cats and usually includes elements of growling, hissing, spitting, attacking, chasing, and biting. ICA may also include elements of territorial aggression, redirected aggression, or fear aggression.

Status-induced aggression

Status-related aggression in cats has not been well studied or accepted in behavioral medicine but has most often been associated with densely housed cats. Cats in more natural settings tend to maintain their relationships through scent marking rather than aggression.

Inter-dog aggression – household (IDA-H)

Inter-dog aggression – household (IDA-H), (sometimes called *sibling rivalry*) is aggression between dogs living in the same household or social group. "IDA-H" is not a diagnosis but a description. Several different types of aggression (some occurring simultaneously) can be exhibited between dogs in the same household, including fear, redirected, or idiopathic aggression (see descriptions). Other types of aggression that may cause IDA-H include the following.

Alliance-induced aggression

Alliance-induced aggression refers to aggression between dogs in the same household that fight only in the proximity of the pet owner. Usually the more fearful and most owner-dependent dog becomes anxious when the other dog approaches the owner and consequently the less confident dog aggresses. If the owner leaves before it progresses to a full fight, the aggression usually subsides. This type of aggression is often inadvertently conditioned by the owner's attention.

Status-induced aggression

Status-induced aggression refers to aggression between dogs in the same household in which the relationship between the dogs is unclear. Fighting often occurs when the social relationship has changed between the dogs. The owner frequently intercedes in aggressive situations supporting the dog that would without interference likely lose the resource or conflict. The aggression is often reinforced in the less confident dog by the owner coddling or petting while often punishing the more confident dog, causing confusion and conflict in the dogs' relationship.

Learned aggression

All types of aggression have some degree of learning involved. The larger the learning component, the better the prognosis because alternate "coping mechanisms" can be taught to the animal. Aggression is conditioned through positive reinforcement (i.e, owner picks up the pet), negative reinforcement (i.e., fear or conflict-provoking stimulus retreats) and classical conditioning (veterinary clinic = pain).

Learned aggression and lack of bite inhibition is often taught to dogs in protection training or protection sports. If taught properly, it is actually a "game of tug" the dog plays with excellent cue stimulus control. In this context the motivation is not fear but instead play and high arousal.

Maternal/hormonal induced aggression

Maternal aggression occurs when a bitch defends her puppies from people or other animals. It is considered to be normal behavior to a degree and usually is not treated as much as managed (removing the bitch before the puppies are handled).

Play-induced aggression

Canine mouthing and play biting are considered normal forms of interactions and communication for dogs but can become problematic when directed toward humans. Although not technically considered true aggression, over-exuberant play can be damaging to the human–animal bond. Often the human response reinforces the behavior (i.e., attention is given) or the play escalates to the point when the owner attempts to punish the behavior, placing the dog in (the dog's perspective) a conflicting situation of uncertainty and high arousal. Inappropriate play can then become a precursor to a more serious type of aggression, that is, conflict-induced aggression.

Feline play-induced aggression involves unsolicited attacks by a young cat targeting people or other cats within the home. It is considered a type of redirected predatory behavior, which may include hiding, chasing, stalking, and pouncing behaviors. Cats that display play-induced aggression are usually young and energetic, taken from their litter early (or orphaned) and living in single-cat households (when directed toward owners).

Redirected aggression

Redirected aggression is incidental to another form of aggression or emotional arousal. It occurs when a dog or cat cannot reach the target of its aggression and out of frustration changes its focus of aggression to an object, person, or other animal that is not the stimulus for the aggressive arousal.

Redirected aggression is very serious because the target of the aggression usually cannot modify their behavior to prevent the aggression. They are "collateral" damage in the aggressive episode.

Stimuli that may elicit redirected aggression in cats can be other cats, odors, noises, unfamiliar people, unfamiliar places, or pain. It frequently begins when a cat sees a cat outside the window or smells another cat. The aggression is then redirected toward another cat or person in the household. ICA can begin between two cats that live together as a result of redirected aggression and likely will not resolve without treatment.

Common triggers in dogs may include barking at fence lines, ringing of the doorbell, or being restrained on a leash. Redirected aggression can start IDA-H (sibling rivalry) when the "victim" dog (dog toward which aggression is being redirected) begins to anticipate the attack and fights back.

Territorial aggression

Dogs are genetically programmed to be territorial. Territorial aggression refers to aggression directed toward people or animals that are not part of the dog's immediate social group or are unfamiliar to them, when they enter the dog's perceived territory. The classic definition of territorial aggression refers to the territory being a fixed location (i.e., house, room, yard, and bed). In some literature, a mobile territory around the dog (i.e., leash, proximity to owner) is also referred to as a territory. However, a mobile territory is probably best described as just fear-based aggression in that specific context. Territorial aggression is influenced by breed, age, sex, and socialization experience. Excitement and arousal increase the aggressive behavior. Fear is an underlying component with territorial aggression and can be observed when a dog approaches and withdraws but as the person turns to leave (and becomes less threatening through the dog's eyes), the dog's territorial aggression outweighs the fear and a bite may occur to the person's back side. Fear can also be seen when dogs seem offensively aggressive through a door or window but become fearful or defensively aggressive once the door is opened.

There is also a strong learning component to territorial aggression. When the behavior is practiced it is almost always negatively reinforced by the threat (approaching person or animal) going away.

Territorial aggression in cats is most often directed toward other cats, known or unknown, rather than humans. It occurs most commonly between male cats and in high cat density areas. It can also occur when a new cat is introduced to the household or when a resident cat returns home from the veterinary hospital because it is not recognized by the other cats. Body language includes staring at the other cat, attack, chase, and paw blows. Signs of fear in the victim may trigger an attack.

Ingestive disorders
Coprophagia
Coprophagia is the ingestion of feces. It is seen most often in dogs either eating their own feces or the feces of other animals. Engaging in coprophagia is normal in most dogs although contributing factors include normal maternal behavior, puppy exploratory behavior, dietary preference, hunger, or attention-seeking behavior. Coprophagia can be a coping mechanism for high-anxiety dogs and has been identified as an oral manifestation of compulsive disorder.

Pica
Pica is generally described as the ingestion of inanimate objects. Although young animals may destroy objects in their explorations, most do not ingest objects, unlike animals that suffer from pica. Forms of pica include wool sucking in cats (sucking on fabric), rock chewing and swallowing, soil eating, or other oral fixation. Some forms of pica may be considered compulsive disorders (see section titled **Compulsive Disorders**).

Predatory behavior
Predatory behaviors refer to a sequence of behaviors that is associated with the process of catching and killing of another animal for consumption. The canine sequence may include orient, eye-stalk, chase, grab-bite, kill-bite, dissect, consume (Coppinger and Coppinger, 2001). It is linked to normal survival behavior and therefore "hardwired" in the brain. It is a highly genetically controlled behavior that is coordinated by the appetite and satiety centers of the brain; therefore bites are usually not inhibited during a predatory attack. Through learning, predatory aggression can be redirected toward conspecifics as with dog fighting circumstances. In dogs, excitement and social facilitation can exacerbate predatory aggression; therefore groups of dogs are more dangerous.

- Bites are usually not inhibited during a predatory attack.

As discussed in Chapter 3, manipulating, killing, and ingesting prey is a learned behavior in cats. The chase and catching of prey is an innate behavior. Cats with access to small animals (rabbits, mice, and birds) may stalk and injure or ingest them.

Elimination
House soiling
House soiling refers to elimination (either urine or stool) in locations the pet owner finds unacceptable or inappropriate. Inappropriate elimination is the most common behavioral reason pets are relinquished to shelters (Salman *et al.*, 2000). Elimination problems can occur for multiple reasons, including medical reasons, ineffective house training or litter box training, urine marking (see later text), separation anxiety (distress), social or environmental stressors, cognitive dysfunction, fear, extreme appeasement, or psychogenic polydipsia.

House soiling by cats usually occurs because of two primary reasons: litterbox aversion or a substrate preference.

Urine marking
Marking is a normal communicative method to call attention to objects, individuals, or an area and is frequently a sign of anxiety in both dogs and cats. Marking in the dog can take the form of visual marks created by a dog pawing at the ground or disposition of chemical cues processed through the olfactory system. Urine marking is the most common cause pet owners seek assistance for marking behaviors. Territorial urine marking is most prevalent in intact males or females.

Urine marking in cats is sometimes called "spraying" because the cat backs up to a vertical surface (less commonly on horizontal surfaces) with its tail straight up and a twitching tip. Some cats mark by urinating, emptying the bladder, or by defecating (middening). It was previously believed the volume of urine when marking was smaller than the volume of urine during house soiling, but a recent small pilot study done by Jacqueline Neilson, DVM, DACVB found the volume of urine amounts when spraying were similar to the amounts found when eliminating (i.e., large amounts of sprayed urine).

Urine marking in both dogs and cats frequently reflects environmental stress or anxiety.

> • Urine marking in both dogs and cats frequently reflects environmental stress or anxiety.

Excitement urination

Excitement urination occurs in dogs that are overly aroused and can also be seen when a dog is in a motivational conflict, that is, the dog is excited to greet people at the door but also uncertain. Excitement urination is different from extreme appeasement urination in that appeasement behaviors are usually not shown at the same time.

Extreme appeasement urination

Extreme appeasement urination is not truly an elimination problem as much as a fear or lack of confidence issue. Appeasement urination occurs when the dog attempts to avoid a conflict by defusing the situation with the normal canine appeasement behavior of urinating small amounts. The dog is uncertain and attempting to communicate he is not a threat.

Anxiety disorders

Anxiety – It is an overwhelming sense of apprehension in reaction to a prospective or imagined danger or uncertainty.

> • Anxiety – It is an overwhelming sense of apprehension in reaction to a prospective or imagined danger or uncertainty.

Fear – It is a combination of physical, emotional, and physiological responses to a threatening stimulus or situation in preparation for flight, fight, or freezing, which in the wild would protect the animal from harm. Abnormal fear occurs when little or no real danger threatens.

> • Fear – It is a combination of physical, emotional, and physiological responses to a threatening stimulus or situation in preparation for flight, fight, or freezing, which in the wild would protect the animal from harm.
>
> • Abnormal fear occurs when little or no real danger threatens.

Panic – It is a sudden surge of acute terror.

> • Panic – It is a sudden surge of acute terror.

Phobia – It is an intense, maladaptive and unreasonable fear of something or a situation that far exceeds the actual danger or harm that is possible.

> • Phobia – It is an intense, maladaptive and unreasonable fear of something or a situation that far exceeds the actual danger or harm that is possible.

Generalized anxiety

Anxiety can occur in specific situations but when it becomes extreme, continuous, and the triggering factors are numerous or nonevident, it becomes generalized anxiety. Pets that suffer from generalized anxiety are often hypervigilant, have difficulty learning, are overreactive to stimuli and unable to adapt to new situations.

Global fear

Global fear is frequently seen in pet-mill animals as a severe genetic fear complicated by complete lack of experience and abnormal development. Global fear often includes fear of all new people, environments, objects, and noises. Animals frequently demonstrate learned helplessness and have difficulty learning.

Separation anxiety/distress

Dogs and cats are social animals and when they are separated from their attachment figure some degree of anxiety may occur. Signs of separation anxiety may include (only when the owner is absent) destruction at doors, general destruction in the home, rearranging of objects, house soiling, excessive salivation, distress vocalization, or self-trauma. Pet owners are placed in a deep emotional paradox. Pet owners report a high emotional value to their pet, often stating their pet is "perfect 95% of the time." Pet owners must then deal with the emotional and monetary cost of the pet's disorder.

Sound/thunderstorm phobia

Sound and thunderstorm phobias often occur in conjunction with each other or develop later. There is a genetic predisposition but phobias can also occur because of a traumatic experience and learning. Sound and thunderstorm phobias are often comorbid diagnoses with separation anxiety. The dog or cat may have a fear of thunderstorms and then experiences a storm when the owners are away. The pet then begins to associate being left alone with the potential for fear-inducing events (thunderstorms). There is evidence that the occurrence of separation anxiety or sound/thunderstorm phobias increases the likelihood that the other disorder will occur. Sound/thunderstorm phobia likely also occurs in cats although symptoms may be less profound and go unnoticed by pet owners.

Acute conflict behaviors, stereotypical behaviors, and compulsive disorders
Acute conflict behaviors

Acute conflict behaviors are an indication of conflict and stress in the environment and can be a foreshadowing of a stereotypy or compulsive disorder. They are performed in response to a specific trigger. For example, the doorbell rings and the dog runs to the door and spins in circles at the door until the person comes inside.

Stereotypical behaviors

An acute conflict behavior could develop into a stereotypical behavior. A stereotypical behavior is similar to an acute conflict behavior but tends to develop because of a more chronic stressor. For example, a lion may pace a path in an enclosure due to the restrictive nature of the environment. A stereotypic behavior is being displayed. If the lion is taken out of the context the behavior does not occur.

A stereotypical behavior is characterized by a repetitive and invariant locomotor pattern that is not a goal-oriented behavior.

Compulsive disorder

Compulsive disorders include behaviors that are usually repetitive, exaggerated, or sustained and are brought on by conflict and stress, but are then shown outside of the original context. A compulsive disorder is characterized by being a goal-oriented behavior that may be more variable in form. Compulsive disorders may be diagnosed when the presenting behaviors are pronounced and interfere with the pet's functioning behaviors. A genetic predisposition is likely present in any case of compulsive disorder but owner attention may reinforce existing compulsive behaviors. Treatment includes improving consistency in the animal's environment, behavior modification, and usually pharmacological intervention.

Compulsive behaviors are categorized into five groups.

Locomotion – tail chasing, spinning, circling, freezing, pouncing, skin rippling.
Oral – self-licking or chewing, air or nose flicking, pica, coprophagia, flank sucking, psychogenic alopecia, wool or fabric sucking, licking objects, polydypsia or polyphagia.
Vocalization – repetitive barking, meowing, whining, howling, and so on.
Hallucinatory – fly snapping, shadow and light chasing, air licking.
Aggressive – self-directed aggression or aggression toward an inanimate object.

Other
Cognitive dysfunction syndrome

Cognitive dysfunction is a progressive organic brain disorder that affects behavior. A decline in neurons, decrease in cerebral vascular blood flow, or increase of neurotoxin deposits alters awareness, decreases responsiveness to stimuli, and decreases the ability to learn and remember. Typical clinical signs include the following:

Disorientation.
Interactions with humans and other animals may be altered.
Sleep/wake cycles are altered.
House training may lapse.
Activity is altered.

Early diagnosis and intervention have been proven to slow the progression of the disease and sometimes alleviate early signs, thus providing improved quality of life for the pet and owner.

Hyperexcitability or hyperactive

Hyperexcitable dogs and cats are in a chronic state of excitement and tend to over-respond to even mild stimuli and show extreme lack of impulse control. Pet owners frequently also note inappropriate play and attention-seeking behaviors. Hyperexcitability exacerbates all other behavior problems and disorders. If a dog is hyperexcitable and has other behavior problems or disorders, the hyperexcitability must be addressed first. Hyperexcitability was found to be a risk factor for a dog to develop conflict-induced aggression (Guy *et al.*, 2001).

Conditioned unwanted behavior

Conditioned unwanted behaviors are not a behavior disorder but are frequently a concern to pet owners and complicate behavior disorders. Every behavior disorder described in this text has some level of conditioning involved. The veterinary technician should be fluent at functionally assessing a behavior's antecedents and consequences to direct the pet owner in teaching only the desired behaviors and explaining the extinction process.

REFERENCES for the above section of diagnosis terminology: (Horwitz and Neilson, 2007, Horwitz *et al.*, 2009; Luescher and Martin, 2010; Landsberg *et al.*, 2013)

Common veterinarian-prescribed behavioral treatments

This section is meant to describe specific aspects of the treatment plan the veterinarian may prescribe. We have intentionally not included individual treatment plans for specific disorders. It is the veterinarian's responsibility to determine what aspects of treatment will be included in the treatment plan, although the technician's insights and feedback will be integral in the development of the plan.

The technician must understand all aspects of the treatment, including the scientific basis for each recommendation, the goal or reason for each recommendation, the proper application of each recommendation and have the ability to teach the pet owner how to apply the prescribed techniques. Describing and demonstrating the techniques (when possible) with the pet owner can alert the technician to potential concerns or challenges the pet owner may have after leaving the veterinary hospital. Techniques may need to be individualized to integrate more successfully into the pet owner's lifestyle.

Treatment plans are multifaceted and usually start with management, then address the animal's temperament (fear, hyperexcitability, etc.) followed by addressing the specific problem behaviors. Below is an example of a treatment plan that might be presented to the veterinary technician to assist the pet owner in understanding and applying.

Diagnosis: Fear-based aggression toward men and general anxiety.

Management: Prevent access to men.

Temperament: Cease punishment; interact in a cue–response–reward format, decrease anxiety with medication.

Behavior modification and training: counter-conditioning (CC) to men, begin clicker training, teach "go to a mat," teach targeting to hand, fit with a head collar, demonstrate response substitution (RS) on walks.

The veterinary technician then instructs the pet owner how each aspect of the treatment plan fits into the treatment process (i.e., ignoring "Fluffy" will decrease her excitability which will make it easier for her to learn), the function of each aspect of the treatment process, how it is to be applied, and how to make it fit into their lifestyle. Appropriate goals and expectations should be considered and discussed.

Most treatment plans will include management techniques, the specific training style to be used, training of specific behaviors, behavior modification, and specific recommended training tools. If pharmacological treatment is included (see Chapter 9), the veterinary technician should discuss potential side effects and proper administration of the medication.

Management

Management is a method of manipulating the environment so the animal is less likely to perform the unwanted behavior or the unwanted behavior is lessened in intensity while behavior modification is being instituted or the new behavior is being trained.

In some cases, especially in cases of aggression, management can be a key point in keeping the client safe and preventing further damage to the human–animal bond until the behavior can be addressed and a treatment plan can be created.

In situations where acute management is required to prevent all chances of the behavior from occurring until the pet and owner can be seen for a consultation, the following management techniques may need to be considered:

– Removing the pet from the home temporarily.
– Removing specific people or pets from the home temporarily.
– Only specific people are allowed to interact with the pet.
– Confining the pet behind a gate or exercise pen and only allowing specific interactions by specific people at specific times.

Avoiding triggers

It is important to avoid eliciting situations or known triggers of the behavior while behavior modification and treatment are being instituted. Avoiding triggers will decrease the chances of the unwanted behavior from continuing to be practiced while training and behavior modification are being integrated into the treatment plan. It is also important to avoid triggers (especially in aggression cases) to keep the target of the aggression safe and to prevent further damage to the human–animal bond.

Specific triggers (when known) should be determined during the assessment and history-taking processes. Once specific triggers are identified, the veterinary technician can assist the pet owner in specific methods for avoiding those triggers. For example, if aggression is likely to occur when the pet is groomed, they are asked to avoid all grooming while the treatment plan is being instituted. If the patient becomes aggressive when disturbed while on the couch, the owner is instructed to limit the patient's access to the couch area to avoid the conflict. In situations where the patient is only aggressive to one family member, that family member is asked to stop all interaction with the patient until after a diagnosis and treatment plan is created. Another example would be walking a dog early in the morning to avoid meeting strangers on walks or avoiding walking in high-density dog areas. The veterinary technician should problem-solve with the pet owner to make sure the avoidance of triggers is manageable for the pet owner.

Goals:

– Keeps the pet and pet owner safe.
– Decreases stress for both the pet and pet owner.
– Avoids confrontations (prevent further damage to the human–animal bond).
– Keeps the patient from continuing to practice the unwanted behavior. By avoiding triggers, the patient is no longer conditioned by the undesirable behavior, producing some degree of relief from the eliciting stimulus.

If triggers for the behavior cannot be ascertained or predicted, the pet owner may be asked to interact with the patient as little as possible until the behavior consultation.

Ignore attention-seeking behaviors

A treatment plan may indicate the need for the owner to avoid reinforcing attention-seeking behaviors. Ignoring means not looking at, talking to, or touching the pet and is often one of the difficult aspects of treatment for pet owners. Most pet owners do not realize they are rewarding attention-seeking or unwanted behaviors with their attention and it should not be assumed that asking a pet owner to ignore unwanted behaviors is self-explanatory. They often do not notice until it is pointed out to them that they are touching, talking, or even looking at their pet when it seeks attention. Pet owners are asked to ignore their pet during behavior consultations so the dependence and intensity of attention-seeking behaviors of the patient can be determined during the consultation. It is also an accurate method for determining how difficult it may be for the pet owner to ignore their pet at home. During a consultation, the pet owner may look at the pet and say "I can't pet you, I am ignoring you" without realizing he/she has just reinforced the pet's behavior. The veterinary technician can give the client specific instructions such as, "Cross your arms and pretend he is invisible" or "Stand up and look straight ahead if he jumps into your lap." Some pet owners may be taught to read a magazine instead of looking at their pet. If the pet owner has difficulty following instructions a TAG Point (see Chapter 5) maybe used. Example: When he barks at you, the Tag Point is "Look at me." The technician should shape the pet owner's behavior and reinforce any initial attempt at ignoring. If multiple family members are present, they can be taught to reinforce each other for ignoring the pet.

Owners should be advised that the behavior will likely worsen (extinction burst or frustration effect) before improving and that is a predictable part of the learning process. They should also be advised that the ignoring of attention-seeking behaviors does not mean ignoring the needs of the pet. If the dog is asking to be let outside to relieve himself, he should not be ignored. This is normal communication of basic needs.

Ignoring their pet is often an extremely difficult and an emotion-laden request for clients. It is imperative the pet owner understand how this aspect will affect the treatment process and that it is only a temporary part of treatment. Explaining that their pet may have an unhealthy dependency on them and that ignoring the excessive attention seeking behavior will help to improve the pet's confidence is often helpful. Instruct the client with empathy, compassion, and understanding.

Ask the pet owners when it will be the most difficult for them to ignore the pet and then give them specific instructions for those situations. For instance, if they indicate ignoring the pet in the evening when it is usually allowed in their lap is difficult, they can be instructed to do training exercises during the time they would have given the pet less-structured attention. Emphasize they may interact during training sessions as much as they like and may reinforce their pet with attention during those sessions. They may also reinforce calm behavior and independence by interacting with the pet. Have the owners focus on interacting with the pet when the pet is ignoring them and is calm.

Goals:

- Decrease hyper-excitablity.
- Decrease attention-seeking behaviors.
- Increase pet owner consistency and predictability.
- Increase the pet's independence.
- Reinforce calm behavior.

Ignore at specific times

The treatment plan may require the pet owner to ignore the pet only at specific times, such as prior to leaving or when returning, when treating separation anxiety. The veterinary technician should assist the pet owner in determining how to change their behaviors during the required times. For example, instead of reassuring the pet before leaving, give the pet an interactive toy. The pet owner may be asked to ignore specific pets when other pets are near, when treating IDA-H.

Goals:

- Decrease dependency on the pet owner.
- Decrease over-arousal of the pet during specific times.
- Remove inadvertent reinforcing of unwanted behaviors.
- Decreasing an alliance with the pet owner when treating IDA-H.

Cue→response→reward interactions

Pet owners frequently interact with their pet casually and randomly throughout the day, speaking to them in sentences and touching them. These casual interactions are usually inconsistent (from the animal's perspective) and often inadvertently condition unwanted attention-seeking behaviors. Pets that do not exhibit anxiety or problematic behaviors can adjust to these inconsistent interactions but pets with anxiety and/or aggression issues frequently demonstrate increased anxiety, hyperactivity, and over-dependence on the owner. In those cases, the veterinarian may include in the treatment plan more consistent interactions such as a cue→response→reward interaction.

Cue→response→reward interaction requires the owners to give the animal a cue for a previously trained foundation behavior (i.e., "sit," "down," "come," "go to your bed," "watch me") when the dog is not initiating attention on its own. The owner is to give the cue, wait for the desired response, and then reward the behavior. The reward may be attention, food, or another desired reinforcer. Frequently, the veterinary technician must

first teach cued foundation behaviors (see later in this chapter) before cue→response→reward interactions can occur because the pet owner may not have a reliable behavior on cue (Table 8.2).

It should be noted that cue→response→reward interactions are quite different from other historically recommended interactions commonly called *Nothing-in-Life-is-Free* (NLIF), *learn to earn*, and *deference protocols*. The aforementioned techniques are meant to change the animal's behavior by clarifying the "social status" between owner and pet. A cue→response→reward (CRR) interaction places focus on changing the owner's behavior to increase consistency and predictability in the relationship. This is an important differentiation because any type of social dominance or "pack mentality" will only complicate and likely be of detriment to the treatment plan (Table 8.3).

Goals:

- Increase owner predictability.
- Decrease the chance of reinforcing attention-seeking behaviors.
- Pet owner focuses on desired behavior.
- Decrease over-dependence on pet owner.
- Decrease hyperexcitability and anxiety.

Change primary caregiver

Changing who takes primary husbandry care of the pet may be recommended when it is determined there is an over-dependence on one member of the household. It may also be recommended when a positive association toward an "unfavored" household member is being developed.

Goals:

- Decrease over-dependence on a family member.
- Increase a positive association with a family member.

Environmental modifications

Physical changes to the environment to decrease the chance of the unwanted behavior occurring are usually the first consideration in all treatment plans. Environmental modifications may include placement of barriers including outside fences, changing feeding areas, changing locations of litter boxes, covering windows with film, moving furniture to prevent access to areas, utilizing gates at doorways, and so on. The veterinary technician along with the veterinarian and pet owner should determine appropriate, functional, and acceptable environmental modification that will fit into the pet owner's lifestyle.

Goals:

- Prevent unwanted behavior from occurring.
- Decrease triggers.

Table 8.2 Cue → Response → Reward possible responses.

Response to cue	Pet owner's response	How to proceed
Behavior offered	Reinforce behavior	Continue with interaction
No response	Wait and cue the behavior again	If still no response, ask for another cued behavior and proceed – discuss with veterinary technician to determine if the behavior is under stimulus control
Cued behavior offered before cue given	Ask for another cued behavior	Reinforce the behavior
Animal becomes aggressive when cue is given	Avoid reacting in any way. Remain calm and end the interaction with as little conflict as possible	Call to discuss with veterinary technician

Table 8.3 A comparison between NLIF and C→R→R interactions.

NLIF	Cue→Response→Reward
Based on changing the dog's attitude	Based on changing the owner's behavior
Goal is to clarify social status	Goal is to increase predictability of owner
No scientific basis	Based on laws of learning
Focus on gaining control over the dog	Giving control to the dog
Strives to create deference	Strives to create meaningful consequences
Accepts person as "leader"	Learns to trust people
About "obeying"	About choosing

Crate confinement or other confinement

Crate or other confinement (exercise pens, rooms, etc.) is used as a management technique to prevent unwanted behavior or to prevent the patient from access to a trigger (i.e., avoiding guests). Confinement should not be used as a punishment or associated with an aversive (yelling, physical punishment, etc.).

Conditioning to confinement is discussed in Chapter 7 in detail.

The fundamental to training an animal to confinement is to classically associate the confinement area with something pleasant. Suggestions could include doing positive-based training session in the confinement area, feeding in the area, giving attention to the pet only when it is in the area (including play time), or allowing the pet to play with their favorite enrichment toy only while in the area.

If the crate or other confinement area has previously been associated with a negative emotional response, the following technique may be helpful.

Crate (or other confinement) reconditioning

If the animal has not generalized the negative emotional response to all confinement areas, the lack of generalization can be utilized when reconditioning to confinement.

Step 1: The "bad crate" is the crate that has been associated in the past with a negative emotional response. Create a "good crate" by making it look and seem as different as possible from the previously negatively associated crate. For example, if a plastic crate was used in the past, use a wire crate as the "good crate." Move the crate to a different room or area of the house. If at any time the pet must be crated while the "good crate" is being conditioned, use the "bad" crate, which already has a negative association.

Step 2: Shape the behavior "go in" at a nonstressful starting point. If the dog shows any anxiety about interacting with the "good crate," begin with teaching "go in" by covering a chair or table and shaping going into the covered area and place the behavior on cue.

Step 3: Once the cue of "go in" has been associated with a positive emotional response (clicker training and treats) it can then be given when shaping to go into the "good crate." Once the pet has been shaped to readily "go in" into the "good crate," continue to condition the crate as you would with a new puppy (see Chapter 7).

Step 4: Do not use the "good crate" at any time anxiety might occur (thunderstorms, fireworks, owner gone too long) until treatment has progressed (i.e., medications have taken effect).

Goals:
– Safety
– Avoiding triggers
– Preventing destruction
– Housetraining

Tethering

Tethering is another type of confinement that allows the pet to be supervised while in the environment with the family. Tethering is frequently recommended when counter-conditioning dogs within the same household to each other by tethering and training both dogs in the same room. Treats are tossed to the dog that is training and to the other dog for not reacting or for relaxation. Tethering is also frequently used for rehousetraining and is always recommended as a safety measure when the pet owner is teaching relinquishment exercises to a dog that has shown possessive aggression.

The animal also may be tethered to the pet owner with a waist leash or may drag a line (see section titled **Training tools**), allowing the pet owner to pick up the drag line to redirect the animal and do RS if the animal becomes reactive or aggressive.

Interactive toys can be tethered in confinement areas to encourage the pet to interact with the toy away from the pet owner, increasing independence from the owner.

Goals:
– Active supervision
– Safety
– Independence training (tethered toy)
– Assists with response substitution (RS) (dragline)

Dietary changes

Behavior is directly affected by diet, therefore dietary changes and/or the inclusion of supplements may be recommended by the veterinarian for various behavioral reasons including aggression, difficulty in training, coprophagia, and cognitive dysfunction. (Landsberg et al., 2013).

The veterinary technician should counsel the pet owner on how to properly change diets and administer any supplements.

Goal:
– Organic benefits to brain chemistry.

Regular schedule

Predictable and consistent timing of meals, play time, training, and walks helps to decrease anxiety and hyperexcitability.

Regular schedules have been found to be beneficial in general and as a preventive measure, as noted in Chapter 7.

Goals:
– Increase predictability and consistency.
– Decrease anxiety and hyperexcitability.

Meal feed twice daily

A case load analysis done by Dr. Andrew Luescher at the Ontario Veterinary College showed that dogs that were on ad lib feeding, and switched to twice daily meal feeding had a better prognosis (Luescher, 2010). Meal feeding also makes defecation more predictable and allows training to occur before meals.

Goals:
– Increases general predictability.
– Decreases anxiety and hyperexcitability.
– Increases desire for food rewards in training.
– Makes defecation more predictable.

Mental stimulation

Human studies have shown learning and brain exercises delay the onset of dementia. Canine research has found similar results and noted that mental stimulation is essential for a high quality of life and can include training walks, puzzle toys, interactive food toys (see section titled Training tools), and so on (Landsberg et al., 2013).

Mental stimulation is often recommended to prevent destructive behaviors due to lack of stimulation, improve focus and concentration, and increase trainability.

Goals:
– Improve quality of life.
– Slow cognitive dysfunction.
– Decrease destruction due to lack of stimulation.
– Increase concentration, focus, and trainability.

Walking off property

Walks off the property reduce anxiety levels and dogs that were walked regularly were shown to have less of a problem with aggression (Luescher, 2010). Owners should be encouraged to walk their dog off the property twice daily for 15–20 min. Walking dogs off the property is believed to decrease hyperexcitability, territorial aggression, and general reactivity. Unfortunately, many owners do not walk their dog off the property because they feel the dog gets enough exercise in the backyard. This thought process overlooks the second and possibly most important benefit to walking the dog off the property, which is the mental stimulation the dog receives from visual, olfactory, and auditory stimulation (see section titled **SEEKING system**). Owners should therefore be informed that even if their dog has a large yard, walking off their property is very important for the mental stimulation it provides the dog.

Some patients may require fitting with a no-pull harness or head halter to decrease pulling or if RS on walks is required. The veterinary technician can also teach cues for loose leash walking beside the pet owner and another cue "to go play" or sniff. Predictability is increased by giving the dog a cue for when it is acceptable to sniff and another cue for walking politely. Cues are given just before the behavior, "go play" – dogs sniffs, followed by "let's go" and the dog is reinforced for coming back to the side of the pet owner with a treat or by being allowed to go sniff again.

Goals and benefits:
– decrease anxiety
– decrease hyper-excitability
– decrease reactivity
– increases mental stimulation
– provides social interaction with the handler

Aerobic exercise

The goal of aerobic exercise is different from the goal of walking the dog off property. Aerobic exercise is exercise such as brisk walking that increases oxygen consumption. Increased aerobic exercise has been shown to improve mood, decrease depression, reduce stress, and increase the ability to cope with stress in humans (Psychology, 2007–2012). Aerobic exercise is associated with the production of endorphins. Some researchers have suggested that neurochemicals such as epinephrine, serotonin, and dopamine also contribute to elevated mood. Aerobic exercise has also been found to have antidepressant type actions (Hunsberger *et al.*, 2007). It should be noted that some dogs may become more energetic and over-stimulated by aerobic activity. Providing these dogs with additional mental stimulation via structured positive training and relaxation exercises may help counteract this stimulatory effect.

Aerobic activity in cats can be implemented by playing with the cat with interactive toys such as a feather teaser.

Goals:
– Increase endorphins.
– Decrease anxiety.
– Decrease hyper activity and excitability.
– Decrease reactivity.

Clicker training

Clicker training is an excellent tool for increasing mental stimulation and likely activates what Dr. Jaak Panksepp calls the SEEKING system.

SEEKING system

Panksepp believes neurochemistries lead companion animals to energetically investigate and explore their world in the attempt to seek available resources and to make sense of environmental contingencies. Others have called the system "foraging/expectancy system",

"behavioral activation system" (Gray, 1990) and the "behavioral facilitation system" (Depue and Iacono, 1989). Panksepp believes the SEEKING system contributes to the feelings of engagement and excitement when resources are sought (Ahn and Picard, 2006) and that the basic impulse to investigate and make sense of the environment emerges from circuits in the lateral hypothalamic corridor of the brain (Panksepp, 1998). This system drives human complexities such as persistent feelings of interest, anticipation, and curiosity. The SEEKING system is what is driving you to read this text.

Panksepp is convinced clicker training (and other mentally stimulating activities) are evidence of the SEEKING system in action (Pryor, 2009). This is not only in relationship to the "trainee" but also to the person training the animal. For example, the SEEKING system is activated when working closely with an animal to solve a training issue or when trying to determine the next successive approximation to reinforce. It is a puzzle that needs to be understood, creating excitement and enthusiasm. Panksepp's explanation makes it clear a trainer using a clicker and trainee are frequently "in-tune" during a training session; both are in the midst of the SEEKING system.

Punishment switches the learner away from the hypothalamus and SEEKING system to the amygdala's path of avoidance and fear (Pryor, 2009).

Clicker training and the practical applications will be discussed in detail in the section titled **Training techniques**.

Goals and benefits:
– Increase pet owner predictability.
– Improve communication between pet and pet owner.
– Increase or repair the human–animal bond.
– Decrease hyperexcitability.
– Increase concentration and retention.
– Teach foundation and complex behaviors that can be used during CC/RS/systematic desensitization(DS) exercises.
– Keep the pet owner safe during training (hands off).

Training techniques

The American Veterinary Society of Animal Behavior recommends training techniques that focus on reinforcing desired behavior and removing reinforcers for undesirable behaviors. Focus should be on addressing the emotional state and environmental conditions driving the undesirable behavior rather than punishing unwanted behavior (Behavior, 2007).

In addition:

1. An animal's behavior is often a "coping" mechanism for an adverse emotional state. If the motivating emotion is addressed, often the undesirable behavior is diminished or eradicated. Utilizing training techniques that positively affect the emotional state of the animal should be used when applying behavior modification techniques.

2. The training techniques should promote and protect the human–animal bond and foster a **healthy** relationship between the pet and pet owner (see Table 4.1). Often the relationship between the pet owner and the pet is strained or damaged with behavior concerns when they approach a veterinary professional. Training techniques that build trust and predictability will begin to heal a damaged relationship.

3. The technique should increase confidence in both the animal and the pet owner. A symbiotic relationship of mutualism between learner and trainer should be fostered. Training is a team activity that should always focus on success. If success is not occurring, the training should be modified to increase success. Learner and trainer should not focus on unwanted behavior or failure. The *information* the animal is giving should be taken into consideration and the training should be modified based on this information. For example, if the dog is unable to respond to a known cue, recognize that the situation may be too distracting and it has not been trained to fluency. Take that information and adapt the environment to help the animal be successful. Then make a training plan to build in distractions more gradually.

4. The training technique should have a low potential for adverse side effects. Learning should be fun, enjoyable, and not something that causes anxiety or fear. Fear of punishment or failure makes learning difficult or impossible.

5. The training techniques should be based on sound principles of learning and scientific data rather than anecdotal experiences. By understanding the scientific basis for techniques, the trainer has the ability to problem solve a training challenge and resolve it in a positive manner. Utilizing techniques on the grounds that they have proved successful in the past without understanding the scientific principles guiding the techniques is neither professional nor recommended (Box 8.1).

> • An animal's behavior is often a "coping" mechanism for an adverse emotional state.

BOX 8.1: GUIDELINES FOR CHOOSING A TRAINING TECHNIQUE.

The training technique should

positively affect the emotional state of the animal,
focus on desired behavior and success,
promote, protect, and foster a healthy relationship between pet and owner,
increase confidence for both the pet and the owner,
have a low potential for adverse side effects,
be based on scientific principles of learning and scientific data.

Why punishment is not recommended in training or the application of behavior modification

Punishment is a complex and advanced tool. It is generally misunderstood, applied improperly, and much overused. When punishment is applied incorrectly or inappropriately it becomes abusive.

> • When punishment is applied incorrectly or inappropriately it becomes abusive.

Punishment, specifically corporal punishment, is defined as the use of physical force with the intention of causing pain but not injury, with the purpose of changing behavior (Mulvaney and Mebert, 2007) and usually includes the use of training tools such as choke, shock, and prong collars.

Punishment-focused training is never included as part of a treatment plan and rarely recommended in behavior modification for the following reasons.

Poor learning and cognition

Research has found the unintended consequences of corporal punishment in children to include increased aggression, depression, lower self-esteem, and poorer psychological and cognitive functioning (Strassberg *et al.*, 1994; Gershoff, 2002). Another study showed children who were spanked had significantly lower IQs than those who were not spanked (Straus and

Paschall, 2009). Dr. Murray Straus reports "children who were spanked the most fell behind the average IQ development curve, and those who were never spanked advanced ahead of the average. The more the spanking, the slower the development of the child's mental ability. But even small amounts of spanking made a difference." Dr. Straus suggested the correlation between corporal punishment and lower IQ may be attributed to the stress and fear punishment causes.

Criteria for effective punishment are difficult to meet

As stated earlier, punishment is a complex and advanced tool. ALL of the following criteria must be met for punishment to be effective and must be successfully met by the pet owner.

The animal's motivation strength is not too high

The stronger the motivation to perform the behavior, the less likely punishment will work. Strong innate behaviors such as aggression (a defense mechanism), chasing, and hunting are particularly difficult to decrease with punishment.

All animals, including humans, use a limited number of strategies to deal with dangerous situations, including escaping or avoiding, freezing, defensive aggression ("fighting back") or appeasement. Underlying physiological changes during stressful situations are similar across species. Soldiers injured in battle fail to notice the injuries while in a traumatic experience. A rat exposed to a cat will not notice painful heat applied to its tail. The cat poses a more immediate and significant danger. In both humans and animals, stress-induced analgesia occurs as a consequence of the activation of the brain's natural opiate system (LeDoux, 1996). The activation of opiates may be the reason some dogs do not respond to extreme physical punishment when motivation or emotional response is high. When fear is the motivating factor, it is unlikely animals will feel the aversive unless at an extreme, intense, or inhumane level.

In addition, punishment cannot reduce any behavior that is naturally induced by punishment.

Examples:
– A dog runs through the invisible fence to chase a rabbit because of a strong innate motivation.
– A dog has a very strong motivation to aggress and is severely punished for aggressing; then when the trigger or target of the aggression approaches, it will likely still be aggressive but also fearful. The fear and the aggression do not cancel each other out but instead compete with each other, creating severe acute internal conflict in the animal.
– A dog urinates when punished – it will not decrease if punished for urinating and the punishment will likely make the urination worse.

Always contingent on behavior and only associated with the behavior

The punishment must occur every time the behavior occurs and should be associated with the behavior and not other people or animals. This is why remote punishment may be recommended in some treatment plans. See the section titled **Remote punishment**.

Proper intensity

The intensity of the punishment must be high enough to interrupt the behavior immediately after application of the punishment but should not be so intense as to create intense fear. Motivation strength or high emotional state (higher motivation requires a higher level of punishment) must be seriously considered. If the motivation or emotional state is high, the intensity level of the punishment may reach inhumane and cruel levels to become effective, if effective at all. At such levels, animals will learn nothing.

If the intensity of the punishment is too low, the animal will get habituated to the punishment. Eventually harsh or cruel punishment will be required to stop the undesired behavior.

Timing

For punishment to be effective, it must be delivered within 0.5 s of the undesired behavior. The ideal time to apply punishment is just as the behavior begins. Any delay will cause punishment to be ineffective. When delivered late, it is no longer associated with the undesirable behavior and likely becomes associated with something else in the environment. For example, a dog eliminates on the floor when left alone. The pet owner returns home and punishes the dog. The dog then shows appeasement behaviors (often described by pet owners as "looking guilty") when the pet owner returns home because the dog has associated urine on the floor as the cue the pet owner will punish him. The behavior of eliminating on the floor was not punished, it was reinforced by the feeling of relief when the pet eliminated.

Alternative behavior choice

Behavior is usually performed to reach a goal or reward. Therefore an alternative behavior should be taught and rewarded in the place of the undesirable behavior that is to be punished. The alternative behavior should be taught and placed on cue and fluent before being used as an alternative choice. Example: If a dog is punished for jumping up by the stranger turning away, it should alternatively be taught to sit to greet strangers.

Punishment (including negative punishment, see Chapter 6) should significantly decrease the behavior within three to four applications. If the behavior is not significantly diminished within three to four applications, the punishment should immediately be ceased and the criteria reviewed.

Punishment is counter-productive to treatment

Fear is a defense system that produces responses that maximize survival. Those responses "represent the operation of brain systems that have been programmed by evolution to deal with danger in routine ways. Although we can become conscious of the operation of the defense system, especially when it leads to behavioral expressions, the system operates independently of consciousness" (LeDoux, 1996). In other words, punishing an animal's method for coping with a highly emotional situation (fear provoking) without addressing the underlying emotional state is neither appropriate nor humane and will likely not be successful in reaching the desired goal behavior.

Example 1: A dog growls when being touched on its head because a past otitis has created a negative emotional response to having his ears touched. The growling is a "coping" mechanism to make the fear-provoking stimulus retreat. Punishing the growling may decrease the behavior (growling) but does not address the underlying anxiety of being touched on the head and will likely increase overall anxiety.

Example 2: A child seeks out a parent and says he/she is afraid there is a "monster in the closet." If the parent were to spank the child it may decrease the coping mechanism of going to the parent for consoling but do nothing to decrease the fear of the "monster."

The AVSAB Position Statement (http://avsabonline.org/resources/position-statements) states that punishment should not be used as a first-line or early use treatment for problem behaviors "due to potential adverse effects which include but are not limited to: inhibition of learning, increased fear-related and aggressive behaviors, and injury to animals and people interacting with animals"(Behavior, 2007).

> • The AVSAB Position Statement (http://avsabonline.org/resources/position-statements) states that punishment should not be used as a first-line or early use treatment for problem behaviors "due to potential adverse effects which include but are not limited to: inhibition of learning, increased fear-related and aggressive behaviors, and injury to animals and people interacting with animals" (Behavior, 2007).

Punishment is not generally recommended for training or in the application of behavior modification for the following reasons:

- Slows learning and cognition.
- Increases fear and fear-based aggression.
- Is very difficult to apply consistently and therefore becomes unpredictable.
- Inadvertent or unintended negative associations are made, including toward the pet owner, other animals, other people and the environment. In this regard, punishment is more like a bomb going off than a solution that pinpoints the exact issues.
- Confrontational – Owner applied punishment is almost always confrontational and is directly correlated to the development of conflict-induced aggression. Confrontation often leads to aggression, putting the pet and the pet owner in danger and further damaging the human–animal bond.

When treating behavioral disorders it is imperative to decrease fear, unpredictability, and confrontations.

> • When treating behavioral disorders it is imperative to decrease fear, unpredictability, and confrontations.

Generally positive punishment is not effective for problem behaviors because all criteria for punishment cannot be met.

> • Generally positive punishment is not effective for problem behaviors because all criteria for punishment cannot be met.

Why the prevalence of punishment-based training and domination techniques persist

Punishment is a complex technique and it is often misunderstand and frequently overused (Luescher and

Shaw, 2007). With the knowledge of potential side effects, why does punishment remain so prevalent in the animal training world? The answers may lie in two historical experiments.

In 1961, Yale University psychologist Stanley Milgram created an experiment to test how much pain an ordinary citizen ("teacher") would inflict on another person ("learner") because he was ordered to by an authority figure ("experimenter") (Milgram, 1963). The experiment consisted of the "experimenter" instructing the "teacher" to administer electric shocks to the "learner" for incorrect answers. Unbeknown to the "teacher," the "learner" was not really receiving shocks but was acting as if he had. The "teacher" was told to move one level higher on the shock generator each time the learner flashed a wrong answer. The shock generator indicated available voltage from 15 to 450 V. Additional verbal designations included slight shock, moderate shock, extreme intensity shock, danger: severe shock and lastly two switches labeled "xxx." At 300 "fake" voltage level, the acting "learner" was to pound on the wall to make sure the "teacher" was aware of the discomfort being caused. At 325 V, the "learner" stopped answering questions and the "teacher" was told to treat each non-answer as a wrong answer, increasing the voltage. Sometimes the "teacher" asked the "experimenter" if the "learner was liable to suffer permanent physical injury" and the experimenter said, "Although the shocks may be painful, there is no permanent tissue damage, so please go on."

The results were astounding and not predicted. Of the 40 "teachers", 14 refused to continue the experiment past 375 V, the point the "student" banged on the wall. The 26 remaining "teachers" followed the "experimenter's" direction until they reached the most potent shock available, two steps beyond the designation: danger: severe shock. Some expressed reluctance to administer shocks over the 300-V level yet complied with the authority of the "experimenter." Milgram believed two findings were surprising. The first was in regard to the strength of obedient tendencies even in the fundamental breach of moral conduct to hurt another. To disobey the "experimenter" would have not resulted in a punishment to the "teacher" yet 26 subjects abandoned their own personal values to follow the direction of the authority figure. The second was the amount of stress the experimenter caused to the "teacher." Many showed severe tension and emotional strain, yet continued as directed (Ksenych and Liu, 1992).

The second experiment was the 1971 Stanford Prison Experiment conducted by psychology professor Philip Zimbardo, which tested the psychological effects of becoming a prisoner or prison guard. Dramatic, albeit controversial, results were found in both the behavior of the "prisoners" and "guards".

A mock prison was created in the Stanford psychology building. Twenty-four male undergraduates were chosen for their lack of psychological issues, crime history, and medical disabilities. A flip of a coin determined which 12 would become "guards" and which 12 would become "prisoners".

The guards were given little instruction but were told to do whatever they thought was necessary to maintain law and order and to gain the respect of the prisoners. The guards created punishment techniques which included verbal harassment, humiliation, isolation, spray from a fire extinguisher, forcing prisoners to do repetitive menial work such as cleaning toilet bowls with their bare hands, placing bags over prisoners' heads, and requiring prisoners to do jumping jacks and push-ups while weight was put on the their back. Punishment was imposed for infractions including disrespect or disobedience from the prisoners. As the experiment progressed, the guards began to see the prisoners as "troublemakers" who were out to get them and consequently steadily increased their coercive aggressive tactics. Prisoners became distressed and fatigued. Acute emotional disturbances, disorganized thinking, uncontrollable crying, and rage appeared in the prisoners.

Three types of guards were identified. Some of the guards were "tough but fair," others were "good guys" who rarely punished the prisoners. One-third of the guards were hostile, arbitrary, and inventive in the different forms of punishment administered. Initially some prisoners rebelled and fought the guards. Others developed psychosomatic illness or broke down emotionally. Some tried to cope by attempting to do whatever the guards asked, to please them. In the end, the guards won total control and commanded blind and unquestioning obedience from each prisoner.

On the sixth day of the proposed 14-day experiment, the study was ended as the prisoners were withdrawing and behaving pathologically and some guards were behaving sadistically. The "good guy" guards were beginning to feel helpless although no guards quit the study, called in sick, requested to leave early, or requested pay for overtime work.

What implications could the Milgram's behavioral study of obedience and the Stanford Prison Experiment have on teaching people to train dogs?

Pet dog owners seek veterinary professionals and dog trainers to give them advice on how to teach their pet. Many of these novice dog owners are advised to use punishment techniques, techniques they may feel quite uncomfortable administering but they often continue with the recommended techniques. Could the veterinary professional or dog trainer take on the role of "experimenter," the pet owner the role of "teacher" and dog the role of "learner" as in the Milgram experiment? Most clients seen at the Animal Behavior Clinic at Purdue University were relieved when they were told they should no longer use the choke collar, pinch collar, or domination techniques they were advised to use by their veterinary professional or trainer.

The Stanford Prison Experiment demonstrated that when given the ability to punish, dominate, and control another, it was reinforcing to some of the guards. Control is a primary reinforcer. Punishment-based and dominance-type training is reinforcing to the person training the animal.

Some owners may use punishment techniques because they do not have the knowledge or understanding of alternative methods. Some may go to a professional who advocates punishment-based techniques and because that professional is an authoritative figure, they comply even if they may not feel comfortable with the techniques. Some professionals may recommend a complete authoritarian relationship between pet and pet owners that includes complete obedience at all times. Such a recommendation does not build a symbiotic relationship and sets up both pet and owner for failure.

Veterinary technicians must be aware of different training styles and recommend pet owners to qualified trainers who use the most up-to-date, relationship-building, and scientifically based training styles available.

Lure reward training

Lure reward training is a style of training that consists of giving a cue for a behavior ("sit"), luring or prompting (in a nonconfrontational manner) the behavior (treat held over the animal's head) and rewarding the behavior (sit).

For the cue to become the discriminative stimulus for the behavior, it is important the cue be given before the lure, otherwise the cue may be overshadowed by the hand movement of the lure. This can be tested by asking the dog to "sit" with no hand movement; if the "sit" does not occur, imitate the hand signal moving over the head as if using a lure without saying the word "sit." If the dog sits without the verbal "sit," it indicates the cue is the hand movement/lure rather than the verbal "sit" cue.

The advantage of lure reward training is that if done properly and without confrontation it is a technique that can be used by almost all pet owners including children.

The challenge is teaching owners how to successfully fade the lure from the behavior either by placing the behavior on a verbal cue or fading the movement of the lure into a hand signal as a cue for the behavior. Otherwise the behavior may only occur when the pet owner uses a treat as the lure.

Lure reward training may be recommended as the training style of choice if the pet owner has difficulty using a marker or if minimal and less precise training is required. Although when dealing with animals with significant fear and anxiety issues, you are likely to encounter some that are not trusting of being reached for or even handed a treat. Lure reward training may be perceived as threatening to the animal.

Event marker (clicker) training

The following text will use "event marker," "marker" and "clicker," and "conditioned reinforcer" interchangeably.

This section will only discuss positive reinforcement markers and not punishment markers.

Marker training is a cross-species communication technology that allows us to communicate clearly and precisely with animals. It is a system of using positive reinforcement in conjunction with a consistent event marker (usually a clicker). The sound of a clicker is both a conditioned reinforcer (see Chapter 6) and a signal marking a desired behavior.

The fundamentals of marker training can be broken down into three steps: observe the behavior, mark the behavior, and reinforce the desired behavior. More advanced and necessary steps including cueing and fluency are discussed later in this chapter.

Benefits of clicker training, both in training and in the application of behavior modification techniques
Accelerated learning
A small research project done in 2006 tested the difference between a verbal- and clicker-type marker with regard to a comparison of training time and the number of required reinforcements. They found that training with a clicker as the event marker not only reduced the required amount of training time, but also fewer reinforcements were needed to successfully teach the behavior. The results of this study suggest that the clicker provides more accurate information than the verbal bridging stimulus, thereby increasing rate of

reinforcement and decreasing the amount of required training time (Wood, 2008).

Improved retention time

The phenomenon of long retention has been abundantly proven with conditioned punishers. Conditioned reinforcers (a clicker for this discussion) are known to take parallel pathways in the brain and behave like conditioned punishers, while triggering different brain chemicals and emotions than punishers.

In practice, if the click is indeed a conditioned reinforcer and is being used correctly as a marker, the association will be retained permanently unless the training is extinguished (Pryor, 2009).

Hands-off and nonthreatening

Many patients suffering from behavior disorders require a nonthreatening and hands-off approach to training, especially when there is a history of aversive training in the animal's past. It also allows the pet owner to train from a distance, which is often helpful when working with a very fearful or aggressive animal. One family member can mark a behavior while another reinforces it. This allows the elderly or very young children to assist in the training process (Figure 8.2).

Marker training as a tool in behavior modification

A marker can be used in behavior modification to change the emotional response to a stimulus, teach an alternate response, and clearly mark subtle steps in a desensitization program.

See details about using a marker in behavior modification later in this chapter.

Strengthens the human–animal bond

As mentioned earlier in this chapter, punishment-based techniques are usually administered inconsistently and unpredictably, creating a relationship based on stress. Clicker training is very consistent and predictable. Nothing "bad" happens and a bond built on a foundation of trust and teamwork flourishes. The animal's responsibility is to offer behavior and the trainer's responsibility is to choose the behavior to be marked and reinforced. It is a team approach. One member of the team is not more important than the other. Owners quickly realize their pet is offering behaviors to get them to click. Frequently owners realize they have drastically underestimated the intelligence of the animal and a new relationship founded upon mutual respect, trust, and understanding is created.

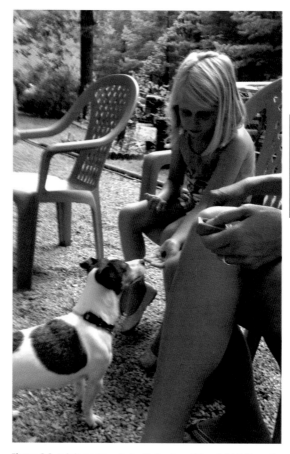

Figure 8.2 Adult marking desired behavior while a child delivers the reinforcement.

Assists in repairing the human–animal bond

Often the human–animal bond has been damaged in cases of aggression directed toward the owner. The target of the aggression may no longer trust the pet and the pet may not trust the person because of past communication inconsistencies (specifically if punishment was previously used). Because clicker training is hands-off, consistent, and focuses on desired behavior, it can be the first step in rebuilding a damaged relationship.

Builds confidence and creativity

Clicker training does not initially require a relationship of trust but rather builds that relationship. Fearful animals become curious, enthusiastic, and more outgoing. The animal learns the click is reinforcing because it is assured a reward will follow. The click is also reinforcing because it gives the animal information. Knowing "what will happen next" and trusting that it will be a pleasant experience creates a confidence and tolerance for even slightly stressful experiences. The animal gains some degree of environmental predictability, which is beneficial to all animals but especially to animals with fear or anxiety issues.

Challenges:

– Some pet owners, either due to physical or mental restraints, may have difficulty accurately using a clicker. In such cases, another person can mark the behavior and the challenged pet owner can toss the reinforcement. Another solution would be to teach the pet owner to use a word as the marker. Although less accurate than a clicker, it could still be a practical choice for some pet owners.
– Deaf animals or geriatric patients that are losing their hearing may require a more creative marker such as a light or hand signal.
– Some sound-sensitive animals may require desensitization to the clicker by using a modified clicker initially (see Figure 8.15).

Other training

The following are not training styles or techniques but rather sports or activities that may be recommended in a prescribed treatment plan.

Agility training

Agility training is a dog sport that combines physical and mental skills as the handler directs the dog through a sequence of obstacles such as tunnels, hoops, weave poles, and seesaws with voice and hand cues and without touching the dog or the equipment (Figure 8.3).

When agility training is combined with clicker training, dogs with low confidence learn to interact with novel objects, increasing their confidence in a variety of settings and that confidence begins to permeate other areas of their life. They become more likely to approach and investigate novel objects, including people and other dogs in other situations once a strong reinforcement history for investigating unfamiliar items and situations has been developed. Novel items that were previously a cause for concern begin to represent an opportunity to earn rewards.

Additionally, agility training strengthens the bond between dog and human as the handler and pet learn to read one another on a unique and deeply satisfying level, communicating well beyond basic cues such as "sit," "stay," and "down."

Disadvantage:

– Some patients may not be able to compete or train, unless in a controlled environment specific to their needs.

Figure 8.3 Agility training is beneficial for both aerobic exercise and mental stimulation. Photo courtesy of Tia Guest, KPA-CTP. Photo credit to www.fastclicksphoto.com.

Concept training

Concept training is a new and advanced training model that infers a general or abstract idea from specific occurrences and teaches the ability to see connections and patterns in a situation.

Examples of concept training include

Discrimination – Discrimination training uses cues (discriminative stimulus) to teach an animal to discriminate between objects (Figure 8.4). This technique is used often in service dog training to teach the name of specific objects such as "shoe," "purse," and so on.

Modifiers – Modifier cues limit or qualify another cue. Examples of modifier cues are left/right, up/down, in/out, and large/small, and are combined with another cue. Example: Ball – big – get it.

Match to sample – Match to sample has been used in bomb and narcotic dog training and is now being used in some service dog programs. The animal is shown an object and then must locate a matching object.

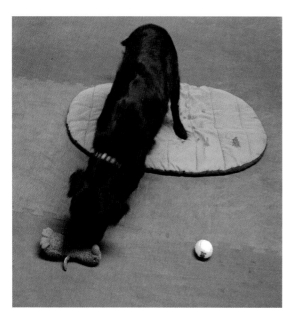

Figure 8.4 "Luna" discriminating between objects. Photo courtesy of Susan Kennedy, KPA-CTP.

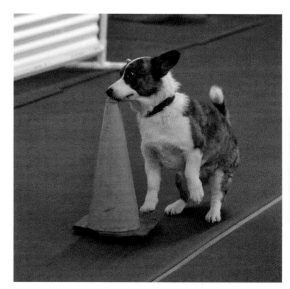

Figure 8.5 "Siren" alerts while doing Nose Work®. Photo courtesy of Becky Hart.

"Show me something new" – The idea of "Show me something new" originated from a dolphin research project by Karen Pryor and later to 101 things to do with a box in dog training. The animal is not cued to perform a specific behavior in relationship to the box (or any other item) but is only reinforced for each novel behavior it chooses.

Although concept training is in its beginning in the companion animal training area, this type of training may become a staple for slowing cognitive dysfunction and when working with animals that require a more challenging form of mental stimulation. Concept training is also stimulating to the trainer because it breaks up the monotony of typical foundation training.

K9 Nose Work®

K9 Nose Work®, an activity and sport inspired by working scent-detection dogs, teaches dogs to find a specific odor (e.g., birch, anise, and/or clove) and locate its source (Figure 8.5).

Developed by Ron Gaunt, Amy Herot, and Jill Marie O'Brien, Nose Work was designed to help most dogs have fun and succeed in an activity that allows them to use their most acute sense – olfaction.

The activity was designed to be inclusive to dogs with issues that might normally preclude them from participating in other group activities. Dogs work one at a time, and while one dog is out of his crate, the

other dogs are covered in their crates or confined in another area. Dogs are unable to see each other and no aversives or punishments are allowed in class. Because emphasis is placed on controlling the environment and not the dog (e.g., using a leash or blocking off an area where you do not want the dog to search), each class or lesson becomes a safe zone where the dogs do not have to worry about either intentional or inadvertent corrections.

Many patients have had their lives shrink because they are not successful in the world at large. A controlled K9 Nose Work setting taught by a National Association of Canine Scent Work certified or associate instructor (CNWI or ANWI) can provide the opportunity for some fearful or aggressive patients to gain confidence and socialize within a safe environment where they also have a chance to fulfill a natural drive and solve puzzles. It also allows geriatric patients to remain mentally active. The benefits of Nose work are also often advantageous for problem prevention and intervention treatment plans (Box 8.2).

BOX 8.2: BENEFITS OF NOSE WORK® TO THE BEHAVIOR PATIENT.

Increases confidence and sociability
Increases mental stimulation

The dog learns an activity that may be more comforting than scanning in times of stress

Raises the arousal threshold (it takes longer to become frustrated or aroused)

Improves the ability to focus on a task

Strengthens the owner–pet bond (often damaged by repeated "failures" in other activities)

Provides passive CC to other dogs, people, and the environment

Training tools

Training tools are used to temporarily or permanently assist with changing behavior. There are a myriad of behavior tools and equipment veterinary technicians can call upon to help owners work with their pets. No single piece of equipment is suitable for every situation. Therefore, one should carefully consider the animal, the owner, and the problem before reaching into their toolbox.

Animals exhibit individual reactions that are based upon a combination of genetics and learning. Although you cannot change the genetic component, with the aid of appropriate equipment, skill, and knowledge in using them, it is possible to manage and then teach the animal an alternative, more acceptable response.

Successful resolution of a problem behavior entails evaluating and recognizing why the animal performs the behavior (see section titled **Functional behavior analysis**) and then applying the principles of management and training to encourage an appropriate response.

Owners must become knowledgeable about the safe and effective application and use of equipment before beginning any behavior modification that will include the use of that equipment. Training equipment is comparable to a surgical instrument – it can be used effectively and without adverse effects if applied properly. It is often helpful to train the pet first and acclimate it to the training tool, then turn attention to teaching the pet owner. Initially, it may be beneficial to demonstrate with a stuffed animal, and then introduce the pet. If multiple pet owners are present, one pet owner can then demonstrate teaching the technique to the others, with the technician's input and guidance. This technique often builds a pet owner's confidence level by watching it, doing it, and then teaching it.

Introducing a training tool to pet owners without teaching them the proper use will likely cause the tool to be reported by them as ineffective or cause the problem to worsen.

It is equally important for owners to understand the importance for all interactions with training tools to include positive, relationship-building methods that avoid causing confrontation or fear-induced behaviors, which would be detrimental to the treatment plan.

The appropriate use and application of any training tool is frequently crucial in regard to the outcome of some cases. For example, in the case of owner-directed aggression, a head halter and dragline may be imperative to avoid further overt aggression toward the owner and prevent further deterioration of the human–animal bond while the treatment plan is introduced.

In such a situation, a training tool such as a head halter and dragline would allow the pet owner to intervene safely, prompt another behavior (i.e. attention), and then increase distance from the provoking stimulus. Without such training tools, it could be nearly impossible to redirect some animals without increasing their fear.

Example: A dog diagnosed with owner-directed, conflict-induced aggression may guard space or objects. In this situation, the pet owner may need to intervene in an emergency situation to remove an item and a head halter and dragline may be required to prompt the behavior of leaving the object, which can then be reinforced.

In any situation, a training tool should be used only to manage a behavior, prompt an appropriate response that can be reinforced, or intervene in an emergency situation (i.e., stimulus suddenly appears and an aggressive reaction is occurring).

In cases where episodes of intervention are occurring frequently, management and other aspects of the treatment plan should be reassessed.

Example: An unplanned visitor rings the doorbell, the dog charges to the door barking, the pet owner cues "come" and prompts the dog to turn toward him/her with a dragline and head halter. The behavior of turning attention toward the pet owner can then be reinforced with a treat. The doorbell should be disconnected and access to the front door should be managed with barriers.

As treatment progresses (i.e., medications reach therapeutic levels, management and behavior modification techniques have been successfully implemented, and the pet owner begins to gain confidence) the dependence on some tools, such as head halters, should lessen quickly. While in severe cases or in situations in which the pet owner would prefer to rely on the training tool, they may always be required to some degree.

Listed below is a small sampling of the equipment that may be part of a prescribed treatment plan and tools the behavior technicians commonly rely upon when working to manage and change behavior while at the same time maintaining safety. Please note, this list is not all-inclusive.

Head halters

There are several different types of head halters currently available, each with its own pros and cons. This section will not discuss specific brands but will instead focus on the general concept of head halters.

Most head halters (also referred to as head collars) have a loop that encompasses the muzzle and a strap that fastens around the neck. When head collars were originally marketed in 1987, it was thought there was a "pack instinct" relationship to the head collar. It is now known that is entirely incorrect. Rather, head halters work by applying pressure behind the neck and around the muzzle so that the dog can be encouraged to display the chosen response by prompting a head turn. The principle is similar to that of a horse halter; where the nose goes, the body follows.

Practical applications and uses

Head halters are suitable for most dogs that pull on-leash, bark at people or other animals, grab hands, clothing, or the leash, jump up on people, or perform other behaviors that require better control.

Head halters employ negative reinforcement (release of tension) and should be paired with positive reinforcement (offering of a treat) to prompt the dog for desired behavior that can be reinforced. For instance, a dog that pulls on the leash and is easily distracted by outside stimuli can be redirected to look at the owner by gently pulling the leash to the side. This will move the dog's head away from whatever has its attention and back toward the owner. A treat is given to the dog as a reward for looking at the owner.

Shaping loose leash walking, reinforcing for attention, and slack in the leash should be taught separately (i.e., without the stimulus present) and then the learned behavior applied in behavior modification.

Many treatment plans include walks off the pet owner's property to increase the pet's mental stimulation and frequently a head halter is required for the pet owner to walk safely.

Example: The pet owner sees an approaching dog in the distance, preferably before the patient does, and if the dog has not been taught a cue for an about turn, the pet owner could use the head halter and leash to quickly but gently turn the dog's head away from the approaching stimulus while increasing distance with fast-paced heeling (see section titled **Response substitution**).

When using a head halter, the leash should always be slack unless the dog is pulling or needs guidance and redirection.

> • When using a head halter, the leash should always be slack unless the dog is pulling or needs guidance and redirection.

Dogs that pull while using a head harness have not been taught properly. The handler has likely continued to walk forward while the leash was taut, therefore reinforcing a taut leash. The leash may also be tight because the stimulus has increased too rapidly or is too close. Shaping loose leash walking, reinforcing for attention, and slack in the leash should be taught separately, without the stimulus present and then instituted as needed.

If the patient pulls ONLY due to a lack of training and is not motivated by an adverse emotional state requiring the pet owner to quickly turn the pet's head away from the stimulus, a no-pull harness may be more applicable and usually requires less acclimation by the pet. The goals for each patient's treatment plan should be considered along with the pet owner's abilities when determining which harness is more appropriate for that patient's specific situation.

As mentioned previously, a head halter is often a necessity for practicing some response substitution, at least initially.

In moments of intervention, it may be necessary to use the head halter to prompt turning away from the stimulus by giving a few short tugs, as if touching someone on the shoulder to gain their attention, and then reinforcing the dog for walking away. Often the best reinforcement for a frightened animal is to increase distance from the fear-provoking stimulus.

Benefits

The use of a head halter can be a quick method (almost instantaneous) for pet owners to walk their dog without pulling, therefore making it more likely the pet owner will walk the dog more frequently. Some head halters can be used for young puppies. This can be useful as a problem prevention tool when the size of the puppy will become out of proportion with the pet owner's abilities to walk the dog (e.g., Great Dane puppy owned by geriatric pet owners).

A head halter allows the handler to turn the dog's eyes, head, and body away from a stimulus without punishing the dog and provides added safety for reactive or aggressive dogs while working to modify their behavior. Head halters are frequently a key to initially and successfully applying RS.

Properly fitted head halters can be worn for long periods of time, which may be necessary in extreme aggression cases, but they should never be left on an unsupervised pet at any time.

Disadvantages and cautionary comments

An introduction and acclimation period is often necessary and may require CC and DS before a head halter can be used properly. If not acclimated properly, if a previous negative association has occurred (some dogs generalize muzzles to the nose strap of the head halter), or if not fitted properly, some animals can find a head halter aversive.

Some dogs seem to have more difficulty acclimating to a head halter than others. Brachycephalic breeds may not be physically able to wear a head halter. Having multiple brands of head halters available will allow testing for the best fit. A head halter can be uncomfortable for a dog suffering from allergies because the nose strap is irritating. In such cases, a different brand of head halter can be tried to improve comfort or a head halter may need to be removed from the treatment plan entirely until the allergy issues are at least somewhat resolved.

Some social stigma to head halters remains (i.e., mistaken for a muzzle). Explaining to pet owners that the head halter is only a temporary tool and that their pet can eat, drink, bark, and even bite (even when fitted properly) while wearing the head halter can sometimes decrease the stigma. Emphasize that their pet may require the head halter only initially, to enable their pet to progress through the treatment plan. One analogy I often use to convince pet owners who are even slightly uncomfortable with their pet wearing the head halter is that of a person walking with a cast as their leg heals. Like a head halter, the cast will hopefully not be needed after the leg heals, although some injuries require an aid for the rest of the person's life. Using the head halter may be a useful tool for the patient's life, and that is neither inappropriate nor unacceptable.

Caution should be taken when working with a pet owner who has done extensive punishment-based training with a choke or pinch collar. Jerking on the leash could be a "muscle memory" behavior and care should be taken to teach the pet owner to never jerk on the leash reflexively. A retractable leash should never be used in conjunction with a head halter. If the dog were to suddenly run to the end of the leash a neck injury could occur.

Some patients with serious handling issues may be extremely difficult to safely and properly fit with a head halter, and may require extensive CC and DS before the head halter can be utilized by the pet owner. In extreme cases, the head halter fitting may either be done as the veterinary technician observes the pet owner and instructs him/her step by step on the fitting and use of the head halter (TAG points would be helpful in this case, see Chapter 5). In severe cases, the head collar first needs to be CC and DS at home before other aspects of the treatment plan are in place (i.e., walking the pet off property). On these occasions, the head halter can be sent home with the pet owner to first CC the head halter and then revisit the situation at a follow-up appointment.

Head halters should never be used as punishment but rather as a prompt to induce a reinforceable desired behavior (like attention or turn away from a stimulus). Often a head halter provides a safe way for the owner to manage the pet on leash while applying behavior modification.

- Head halters should never be used as punishment but rather as a prompt to induce a reinforceable desired behavior (like attention or turn away from a stimulus).

Basket muzzles/other muzzles

It may be assumed many dogs will require wearing a muzzle at some point in their lives. The ability to comfortably wear a muzzle can be critical when treating some behavior disorders and some communities have laws requiring specific breeds of dogs to wear a muzzle whenever out in public.

Muzzles may be used to help keep a dog from biting or causing injury during the treatment process. They can also be used for dogs with coprophagia and pica to prevent the dog from picking up inappropriate items while outside.

The two types of muzzles that will be discussed in this section include nylon and basket muzzles.

Nylon muzzles

Veterinarians and groomers often use nylon muzzles for short procedures. They surround the dogs muzzle and are held in place with two straps that fasten at the back of the neck. Nylon muzzles are easy to size, easy to apply, and equally easy to remove.

Example: A dog with history of aggression has a mat that needs to be trimmed from behind the elbow. A nylon muzzle is applied and the mat is quickly trimmed. One significant disadvantage of nylon muzzles is that the patient's mouth is closed or almost completely closed, thus preventing panting and could result in overheating if used for long periods of time, especially during hot weather, or if used on a struggling dog. Another consideration, depending upon how the muzzle is made, is that the person restraining the dog may accidentally slip a finger through the front opening and a bite can still occur. It is also difficult to use classical CC with a nylon muzzle because often the patient is unable to readily take a treat.

Basket muzzles

The basket muzzle is aptly named. It has a wire or hard plastic basket-type cage that fits over the dog's muzzle and buckles in the back. They come in sizes suitable for any breed of dog. Some basket muzzles have a strap that runs up and over the top of the dog's head and fastens to the strap on the muzzle. This holds the muzzle in place, a feature very useful for dogs with short faces.

Dogs wearing this type of muzzle are able to open and close their mouth to pant and drink water. Basket muzzles often have openings wide enough so the dog can receive treats through the muzzle (Figures 8.6 and 8.7). Food can be placed in the basket muzzle and then stored in the freezer for patients. The basket muzzle becomes a treat delivery device the dog wears on its face.

Basket muzzles can be worn for longer periods of time, but require more work to properly fit the dog. They can be useful when performing DS by giving an added "safety zone" in case a mistake is made during DS and the animal becomes aggressive. This gives the veterinary technician a "buffer" and helps the technician to focus

Figure 8.7 Jerky treats being advanced through a basket muzzle.

on the procedure being desensitized. The basket muzzle may also help pet owners to relax as they implement behavior modification exercises.

Basket muzzles can also be used as a management tool while treatment is being implemented for dogs that compulsively eat unacceptable objects or compulsively self-mutilate.

Example: A dog with a history of pica has had surgery several times due to ingesting rocks from the yard. It has become a contest as the dog attempts to eat the rocks before his owner can intercede. Although the owner must still supervise the dog, it is possible to allow the dog outside for a longer period of time with minimal worry about ingesting inappropriate objects.

Cautions

Muzzling a dog is not a guarantee of safety, and caution should still be exercised when working with an aggressive dog.

Dogs wearing hard basket muzzles can still cause injury by performing a "muzzle punch," an act where the dog forcefully jabs his mouth at a person or other animal. Additionally, the openings in the basket are often wide enough for a finger to slip inside and a bite to occur.

Muzzles should never be considered a replacement for training or safe confinement for aggressive dogs. Instead, they are used to safely implement training and while assessing progress. They are not in themselves the treatment. Simply putting a muzzle on a dog that is aggressive toward strangers and then allowing the dog around strangers (without implementing DS and CC) is inappropriate and is not treating or improving the underlying problem.

Figure 8.6 Dog receiving canned cheese through the basket muzzle.

Body harnesses

Harnesses come in several different styles, depending on the purpose and unique use of the harness. Harnesses described in this section will include a no-pull harness and a standard harness. Each has its own unique use.

No-pull harnesses

No-pull harnesses come in front clip, back clip, and a combination of front and back clips styles. Front clip harnesses attach the leash to a clip that is in the middle of the harness across the front of the dog in the thoracic inlet area. They stop pulling by steering the dog to the side and directing their attention back to the owner. To explain the physics of how it works, you might compare it to a line on the bow of a boat. No matter which direction the water flows, the boat pivots around to face front. Back clip no-pull harnesses have a martingale-type loop in the middle of the harness with a ring that clips between the dog's shoulders. When the dog pulls on the leash, the loop tightens up and applies pressure on the dog's chest and between the shoulder blades. There are also harnesses that combine front and back clips.

The no-pull harness is a good choice for dogs that pull hard but do not require their heads being turned toward the pet owner during behavior modification. A no-pull style harness may be beneficial to dogs with medical problems impacting their neck area. Usually no acclimation period is needed to condition the dog to the harness. Just connect the leash and go.

Considerations

No-pull harnesses can be difficult to fit properly. If a dog is not fit properly, or if the dog is taken for a run while wearing a no-pull, the harness may rub and cause sores to develop under the dog's front legs. Some dogs learn to pull through the harnesses. The biggest drawback to a no-pull harness is that it provides no or little benefit for overly reactive dogs and dogs that jump or mouth because the dog is difficult to redirect without controlling its head. Front clip harnesses are not a good choice for dogs that like to grab the leash simply because the leash is easy for them to reach. Wiggly dogs or dogs with short legs can sometimes slip out of a harness.

Standard harnesses

Standard harnesses provide no control against pulling and clip in the back.

Standard harnesses can be used for small dogs with neck, spine, or trachea problems. Many cat owners relish the idea of allowing their cats to enjoy the great outdoors, but are unsure about how to accomplish it safely.

Cats can easily be taught to walk on a leash. There are harnesses specifically created that allow cats outside time while minimizing the chance of escape.

Standard harnesses function similarly to those used for training sled dogs. They use the dog's opposition reflex to encourage pulling and some animals are able to slip out of a standard harness.

Treats

The importance of treats and the way they are used cannot be stressed enough. Owners often select a treat "they" consider desirable only to discover the animal does not share their opinion (see section titled **Determining a reinforcement hierarchy**). The value of a treat is determined by the animal.

Practical applications and uses

Treats can be used as a distraction, or to develop positive associations during a procedure. Some popular and easy-to-keep options for dogs include peanut butter, cream cheese, string cheese, canned dog food, canned cat food, canned baby food, canned chicken, and hot dogs. Cats often enjoy dry/soft cat treats, canned cat food, baby food, tuna, sardines, and chopped chicken. Technicians can use tongue depressors, popsicle sticks, and empty syringe cases as treat-dispensing tools in addition to hand-feeding treats (Figure 8.8).

Example 1: If a pet is sensitive to having its feet handled, begin by briefly touching a toe while feeding a high-value treat. Repeat this process several times. The next step is to touch the pet's foot and quickly treat. Once the animal is looking forward to having his foot touched so he can get a treat, begin to maintain contact a little longer before treating. Slowly work up to holding the paw, then giving gentle squeezes, and eventually

Figure 8.8 An empty 12-cc syringe case can be recycled as a treat dispenser.

touching between his toes. How much time this takes depends upon the animal and past learning history.

Example 2: When vaccinating a cat, it may be helpful to allow it to lick a treat off a tongue depressor or the exam table, thus providing a distraction.

Considerations

There are several challenges with using treats. Large quantities of treats can result in weight gain. This can be offset in several ways. Special high-value treats can be given when teaching difficult behavior, while a portion of the pet's regular diet can be fed as a reward for behaviors it already knows. Additionally, once a dog is able to reliably perform a behavior, it is possible to substitute something else the animal likes for food, including play, walks, or petting.

If owners are not careful while training, pets can learn that the cue to performing a behavior is only when the pet owner has treats. This can easily be corrected by instructing the pet owner to train throughout the day without treats in plain sight (i.e., in a container on a shelf).

Treat bags

Treat bags can be a fancy bag that hooks to your belt or something as simple as a carpenter's apron with large pockets. Treats can also be stationed in areas where behavior modification is likely to occur, such as at the front door for quick access (Figure 8.9). Quick reinforcement helps with keeping a high rate of reinforcement, and reminds the pet owner to reinforce behavior. If the apron or bag has multiple pockets, it is easy to separate high-value treats from low-value treats.

Target sticks

A target stick can be commercially made or homemade, using a small dowel rod with a wooden ball fastened to the end.

Targeting is a universal skill that has many different functions and is useful in all animals. Zoos often use targeting on large animals for drawing blood or other husbandry duties that would otherwise require force or use of drugs.

The first step is to teach the pet to touch the stick and immediately reward. The target should be held close to the animal to encourage success but avoid moving the target toward the pet. Instead have the animal move forward to touch the target.

For animals that are fearful or reluctant to touch the target stick, the pet owner can use hands or fingers and then change over to a target stick. It may be necessary to shape the behavior by rewarding any movement toward

Figure 8.9 Station treats for easy and quick access. Treats in a bag at the front door.

the target and increasing the difficulty in incremental amounts.

One of the benefits of targeting is that fearful dogs can transfer touch from someone familiar to a new person or object. Overly reactive dogs use targeting as a way to reorient toward their owners when faced with a distraction. Recalls and loose leash walking can easily be taught with targeting (Figure 8.10).

Figure 8.10 Various target sticks.

Calming cap

Behaviors can be affected by a dog's emotional reaction to people, places, and objects encountered in the environment. Triggers, such as the sight of a person walking by, another dog close to their home, or riding in a car, may result in a sudden and intense fearful or stress-related reaction. Dogs in such a highly aroused state are difficult to work with because they lose the ability to focus on other behaviors that can be rewarded.

Calming caps are lightweight fabric masks with a sheer panel that filters a dog's vision (Figure 8.11). The calming cap addresses sensory overload and maybe helpful in creating a nonstressful starting point for DS to occur. For example, if a dog is triggered by another dog even when it is a block away, a calming cap can be used to decrease the visual aspect of the stimulus, possibly creating a point for DS to occur. This in turn may help lower the dog's arousal response. It is not a blindfold but rather a visual filter – some sight still occurs. Dogs are still able to perform normal behaviors that rely upon vision, such as maneuvering around his environment while on walks.

The calming cap does not "cure" the dog but helps manage the situation while the technician works to modify the underlying cause. It can be used along with a body wrap for dogs with thunderstorm phobia, especially if the problem involves sensitivity to lightning. Success has been reported with some dogs with separation anxiety when the calming cap was included as part of the therapy.

Calming caps are lightweight and offered in various sizes and most dogs can easily be conditioned to wear the calming cap for long periods. This helps the dog to better tolerate longer trips in the car or lengthy periods of stormy weather.

Considerations

Some animals that are globally fearful or have severe anxiety disorders may not do well with a calming cap. Either their anxiety worsens or the animal goes

Figure 8.11 A calming cap can be used as a "visual filter" during behavior modification.

into learned helplessness, which is not beneficial to the application of behavior modification. The calming cap should not be used to place an animal into learned helplessness to expedite a medical treatment.

Anxiety clothing

"Anxiety clothing" relies upon pressure to help calm fearful or anxious dogs and cats. One of the most commonly used brands is the "Thundershirt." A 2011 study conducted by CanCog Technologies and overseen by Veterinary Behaviorist, Gary Landsberg, D.V.M., revealed significant improvements during a thunderstorm test for dogs wearing a Thundershirt.

Some experts believe the success of anxiety clothing is directly related to the calming effect of pressure on the nervous system. It is thought that this pressure is responsible for the release of calming hormones such as endorphins. This concept has been observed in humans for many years.

Examples: Wrapping an infant snuggly in a blanket is frequently used by parents and in hospital nurseries to encourage calmness in fussy infants. Dr. Temple Grandin discovered how applying gentle pressure to the body relieves the anxiety commonly experienced by people with autism.

Anxiety clothing may bring immediate relief to some animals, require several repetitions for other animals, or have no effect. It often is used as an adjunct to behavior modification and can be worn for extended periods of time when necessary.

Considerations

Some anxiety clothing uses velcro as a way to close and connect sections together. Dogs with extreme noise sensitivity may startle at the sound of the velcro being pulled apart and CC and DS to the sound may be required prior to using it on the pet.

Waist leashes, tethers, draglines, long lines
Waist leashes

Waist leashes are multipurpose tools. They can be specially designed leashes that buckle around the waist with a leash that attaches directly to the belt. Waist leashes can simply be a leash that is tied around the owner's waist, or clipped using a strong carabineer.

The waist leash is recommended for puppies or adult dogs that require constant supervision to prevent house soiling or inappropriate chewing. They can also help encourage attention to the owner as the pet learns to watch and anticipate movements. Runners often use them to keep their hands free while jogging with their dogs. Loose leash walking is often taught using a waist leash.

Owners who employ the waist leash for supervision are not forced to hold the leash and thus can go about their normal routine. When used for training, owners learn how to maintain attention without pulling on the leash. When training a dog that has shown reactivity or aggression in public, the waist leash maybe used as a second leash and as a safety back-up.

Considerations

Waist leashes offer many benefits, but also have some drawbacks. Some owners forget they have a dog attached to the end of the leash and may trip over their pet and fall, or step on the pet, causing injury. Very strong dogs may have the ability to pull their owners over when excited.

Tethers

Toy tethers are usually made of plastic coated wire cables with snaps on one or both ends. They are offered in different lengths. Using a wire cable prevents the dog from chewing through the tether. The plastic coating provides protection to nearby objects.

Wall tethers are often used during training and behavior consultation to practice hands-free behaviors, but are also a safety tool during behavior consultations (see section titled "**Staying safe**").

The tether provides an opportunity to safely observe the dog's behavior. It also takes the leash out of the owner's hands, allowing him/her to answer questions and provide information without worrying about the pet.

Short tethers, approximately 3 ft in length, are generally used to prevent dogs from becoming tangled. Anchoring the tether to an eyebolt secured to the wall or floor provides stability when faced with large strong dogs in practice behavior modification sessions.

Considerations

Tethered dogs must always be supervised. Avoid long tethers as it is possible for dogs to become tangled. Check tethers and anchors frequently to detect any weakness. Do not allow dogs to chew on the tether as it can cause harm to teeth.

Draglines

Draglines are often considered interchangeable with long lines. However, there are some differences. Drag lines are used for close work inside the house and tend to be made of a lighter material and are narrower than a regular leash, with a length of no more than 10 ft. Although similar to a regular leash, it has no handle and is much less likely to become snagged on objects.

As the name indicates, the dog drags the leash around with it. It offers an easy way indoors to interrupt undesirable behaviors and gain control of a dog that darts out of open doors, jumps on furniture, or jumps on guests. The owner is quickly able to pick up the leash and guide the dog away from what it is doing. Indoor draglines can be used in combination with head halters to help with directing the dog's attention back to the owner. They are often recommended for dogs that dislike having their collars grabbed.

A benefit of a dragline is that owners never need to physically touch the dog, making it much less likely that any negative association will be made with hands and prevents further injury to the pet owner.

Considerations

Even though these make useful training tools, dogs should never be left unattended when wearing one. It is also important never to grab and yank on the line; they are meant to gently redirect the dog's attention. A dragline may be necessary in the early stages of training. Once the dog is able to respond reliably to the owner even when distracted, a dragline would no longer be necessary for response substitution.

Long lines

Long lines are most frequently used outside. They are usually made of nylon, cotton, or leather and may extend anywhere from 20 ft to 100 ft.

One of the most common uses for a long line is teaching the recall outside, around distractions.

A benefit of long lines is that they provide more room for exploration, while keeping the dog safe and ensuring it will not run away.

Considerations

Long lines should never be used with head halters but instead be fastened to the dog's regular collar or harness.

Owners should never allow the dog to run and "hit" the end of the line. This can cause severe injury to the dog. There is risk a dog could become tangled in a long line and panic.

Additionally, owners should be careful when holding a long line. If the dog begins to run and the owner allows the line to slip through his/her hands, a rope burn can easily occur. This possibility can be greatly decreased by tying knots in the line at several different spots to provide a better grip.

Using a long line when working with an overreactive dog can be dangerous and the pet owner must always be aware of the environment and changes in the environment before the dog does, otherwise it may charge to the end of the leash, injuring itself and the pet owner.

Interactive toys or puzzles

The use of interactive toys or puzzles for preventing behavior problems and disorders has been discussed at length in Chapter 7. Interactive toys and puzzles are frequently recommended in treatment plans as a way of increasing mental stimulation and enrichment. They offer an opportunity to practice a variety of problem-solving techniques and are often recommended in the treatment of separation anxiety and teaching independence from the pet owner.

Pheromones

Pheromones are chemicals released by one animal that send messages to other animals of the same species, using scent. Pheromone-based products for pets were introduced in the US in 2001. They mimic naturally occurring dog- and cat-calming and appeasing pheromones and may relieve stress in pets. Pheromone-based products are available as sprays, plug-in diffusers, and wipes. There are also pheromone collars for dogs.

Feline pheromone products have been recommended to help with marking, spraying, and aggression problems but they are also used to help alleviate stress while traveling, when a cat is being boarded, or during veterinary visits. One of the most recognized feline pheromone products currently on the market is Feliway®. It imitates the F3 facial pheromones cats deposit when cheek rubbing to mark something in the environment as safe and not to be feared.

Canine pheromones are used in adult dogs for stress, separation anxiety, and noise sensitivity to thunderstorms or fireworks. They can be used to help puppies deal with the stress of entering new homes. Dog appeasement pheromones are released by nursing dogs to calm their puppies. The product people are most familiar with is Adaptil™.

As pheromones are species-specific, they should have no impact on other animals exposed to them. Although pheromones may not work in every animal, there are no reports of negative reactions to the products. Therefore, they are considered safe to use in almost any situation where animals experience stress.

Considerations

Pheromones used alone are often not sufficient to ameliorate stress-related behavior. Instead, they should be employed as part of a comprehensive modification plan. It is equally important for animals to first be examined by a veterinarian to rule out medical problems before assuming a situation is behavior-related.

Reward markers

Reward markers are often used without owners even realizing it. There can be multiple reward markers, but the three basic types are the clicker, a verbal marker, and a visual maker. They all communicate to the pet that whatever behavior the animal is doing at that time is correct and a reward is coming. In order for a marker to work, it must be used as the behavior occurs and before the dog has performed a different behavior.

Example: A dog is being taught to sit. As the dog's rear end makes contact with the ground, mark the behavior and reward. The dog has been rewarded for sitting. An easy mistake is for the dog to sit and then immediately stand up before the owner uses the reward marker. If the owner gives the reward marker at that time, the dog is rewarded for standing.

Clickers are devices that make a short, distinct "click" sound. They are often preferred by trainers because they are so precise that it is easy for any animal to hear and understand the behavior that is being rewarded. See section titled **Event marker (clicker) training**.

Verbal markers are probably one of the most widely used tools. Owners often tell their pets "Good dog" or "Good!" when a desired behavior has been performed. When owners use a verbal marker, it is important to select short and distinct words and always follow the word with a reinforcement. To prevent confusing an animal, avoid phrases frequently used in everyday conversations (i.e., yes, okay) and instead select seldom-used words.

Deaf dogs cannot hear audible markers. However, there are several ways to compensate for this situation. Owners may use a pen light or small flashlight, there are vibration collars owners can activate, or even a hand signal such as thumbs up, to signal a well-done behavior.

Visual and sensory markers help owners to easily communicate with a pet that otherwise might be difficult to train. They can be tailored to meet the needs of the situation and the animal.

Remote reward

A remote reward system allows owners to quickly and efficiently reinforce desirable behaviors from a distance, without being directly associated with the process. They are lightweight and portable, so they can easily be used in many different locations. The most recognized of these systems, Treat and Train®, was developed by veterinarian, Dr. Sophia Yin. In a 2008 issue of Applied Animal Behavior Science, Dr. Yin published results of research that appeared to confirm the efficacy of a behavior modification protocol for dogs with a history of excessive barking and jumping that used a remote control food reward dispenser.

The systems employ operant conditioning and shaping to train new desired behaviors. Many provide a strong tone prior to dispensing the treat, so the pet learns that the tone predicts a treat.

The remote reward system is appropriate for use in puppies, adult dogs, kittens and adult cats. It is an effective part of a modification protocol for behaviors like jumping, barking, and door-charging, as well as serving as an aid for working with separation anxiety. Owners of competition and agility dogs have reported improvement in performance using remote reward systems. Remote rewards can help cats and kittens to learn to love their crates and use appropriate areas for scratching.

An example of using a remote reward system: steps to teach a nonaggressive dog proper door greeting behavior

Introduce the dog to the tone/treat combination over several sessions. By dispensing the treats at 5-s intervals, the dog can easily be taught a down-stay on a mat. (If the dog gets up, the tone/treats stop). Once the dog has developed a strong down-stay, it is time to progress with the training. Arrange for a familiar guest to visit your home at a specific time. Place the dog on a down-stay on the mat in front of the Treat and Train® and have the guest ring the doorbell or knock on the door. Immediately use the remote to begin rewarding the dog in the down-stay every 5 s. Open the door and welcome the guest while continuing to reward every 5 s. Maintain the down-stay for 30 s during which the visitor may greet the dog (tone/treat continues). Release the dog after 30 s. If at any time the dog breaks the down/stay, instruct the guest to ignore the dog and stop the treats. Repeat this exercise several times. During this training, it is important to prevent the dog from practicing inappropriate behavior. This can be done using a baby gate, confining the dog in a kennel, or using a tether.

Most remote reward systems are lightweight and portable. Those with a tone mark the appropriate behavior and indicate a treat will follow. With some models it is possible to program automatic ongoing rewards between 3 s and 1 h apart.

Considerations

Most systems require batteries that can go dead in the middle of a training session. Occasionally, there can be a defect in the remote control. Some models may not handle all types of dog food and will become jammed.

Double leashing

Double leashing is used to provide an extra degree of safety to prevent escape and possible injury to the dog.

The double-leash technique is a great tool, especially when working outside. The main leash is attached to the head collar and held by the owner. A second hands-free waist leash is then attached to the dog's harness or buckle collar. In case the dog becomes startled and lunges away, or some type of equipment malfunction happens, there is a backup system to provide security (Figure 8.12).

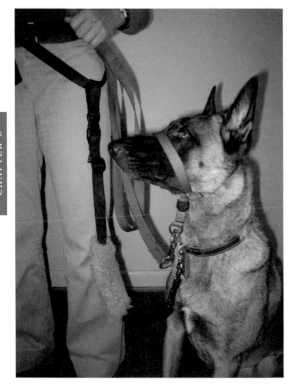

Figure 8.12 A second hands-free waist leash attached to the dog's harness or buckle collar for increased safety.

Figure 8.13 Decoys can be used for assessing behavior and during desensitization.

Decoys

Decoys are life-size stuffed animals that can be used when assessing a dog's level of aggression toward other dogs and are often useful as a nonstressful starting point when practicing DS to other dogs (Figure 8.13).

This chapter has provided information on a few of the most commonly used tools available for technicians working to manage and modify behavior. Technicians can use these items to begin establishing their own individualized tool kit for training.

Marker training techniques and skills

Markers can be used as either a conditioned reinforcer or as a conditioned punisher. This text will focus on the use of a marker as a conditioned reinforcer to teach desired behavior. See Table 8.4 for general guidelines for marker training.

Functional behavior analysis

Dr. Susan Friedman describes applied behavior analysis (ABA) as the technology of behavior change based on the experimentally derived principles of learning and behavior. The primary focus of ABA is to 1) determine the functional relationship between observable behavior and environmental events: What does the animal DO? 2) explain the function of the behavior by its consequences: Why does the animal do that? 3) intervene by redesigning the environment to provide the animal an alternate way to achieve the same purpose served by the problem behavior: What can the animal be taught to do instead? 4) teach new skills to make the problem behavior less likely to occur.

Functional behavior analysis is a technique of assessing the antecedent, behavior, and consequence and then functionally assessing whether the hypothesis about the antecedent and consequence is accurate. Behavior analysis is an essential tool for creating behavior change, whether in teaching a foundation behavior or in addressing problem behaviors (Friedman, 2009a,b).

A veterinary technician (trainer) can influence operant conditioning by influencing the antecedents (what happens prior to the behavior) and the consequences (what occurs immediately following the behavior). The behavior (what the animal DOES) is not manipulated but rather changed by the trainer's influence on antecedents and consequences.

Functional assessment

Dr. Susan Friedman describes the steps in a functional assessment as the following:

(1) Observe and operationally define the target behavior.

   (a) What does the animal do that can be observed and measured?

Table 8.4 General guidelines for marker training.

Mark, then reinforce.	Reinforcement before the click will make the click meaningless.
Keep the treat hand still until after the click.	Movements before the click will overshadow the marker.
If you click you must reinforce.	Not reinforcing after a click will deteriorate the classical association of the marker and reinforcement.
Keep sessions short (2–5 minutes).	Training sessions are intensely mentally stimulating. A 5-min training session can be as mentally stimulating as a 20 min walk.
End session early rather than later.	End session while a high rate of reinforcement is maintained.
Smoothly lower and raise criteria to keep a high rate of reinforcement.	Don't always increase criteria, at times slip back to a lower criterion for reinforcement.
Work on only one new (not on cue) behavior per training session.	This will help to decrease confusion for both the learner and the trainer.
Initially train with low distractions.	Once the behavior is learnt and on cue, begin adding distractions incrementally.
Start to reinforce within ½ second.	Late reinforcement can cause frustration and miscommunication with the learner.
Initially reinforce every desired behavior; once the behavior is on cue, under stimulus control and fluent, reinforce with variable reinforcements and/or intermittently.	Variable reinforcement will maintain the behavior.
Do not use punishment to teach a behavior.	If the expected response does not occur, do not reinforce. The opposite of reinforcement is NO REINFORCMENT See Table 8.9
Test cued behaviors for stimulus control	
Generalize	Once the behavior is on cue, generalize to different people giving the cue and different locations. Begin in most familiar location with low distractions, then add various locations followed by adding low-level distractions.

(2) Identify the distant and immediate physical and environmental antecedents that predict the behavior.

(a) What general conditions or events affect whether the problem behavior occurs; medical or physical problems, sleep cycles, eating routines and diet, daily schedule, etc.?

(b) What are the immediate antecedents (predictors or triggers) for the problem behavior? When, where, and with whom is the behavior problem most likely to occur?

(3) Identify the consequences that maintain the problem behavior, that is, the immediate purpose the behavior serves.

(a) What does the animal gain by behaving in this way, such as attention, an item or activity, or sensory feedback?

(b) What does the animal avoid by behaving in this way, such as particular people, a demand or requests, items or activities, or sensory stimulation?

(c) To what extent does the animal's natural environment support the behavior (i.e., what function might it serve)?

Once the above assessment is complete, intervention can proceed (Friedman, 2009a,b).

Foundation trainer skills
Ability to observe behavior

The skills needed to use a marker successfully are the same qualities required of a good behavior technician: excellent observation of behavior, precision and consistency in training and communication skills, and the ability to be generous with and knowledgeable about reinforcements.

The ability to accurately and objectively observe behavior during training enables the trainer to determine what actions occur naturally by the animal and are therefore more likely to occur in specific situations. The trainer can then capture these naturally occurring behaviors by marking them or by shaping a more complex behavior by incrementally marking more extreme behavior through successive approximations.

Astute observers can note the subtle precursors of the desired behavior (e.g., cat dips its head just before picking up its foot to groom). Lifting of the foot can then be better predicted and consequently improve the marker timing.

Species differences

Before training an animal, as much as possible should be learned about the animal's natural history, social structure, feeding habits, and other naturally occurring

Table 8.5 Species considerations.

Observation	Use in training
What behavior does the animal do naturally?	Identifying naturally occurring behaviors for the species will help identify appropriate behaviors to capture and shape.
Which behaviors occur most frequently?	Choosing a frequently occurring behavior will improve the rate of reinforcement.
Do certain behaviors always lead to other behaviors?	Identify pre-curser behaviors to better predict and time the marker.
How does the animal respond to different sights, sounds?	Species differences in response to sights, sounds, etc will determine an appropriate event marker and assist the trainer in avoiding fear-provoking stimuli in the environment.
What does the animal find reinforcing?	Will help to determine the reinforcement hierarchy for that specific species.
How can that reinforcement be given quickly and efficiently?	The method and delivery of reinforcement will affect the rate of reinforcement.

Figure 8.14 A clicker taped to the handle of a spoon for quick reinforcement for cats and other animals.

behaviors (Ramirez and John G. Shedd Aquarium, 1999).

The laws of learning and marker training techniques discussed in this chapter are the same, regardless of the species being trained but there are differences between species (and between individuals within that species) in regard to their physical abilities and patterns of behavior, reinforcement hierarchy and how reinforcement is delivered (Table 8.5).

Physical abilities and patterns of behavior include the following: What does the animal do naturally? When is its most active time of day? Which behaviors occur most frequently? Do certain behaviors always lead to other behaviors? (i.e., Stretching before yawning, spinning before lying down.) How does the animal respond to different sights, sounds, and environments?

What reinforcement to use and how to deliver the reinforcement also varies between species. For instance, cats tend to take a long time to consume their reinforcement, stopping to groom in between reinforcements. For that reason, a helpful training tool to deliver reinforcement to a cat is a clicker taped to the handle of a spoon, which allows the cat to quickly lick a reinforcement (canned food, tuna, ice cream, etc.) and

then the spoon can quickly be removed to set up for another opportunity to perform behavior (Figure 8.14).

Choosing an appropriate event marker

Conditioned reinforcement markers are used to systematically "explain" or give information about a behavior. During learning of a behavior, the information the marker delivers becomes as important as the reinforcement itself. Once the behavior is under a stimulus-controlled cue and is fluent, the marker is no longer required.

The marker chosen should be able to precisely pinpoint a behavioral moment as it is used to inform the animal that the current criterion of behavior has been met.

The event marker should be brief so only a specific increment of the behavior is marked, for example, a muscle relaxing in the shoulder. The marker should not be something the animal must discriminate from similar stimuli in the environment (Table 8.6). For example, a verbal marker of "yes" must be discriminated from other words the animal hears throughout the day. Although the voice can be used as an event marker when a clicker is not available, it should not be the consistent marker. Research suggested that using the voice as an event marker slowed learning and required more reinforcements than a mechanical marker (Wood, 2008).

The marker should not have a previous association. For example, a whistle that is a cue for "come" should not also be used as a marker. This can occur if a pet owner has improperly used the clicker to "call the dog." Some animals, specifically sound-sensitive animals, may generalize the marker sound to previously negatively associated events. In that case, the technician must determine a different type of event marker (a

Table 8.6 Qualities of an appropriate event marker.

Brief	Only one behavior is isolated
Distinct	Easily noticeable
Different	Not easily confused with other environmental stimuli
Neutral	Has no previous associations
Easy to deliver	Improves speed and accuracy of the event being marked

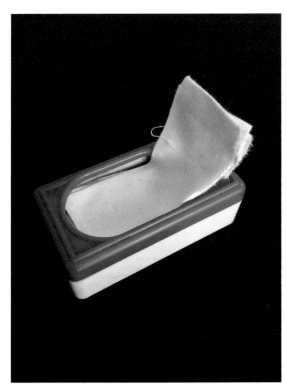

Figure 8.15 Placing tabbed tape pieces on the dimple of the clicker and systematically removing pieces can aid in desensitizing the sound of a clicker for sound-sensitive animals.

flash of light) or desensitize the animal to the marker (Figure 8.15).

The marker must be easy to quickly and efficiently deliver so the desired event or behavior is marked accurately and precisely.

Conditioning the event marker and teaching contingency

The event marker is a conditioned secondary reinforcer that is classically conditioned to an unconditioned reinforcer (UR) (something that is intrinsically reinforcing to the animal) and is therefore under the same requirements for classical conditioning to be effective.

– The presenting order must be correct (i.e., mark then treat). The click must always occur before the unconditioned reinforcer (UR).
– The CR and the UR must occur at a 1:1 ratio (i.e., if you click, you must reward). Because the event marker does not have an intrinsic value to the animal, the 1:1 ratio maintains its reinforcement value.
– Secondary environmental stimuli, such as the trainer's body movements, distractions, and other sounds in the environment should be minimal, decreasing the possibility that the animal will make an association with outside environmental stimuli rather than the sound of the marker. Animals that are astute at noticing the subtle movements of the handler often associate a movement just before a click as the marker; therefore handler movements should remain at a minimum until after the marker, including facial expressions and eye movements.

The conditioning of the marker must occur for it to have intrinsic value to the animal but can often occur within 1–2 clicks. It was once believed conditioning of the marker should be a separate and specific procedure from teaching the animal that the click was contingent on its behavior. It is now understood many animals may learn very quickly that the marker sound means reinforcement and that teaching them that the click is contingent on their behavior can and should occur almost simultaneously with conditioning of the clicker.

When initially conditioning the marker and teaching the animal the marker is contingent on its behavior, it is best to use a variety of very special, flavorful, soft, food treats. Food is most often the chosen UR because it is commonly near the top of most animals' reinforcement hierarchy.

Small (the size of a pea, one lick, etc.), soft food treats can be eaten quickly, so many repetitions of reinforcement can be completed in a short training session. The value of the food reinforcer is not in its size but in the experience itself. For example, people often play penny slots machines for hours. Small food reinforcements also prevent the animal from becoming satiated quickly. Increasing the variety of the food reward improves learning because it maintains interest in the training session. Creating "trail mix" so that the treat hierarchy can be varied smoothly and fluently throughout the training session is helpful.

To teach contingency of the clicker to behavior and classically condition the clicker, follow this process:

- Click and treat 1–2 times for "nothing," just to assess the animal's response to the clicker sound.
- Immediately begin to capture (clicking) some behavior the animal does (i.e. glancing toward the trainer) and follow each click with a treat.

It is important that the animal learns early on that it makes the click happen by doing something. Spending too much time classically conditioning the animal to the clicker (i.e., clicking and treating for no specific behavior) can make teaching the click is contingent on the animal's behavior more difficult.

Targeting is very useful in teaching the animal to offer a behavior and also aids the trainer in practicing accurate timing of the click. The goal behavior is for the animal to touch the end of a target stick (or other target) with their nose, paw, or other body part. Targeting once taught can be used as a prompting technique (detailed below). Most animals will quickly investigate an object held in front of them. A target could also be a spot on the wall or floor, or a specific object lying on the floor. A target could also be a specific object lying on the floor (i.e. a head collar) or a spot on the wall or floor. Practice tip: Multi task by using a training tool, such as head halter or basket muzzle placed on the floor or held in the trainer's hand, as a target when teaching behavior contingency. This process will also help create a positive emotional response to the training tool. At the moment the dog's nose touches the target, the trainer should mark and reinforce the behavior. Eventually the dog will begin following the target because it understands touching the target will be reinforced. The dog then understands that the click is rewarding and it can "earn" the reward by offering a behavior.

> - Practice tip: Multi task by using a training tool, such as head halter or basket muzzle placed on the floor or held in the trainer's hand, as a target when teaching behavior contingency. This process will also help create a positive emotional response to the training tool.

The click has become a conditioned event marker when, after the click, the animal turns toward the trainer for reinforcement, and after eating the treat repeats the behavior (Table 8.7).

Table 8.7 Functions of the event marker.

Function	Message to learner
Precise acoustic event marker	"That's it! What you were doing at that exact moment was what I wanted."
Bridges the event and reinforcement	"Reinforcement is coming."
Click ends the behavior	"Criteria for that repetition have been reached."

> - The click has become a conditioned event marker when, after the click, the animal turns toward the trainer for reinforcement, and after eating the treat repeats the behavior (Table 8.7).

Determining a reinforcement hierarchy

An individual reinforcement hierarchy should be determined for each learner and for specific situations. The hierarchy will vary depending on species of animal, current environmental factors, and the learner's current emotional state. For example, an animal that is highly motivated to chase prey will probably not be reinforced by food in that situation. A fearful animal may not find food reinforcing at the moment it is placed on the examination table but may find the food treat reinforcing when the fearful stimulus is decreased (i.e., when the animal is placed back on the floor). In such a situation, try a higher value reinforcement while it is still on the table; if unsuccessful, remove the animal to the floor and try the reinforcement again. If the animal readily takes the higher level food reinforcement from the table but does so more roughly than previously, do not increase what you are doing but wait until it is taking the treat more gently. If the animal takes the treats without "snatching" them, the procedure may continue. Fearful animals often first grab treats roughly just before they stop taking treats entirely, which is an indication the stress level is too high. If the animal will still not take the high-value reinforcement, the stress in the environment must be decreased before training can commence.

Difficult to perform behaviors or an animal in mild emotional distress must be reinforced with a higher value reinforcement.

> • Difficult to perform behaviors or an animal in mild emotional distress must be reinforced with a higher value reinforcement.

Manipulating motivations

Just as with humans, reinforcement value will be affected by competing motivations. For example, I may want to go for a walk and it is raining outside, therefore I find the smell of fresh baked cookies more reinforcing than walking and I stay in the house and eat the cookies. If it had been sunny outside I may have found the walk more reinforcing than staying in the house to eat the cookies.

Animals are faced with competing motivations that are driven by senses that we humans cannot completely understand. It is critical that the animal's reinforcement hierarchy in various situations be determined and then applied for more effective and faster training.

Astute trainers are able to subtly manipulate motivations.

Example 1: "Todd" is a 2-year old, neutered male, mix breed dog that finds playing with the other dogs at class more reinforcing than food treats. "Todd" pulls at the leash in the attempt to make contact with another dog while his owner pushes a treat into "Todd's" face. The trainer manipulates the reinforcement by asking the pet owner to not feed "Todd" before class, bring steak in the treat pouch, and come to class 20 min early to play with another dog. The motivation to play is decreased while the motivation for the food reward is increased.

Example 2: With a dog that is charging forward toward another dog, the reinforcement type and rate will likely need to be at a higher level, depending on the underlying motivation (excitement, frustration, fear, or a combination thereof). The trainer must be perceptive and increase the value of the reinforcement (i.e, hot dogs) while also decreasing the motivation (i.e., the target dog moves further away). In some cases, until the negative emotional response of a situation is altered, the only reinforcement the animal desires may be increasing distance from the fear-provoking stimulus.

Once it is determined what URs the subject desires, a UR hierarchy can be developed. For example, the tennis ball may be preferred over kibble, but hot dogs may be preferred when a cat is present, and a tennis ball may be more reinforcing than steak when training in the back yard. The top of the hierarchy can be used to train the most difficult task and lower ranking URs can be used for easier tasks or only average responses.

Animals that are the easiest to train are animals that have a vast reinforcement hierarchy and are easily reinforced. For example, the stereotypical Labrador retriever; the UR possibilities for these dogs are endless because there is so much that they want. This is one reason cats can be more difficult to train. Their reinforcement hierarchy is usually smaller and more difficult to determine and manipulate.

Reinforcement schedules

The schedule of reinforcement refers to the pattern of reinforcement that is chosen (see Chapter 6). Continuous reinforcement is best used during the initial stages of training to expedite and solidify learning. A continuous or 1:1 ratio should be maintained during the early stages of teaching the behavior, although the type of reinforcement can and should be varied. For example, a dog may receive a food treat for coming to the owner and other times a toss of a toy may be the reinforcement.

Not all behaviors must be continuously reinforced once they have been well learned (placed on cue, fluent and generalized to multiple situations). Once a behavior is well learned, one usually moves on to an *intermittent reinforcement schedule*, whereby not every correct response is rewarded. The effect of intermittent reinforcement is that the behavior will become resistant to extinction.

Difficult or problem-solving behaviors (tasks that require ingenuity and creativity such as some service animal tasks) or highly desired or valued behaviors should continue to be reinforced continuously.

Most pet owners generally and routinely **under** reinforce desired behaviors and therefore the technician's focus should be more on how the pet owner can continuously reinforce behaviors they like. Using lower ranking reinforcements (petting, talking to the animal, clapping hands, etc.), intermittent reinforcement will occur naturally.

Reinforcement delivery

Delivery of the reinforcer should occur, as a general rule, within 1 s of the marked behavior and before another behavior occurs. Delays will slow the training process considerably.

"Clean" and efficient treat delivery is imperative to making sure the strong association to the marker is maintained. Any unintentional movements by the trainer before the event marker will cause the marker to lose value. Keep the actual delivery of the reinforcement separate from delivery of the event marker. If treat delivery occurs at the same time as the marker, overshadowing will occur, causing the marker to be ineffective because the marker has no predictive value.

> • Keep the actual delivery of the reinforcement separate from delivery of the event marker.

The placement of the treat after the click is also a tool to assist with the next repetition of the behavior. This is different from luring because it comes after the marker and does not prompt the behavior and therefore does not need to be faded (see section titled **Luring – handler prompts**). The strategic placement of the food reward can set the animal up to easily perform another repetition, thus avoiding the performance of other unnecessary behaviors between repetitions.

Example: When teaching a dog to go to a mat or bed, click the dog for looking at the mat on the floor and toss the treat beyond the mat. The dog goes out past the mat to eat the treat. After the dog has completed eating the treat and turns back toward the mat (because the handler is in that direction), click again as it moves toward the mat but before it moves past the mat. Tossing the treat beyond the mat sets the dog up to turn again toward the mat after eating the treat, increasing the likelihood the behavior of approaching the mat can be captured.

Treat delivery from the hand

When delivering food reinforcement from the hand, the animal's head or eyes will often orient toward the treat. Drifting toward the treat can be advantageous when rewarding the animal in a stationary position or when the movements required are in close proximity to the trainer.

For example, a dog is clicked while walking close to the handler on the left side. The treat is delivered by the hand closest to the dog's head (left hand) to encourage staying in that position for the next cue or repetition (Figure 8.16).

Hand delivery of treats can also help to gauge the animal's frustration, excitement, or anxiety level. Animals that have previously taken treats gently but begin to "snatch" or grab roughly at the treat are likely demonstrating an increase in anxiety. Take note and only raise criteria once the animal is again taking the treats gently. Criteria may need to be raised slowly or a break may be necessary.

Precautions:

– Learn the animal's food-guarding history. Some dogs with serious guarding issues may become aggressive when treated from the hand. In such cases, tossing the treat is better until trust by the animal has been gained.

– Some fearful animals may "suddenly" realize they are in close proximity to the technician and find themselves in a motivational conflict (wanting the treat but too close to the veterinary technician) and consequently, feel the need to aggress.

Tossing the treat

As mentioned previously, conscious and accurate placement of the treat allows the trainer to "set up" for the next repetition. When it is advantageous for the dog to work at a distance from the handler or the trainer is working to shape the dog's path, tossing the treat along that path will generate anticipation and increase the likelihood of the behavior. Tossing of the treat may also allow for the additional reinforcement of chasing and "catching" the treat for dogs that enjoy that activity.

For example, teaching a dog to walk onto a scale by tossing the treat onto the scale after clicking the dog for approaching the scale will set up the likelihood of the next criterion, stepping one foot onto the scale.

Precaution:

– Pet owners should be cautious while tossing treats in a household with multiple pets. When teaching something new or if tossing treats during a training session, it is best to place other pets in another area.

Timing

Accurately predicting the behavior and clicking at the precise moment that the behavior occurs is a fundamental and critical skill. Habitually late clicks will communicate inaccurate information to the pet about what is being marked and reinforced. Before timing can be accurate, the trainer must have a clear picture of what the desired behavior is and have a plan for when he/she will click. Being unsure or indecisive of the criteria can often cause the click to be delayed.

Once a behavior is on cue, the click can be incrementally delayed to shape the fluency of duration of the behavior.

Capturing behaviors

Any behavior that can be detected by the human senses can be marked and reinforced.

Figure 8.16 A treat delivered by the hand closest to the dog's head to encourage staying in that position for the next cue or repetition.

> • Any behavior that can be detected by the human senses can be marked and reinforced.

Capturing is the technique of waiting for a behavior to occur and marking the behavior as it happens naturally. For example, "sit" or "down" may be taught by simply marking the behavior when it occurs. Tossing a treat away from the animal will cause the animal to get up from the "sit" or "down," which will create another opportunity for the animal to offer another "sit" or "down." Behaviors like yawning or deep breaths can be captured to encourage relaxation. This is an excellent technique when training fearful or aggressive animals that cannot tolerate close interactions.

> • Behaviors like yawning or deep breaths can be captured to encourage relaxation.

Behaviors such as play bows, sneezing, or scratching are easily captured and can become cute tricks. The challenge of capturing behavior is that many behaviors are not offered frequently and therefore are more difficult to mark and reinforce.

Shaping

Shaping is the process of "building" a behavior by successively reinforcing bits or "criteria" of the behavior that are approximations of the final behavior. The animal's behavior is molded into an end response by the trainer's differential reinforcements of the behavior. The process of differentially rewarding some behaviors and not others is called *successive approximation*.

Gradually the trainer "expects more" (raises criteria) until the desired behavior is reached. For example, to teach a dog to walk backward you would click shifting of the weight backward, any movement of a back or front foot, greater movement of the feet, and so on, until the dog moves backward. An excellent training technique used to teach trainers how to watch for small increments of behavior is to have the trainer sit in a chair with his/her back against the chair at all times; the dog is directly in front of the chair and the trainer must teach the dog to walk backward without allowing his/her own back to leave the chair. Good observational skills and excellent timing are critical in shaping the behavior.

The first approximation of the behavior is initially captured and marked and rewarded several times. Then the criterion for the next approximation is set. In a "perfect" training session, approximations should look as shown in Figure 8.17.

CHAPTER 8

Figure 8.17 Basic shaping plan example for "back up"; in a "perfect" training session approximations occur at each step in a steady incline. Photo courtesy of Melissa Spooner, LVT, VTS (Behavior), BS, KPA-CTP.

In reality, shaping is not usually a steady upward staircase but more comparable to a "dance," with criteria being raised and lowered to keep a steady stream of information flowing to the animal (Figure 8.18). If a criterion is raised too quickly, the response rate of the animal becomes *slower* and the situation becomes increasingly *stressful* for the animal. If pushed to the extreme, an animal may quite simply quit working altogether and show signs of distress and will have to be retrained using more frequent reinforcements. Before this occurs, drop the current criterion to the last successful approximation and continue raising criteria but within smaller increments of the approximations. See general shaping guidelines in Table 8.8.

Creating a shaping plan

A shaping plan is a framework for developing a behavior. The trainer considers potential increments of behavior to reach a criterion and creates successive approximations of the behavior into their plan with the final desired behavior at the top of the staircase. A shaping plan is used to guide the training process and should be reevaluated, assessed, and modified frequently during the shaping process.

As noted previously, shaping of behavior is really a combination of science and art. The trainer must be knowledgeable and subtly raise and lower criteria while keeping a high rate of reinforcement (see subsequent text).

Rate of reinforcement per minute

A high rate of reinforcement (reinforcements per minute) provides the learner with a continuous stream of information over a small period of time, keeping the learner engaged. It can also be used as a guide to the trainer as to when to place a behavior on cue. The rate of reinforcement is highly variable between subjects due to the differences between the speed at which the animal can perform the behavior and the time it takes to reinforce behavior. For example, when training a dog to lie down, a Great Dane will likely receive fewer reinforcements per minute because it takes longer to

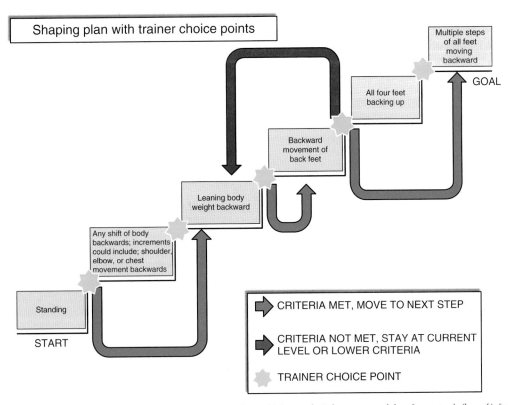

Shaping plan with trainer choice points

Multiple steps
of all feet
moving
backward

GOAL

All four feet
backing up

Backward
movement of
back feet

Leaning body
weight backward

Any shift of body
backwards; increments
could include; shoulder,
elbow, or chest
movement backwards

Standing

START

CRITERIA MET, MOVE TO NEXT STEP

CRITERIA NOT MET, STAY AT CURRENT
LEVEL OR LOWER CRITERIA

TRAINER CHOICE POINT

Figure 8.18 In reality, shaping is a raising and lowering of criteria to keep a high rate of reinforcement and therefore a steady flow of information to the animal. Photo courtesy Melissa Spooner, LVT, VTS (Behavior), BS, KPA-CTP.

assume the down position than it does for a Jack Russell terrier. Therefore, the highest reinforcement rate (rr/minute) that can be successfully achieved for that behavior with that specific animal should be the guide to when to add a cue. Each animal and each behavior should have its own ideal rate of reinforcement per second and be determined by keeping accurate training records. A very general guide is to aim for an rr/minute of around 8–20.

A "jackpot" is a term used to describe giving a high-value reward or several high-value treats in a row to emphasize to the learner the significance of the behavior just performed. It is to be used when a learner masters a particularly difficult behavior or is making an effort to get back into the training game. The problem with a "jackpot" is that if the training session is continued, the subsequent reinforcements for repetitions of the same behavior will be less.

When an animal makes a breakthrough in training, it is a good time to end the training session. End on a good note while the learner is still engaged. However, abrupt discontinuance of a training session can be upsetting to the learner. So, to end a session, scatter several treats on the floor or play a game of tug or fetch. An "end of training" session routine, although not a "jackpot," may look like one in action. So if tempted to give your learner a "jackpot," consider this an appropriate time to give a special reward and take a short break from the training session.

Prompting

Prompting is a (humane) way of inducing a behavior and is often used in the shaping process to cause a specific behavior or criterion of the desired behavior to occur. The most common types of prompts are physical or environmental prompts, luring, and targeting.

The behavior is prompted, marked, and reinforced. The eliciting behavior (prompt) becomes the cue to do the behavior. Later training sessions gradually reduce the intensity of the prompt, eventually fading it entirely and transferring to a different cue or incorporating it into the new cue. For example, movement of a hand

Table 8.8 Shaping guidelines.

Raise criteria in increments small enough so that the subject always has a realistic chance of reinforcement.	Smoothly and fluidly raise and lower criteria so that a high rate of reinforcement can be maintained.
Don't try to shape for multiple criteria simultaneously (i.e. speed and duration).	Create a shaping plan and include the specific criteria for each step. Set your goals for each training session (which criteria you are currently working toward.)
When introducing a new criterion, relax old criteria.	For example, when working on speed of the behavior, do not require the criterion of precision.
Modify your training plan when needed.	Stay ahead of your training subject. Stop and revise the training plan if the training subject suddenly progresses ahead of the plan.
Don't change trainers in a training session.	Multiple trainers can be utilized but do not have multiple trainers training the same task. Different trainers will likely have different criteria and shaping plans, thus creating confusion.
If one shaping plan is not progressing, create another.	There are many ways to "get behavior"; if one plan is not working "think outside the box" and create another plan.
Don't interrupt training sessions abruptly.	Stopping training suddenly can be punishing to the learner. Instead plan an end point and place the start and stopping of training on cue.
If the behavior deteriorates, go back to the beginning of your shaping plan.	Behaviors are likely to regress if marker timing is late or if the criteria are not appropriate. Review and revise your shaping plan.
End sessions on a high note.	Ending sessions on a positive note is reinforcing for both the trainer and the learner.

Modified from 10-laws of shaping by Karen Pryor, K. (1999). Don't Shoot the Dog!: The New Art of Teaching and Training. New York, Bantam Books.

over a puppy's head makes the behavior of bending the rear legs more likely to occur and therefore can be reinforced. The hand movement over the head will continue to be the prompt (cue) until it is transferred to another cue, such as the word "sit."

Physical and environmental prompts

Physical and environmental prompts include such things as touching a puppy's rear to prompt a "sit" (physical prompt) or teaching a dog to heel by walking with the dog next to a wall (environmental prompt). Physical prompts are not commonly recommended because they can cause fear or resistance in some animals, especially animals suffering from fear and anxiety disorders. Environmental prompts can be used to increase the likelihood of a behavior being offered and promote precise muscle memory with early learning and repetitions.

Luring – handler prompts

Luring is an advanced skill and is the process of holding a food treat or toy in front of the dog's nose to guide the dog into the desired position. Examples would include holding a treat over a puppy's nose to guide it into the sit position or throwing treats onto a mat to teach "go to your bed." While luring is a very useful prompting technique, it can have the drawback of the dog becoming so focused on the food treat that he does not think about what he is doing to get the reward. In such cases, a better prompting technique would be targeting.

Luring is an advanced skill because it requires consideration and thought in the training plan as to how the lure will be faded. If a lure is used to prompt the behavior, it should be faded within one or two repetitions.

> • If a lure is used to prompt the behavior, it should be faded within one or two repetitions.

Luring can also be beneficial as a management tool when a dog is in a situation that he is perhaps not equipped to handle. A food lure may distract the dog and allow the handler to move the dog away from the situation.

Targeting

Targeting is the prompting technique of teaching the animal to touch or follow an object such as the trainer's hand, a stick, or other object. Targeting is very useful in teaching a dog to heel at your side by having it touch the target of your hand occasionally as you walk. Targeting can also be used to teach body placement. For example, to get a puppy to step on to the scale to be weighed, the puppy can be taught to target and follow your hand directly onto the scale. Large zoo animals and horses have been taught to target their nose on a spot, which acts as a stationing behavior to aid in medical care.

Targeting is a technique that is very easy and quick to teach. Simply hold the target in front of the animal and click any movement toward the target. Many animals tend to investigate a novel item that appears in their environment and the trainer should be prepared to capture the first investigation of the target. If the animal grabs the target with its mouth, initially mark the behavior but then raise criteria for only nose touches. This might be accomplished by clicking as the animal approaches the target prior to putting his mouth on it. The next step would be to gradually move the target so the animal will follow the target. The animal can also be taught to maintain the target position by the trainer gradually withholding the click for longer durations.

Fading prompts

When a prompt is used, it often becomes the cue or discriminative stimulus for the animal to perform the behavior and therefore it may be desirable to transfer to another cue quickly. Often the ultimate goal is for the behavior to be on a verbal or hand cue, without the prompt being presented. For this reason, when using prompts, a plan should be in place as to how the prompt will be faded. A prompt should only be needed for one to three of the offered behaviors and then quickly faded out. The trainer can then switch back to shaping the behavior if needed after removing the prompt. Tactile prompts are more difficult to fade than visual prompts.

Prompting a behavior is an advanced skill.

> • Prompting a behavior is an advanced skill.

When using a food lure to teach a puppy to lie down, it is useful to gradually decrease the size of the treat held in your hand. Eventually the trainer holds his/her hand in the same luring position but without a treat. This hand movement can then be turned into a hand signal for the down position or transferred to a verbal cue. A target can be faded by gradually decreasing the size of the target.

Cues

This text has attempted to use the word "cue" instead of "command." A cue is simply information, a signal as to which behavior is to be performed at that moment and a promise of a desired result. A command in contrast, has a level of threat involved: do this or else … (Pryor, 2009).

Cues are learned antecedents and discriminative stimuli that predict the potential for positive reinforcement.

Cues give the animal information and provide a common language between trainer and learner. Cues also differentiate between behaviors and are key to building complex behavior chains.

Once the concept of cues has been learned by the animal, it will become easier and faster to associate its behavior with cues.

Cues improve the quality of an animal's life by giving it information; that information is reinforcing in itself. It tells the animal, "Do THIS behavior at THIS moment and the opportunity for reinforcement is in place." Karen Pryor compares cues to a green light at a stop light in *Reaching the Animal Mind*, 2009. "Think about that little sense of joy or relief you feel when the traffic light turns green; that's a cue, identifying a behavior that you want to do. Every cue is a green light, permission to go do the thing it names. The cue thus becomes reinforcing in itself. Any time you give a well-learned cue, you are actually reinforcing what the individual you are cuing happens to be doing at the time."

> • Cues improve the quality of an animal's life by giving it information.

As learning is constantly occurring, any event or situation can become a meaningful and predictive cue or antecedent for other behaviors and consequences. Dogs may show fear reactions only in certain places (if they had previously been rewarded there through escape/avoidance conditioning), or only respond to cues when the pet owner's treat bag is present.

For example, the garage door going up is a cue that you will be entering the house. Seeing a dog in the distance can become a cue to the dog that his choke collar will be jerked. The doorbell cues a person at the door. Often the technician and trainer must analyze behaviors to determine how to manipulate previously associated cues (like the doorbell).

Cues can be predictors of our behavior. For example, when walking with your dog say "left" just before you turn left. After only a few repetitions the dog will associate the verbal "left" with the behavior that is about to occur: the trainer turns. The trainer can then say "left" before turning, pause, and reinforce any left turning movement the dog does. Another example is to say "up" just before picking a dog off the floor. The dog will quickly associate the cue "up" with what you are about to do. If the dog enjoys being picked up, this informational cue will provide the dog with increased predictability and decreased anxiety with the situation, which is very important for fearful or anxious animals.

Cues can also be used to build other behaviors. For example, the known behavior of "down" can be used when shaping "go to a mat" and later faded out so "got to a mat" means go to your mat and lie down without requiring the "down" cue.

Types of cues

Cues should be easy to give consistently, distinct, and easily perceived by the animal and easy to transfer to another cue if needed. Cues can be anything the animal perceives; for example, words, sounds, scents, sight of an object, movement, or an environmental situation can become a cue. Motion cues are usually more salient to the dog and easier to perceive then verbal cues.

How and when to add the cue

A cue can be added when the behavior can be reliably predicted (or prompted) and begins to occur regularly with more intensity and intention. What "regularly" is will be determined by the animal's learning history. A long learning history of clear and properly applied cues will likely make it possible for the animal to generalize the use of cues more quickly. The rr/minute for these animals may be lower than for a novice. A very basic rule of thumb is to add the cue when the rr/minute has reached 8–15 clicks.

The cue is given just before the behavior occurs. The behavior is then rewarded only after the discriminatory stimulus (cue) has been given and not reinforced when the behavior is offered without the cue. Through discrimination, the animal learns the behavior will only be reinforced when the cue precedes the performance of the behavior.

It was once believed a cue should not be added until the behavior was "perfect". As marker-based training has progressed in understanding techniques and as animals have progressed because of better training, it is clear cues are valuable information for the animal and should not be withheld until fluency has been achieved, but added early. Cues can be readily transferred and changed. Thus, a trainer who wants a high degree of precision in a behavior may elect to first use a nonformal cue for a less precise behavior and then transfer to a formal cue for the precise polished behavior.

Example of properly adding a cue:
- Dog offers rear end on the ground, click/treat (C/T).
- Trainer gives the cue "sit" as the dog sits, C/T.
- Trainer gives the cue "sit", just before the dog sits, C/T.
- Trainer gives the cue "sit", before the dog offers the sit, C/T.

– The trainer pauses, if the dog offers the "sit" there is no reinforcement or response from the trainer. The dog gets up from the sit and considers what was different; at that moment the trainer gives the cue "sit" and the dog learns the cue is the key to reinforcement. It is the trainer's responsibility to teach the dog to discriminate when the behavior will be rewarded (cue is given) and when it will not be rewarded (cue not given).The trainer can set the animal up for success by providing the cue frequently: 10–20 repetitions where the cue is given prior to the dog offering the behavior. The trainer pauses slightly and if the dog offers the behavior it is not marked or treated. But then the trainer gives the cue for the behavior, helping the animal discriminate. The dog should be successful more often than not. As the cue is added, the animal's behavior will likely slightly decrease in quality as the animal perceives the addition of the cue and then recognizes its meaning.

Waiting for the cue demonstrates a degree of impulse control, a very valuable and useful skill for companion animals. Once the animal makes the connection and association between the behavior and the cue the animal can be shaped to wait for the cue rather than randomly offering the behavior. The animal learns only behaviors that occur immediately after the cue will be reinforced and other offered behavior will not.

The cue can be strengthened by alternating between different cues (i.e., "sit," "down," "touch"), minimizing cues so they are subtle, removing any prompts, and generalizing the cue to different situations and environments.

Generalization

Generalization is the concept of learning that the cue means the same thing in a multitude of environmental contexts. For example, do the cued behavior regardless of changing variables like location, person giving the cue, and so on. The more generalization is practiced, the faster behaviors are generalized.

Lack of generalization history in regard to problem behaviors and behaviors associated with fear is beneficial when applying behavior modification. A location or situation that looks and feels different from previously associated events is often the first place to apply behavior modification.

Transferring cues

Frequently, cues for a specific behavior will need to be changed. For example, the cue may currently be a hand signal over the dog's head (likely from being prompted with a treat over the head and not faded) and the pet owner would prefer the cue to be verbal.

When transferring cues it is important to give the cues in the correct order. It is very important the two cues, the new cue and the old cue, do not occur simultaneously as the unlearned cue may be blocked.

> - It is very important the two cues, the new cue and the old cue, do not occur simultaneously as the unlearned cue may be blocked.

Example of transferring a hand signal for sit to a verbal cue, "sit"

- New cue "sit" followed by known cue (hand signal), dog sits, C/T. Repeat several times.
- Verbal "sit" pause … old cue (hand signal), behavior, C/T. Repeat several times.
- Verbal "sit", pause, pause, old cue (hand signal), but given more subtly to fade it out, behavior, C/T.
- Verbal "sit", pause, pause, pause, very slight hand signal given, behavior, C/T
- Verbal "sit", pause, pause, pause, dog offers sit without the old cue, C/T.

"Poisoned" cues

Frequently a cue develops a negative emotional association or is "poisoned."

A cue that has been associated with an aversive (whether intentionally or unintentionally) becomes a cue that is no longer "safe" and predictable of a positive outcome. "The cue becomes a conditioned negative reinforcer, signaling the opportunity for avoiding punishment. The shift becomes visible in the learner's attitude, which switches from attentive eagerness to reluctance, often with visible manifestations of stress" (Pryor, 6/25/2002).

"Poisoning" of a cue is commonly seen when treating companion animal behavior problems and disorders. In many situations, the pet owner applies many different training styles, including punishment-based training and is inconsistent with cues and reinforcements. An analogy would be if a person were told, "Go sit in the chair" and every time he/she sat in the chair something "bad" occurred. Soon, when the person heard "Go sit in the chair" he/she would have a negative emotional response to the cue. An example of a pet owner inadvertently "poisoning" a cue would be when the pet owner cued "come" and the dog ran to the pet owner and was then punished (i.e., inappropriately punished for running away). In such situations, the behavior should be

retaught through shaping, capturing, or targeting and a new cue should then be attached to the behavior. As the new positive relationship builds between the pet owner and pet, the new cue can be utilized without association to the previous negative emotional response.

Stimulus control

When a response is under the influence of a cue and meets the following conditions in a training situation, it is considered to be under "stimulus control" and may then be taught to fluency. A behavior cannot become fluent until it is under stimulus control. The cue can now be generalized to new environments and conditions and stimulus control should be retested.

The four conditions for a behavior to be under stimulus control are given in Table 8.9.

Fluency

Fluency refers to the animal's ability to perform a cued behavior with speed and accuracy. Each criterion for fluency should be trained separately. When one criterion of fluency is being shaped, it is necessary to lower criteria for the other aspects of fluency. For instance, when shaping for speed or latency the precision of the behavior may deteriorate (Figure 8.19).

Precision – Precision is how a finished behavior should look. The trainer must first have an image of the precise behavior and then gradually shape the behavior toward those qualifications. For instance, a straight sit with the dog's shoulders by the handler's left knee, head looking straight ahead, and muzzle parallel to the ground.

Low latency – Low latency refers to the lag time between a cue being perceived and the time the animal begins the behavior. Low latency improves attentiveness and is a sign to the trainer that the cue is clearly understood. The animal often generalizes latency and later new cued behaviors will decrease in latency from the beginning. Low latency can be shaped by determining the current average length of latency and then shaping lower latency by C/T only shorter latency.

Speed – Speed of the behavior refers to how quickly the animal performs the behavior. The goal is to have the behavior performed as quickly as possible, with consideration for the animal's physical abilities. Determining the current average speed of the behavior and reinforcing for faster completions of the behavior will shape faster speed of the overall behavior.

Distraction – Distractions, such as the smell of other animals, are a constant occurrence in the environment and may not even be distinguishable to a human.

Table 8.9 Four conditions to test for stimulus control of a trained behavior.

Condition	Description	Example
C = B	Cue given and the desired behavior occurs	Verbal cue, "Sit" = Dog sits
C−B	No cue results in the behavior not being offered	During a training session the sit behavior is not offered without the cue, "sit".
ΔC ≠ B	A different cue is given and it does not result in performance of the behavior being tested	Handler cues "down". The dog does not sit.
C ≠ ΔB	Cue given does not result in a different behavior	Handler cues "sit". The dog does not lie down.

C= cue; B= behavior; C = no cue; B = no behavior; ΔC = different cue; ΔB another behavior; ≠ does not equal.

Figure 8.19 Fluency criterion: precision, latency, speed, distractions, duration, distance. Each criterion of fluency should be shaped separately.

The trainer should identify specific distractions and then introduce them in a controlled manner (sometimes requiring desensitization). The animal is taught to associate the presence of a distraction as an opportunity for reinforcement.

Duration – Duration is the length of time a behavior can be sustained. Duration is gradually shaped by systematically delaying the C/T for longer periods of time. It is important to vary the duration. For example, when working on an average duration of 10 s, some repetitions may take 3 s, others 12 s. When the criteria are varied, the learner is less likely to anticipate the end of a repetition.

Distance – This criterion of fluency usually applies to stationary behaviors such as sit-stay. Cued behavior occurs when the handler gives the cue while at a distance from the animal and the animal responds without approaching the handler. This can be the most difficult aspect of fluency for dogs that have only been trained near their handlers or who are overly attached to the handler and have separation issues. Often when cued from a distance, these animals will run to the handler before performing the behavior. It may be that proximity to the handler has become part of the cue.

Behavior chains

Behaviors chains are behaviors linked together by a sequence of cues. Each behavior has been previously trained, is under stimulus control and trained to the desired level of fluency before it is placed into the chain. Cues for the sequence may be environmental or delivered by the handler. Learned cues are reinforcing and are used to reinforce the previous behavior, therefore creating a behavior chain. Each behavior in the chain is reinforced by the next cue until the last behavior in the chain is marked and reinforced. Each cue in the sequence is both a marker for the current behavior and a cue to perform the next behavior.

Complex chains are commonly required for a sequence of behaviors to be performed. For example, "explosive" dogs must search, locate the bomb, sit, and bark. Service animals must target an item, retrieve the item, and deliver the item to a person's hand (Figure 8.20). Chains of behavior also occur naturally. The dog focuses attention toward a stimulus, the pet owner tightens the leash, the dog aggresses, and the stimulus leaves.

Behavior chains are often assembled by backchaining the behaviors. Each skill in the chain is first taught individually and the last behavior of the sequence is conditioned first. The situation in which the last behavior is performed becomes the discriminatory stimulus for the next behavior. The second to the last behavior is then conditioned, followed by the third to the last behavior, and so on.

Backchaining utilizes the concept that familiar is reinforcing. By adding the last behavior in the chain first, the second to the last behavior in the chain is reinforced by the familiarity of the next behavior. "Knowing what to do next" is very reinforcing to animals.

When the dog has learned the entire chain, the primary reinforcement would only be given at the end

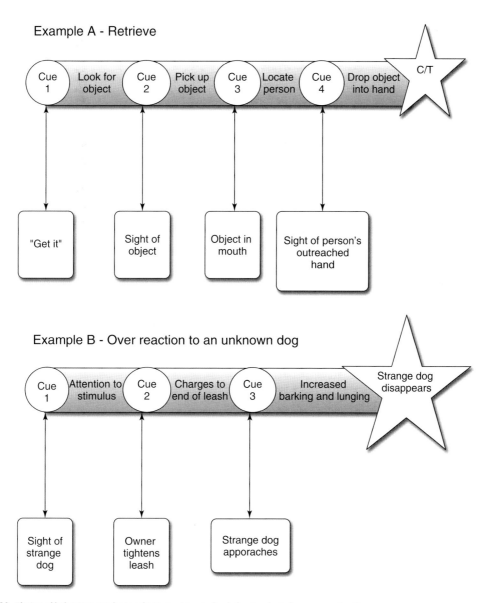

Figure 8.20 Chains of behaviors can be taught to create complex behaviors but also occur naturally.

of the sequence. To prevent breakdown of a chain, it is important to continue to practice components of the chain individually.

Behavior modification

It is the veterinarian's responsibility to diagnose a behavior disorder and prescribe the treatment plan, although input from the entire treatment team (veterinarian, veterinary technician, trainer, and pet owner) is critical for creating a practical and successful plan.

We will first discuss general theoretical concepts and general applications of each technique, followed by specific exercise examples. Commonly prescribed exercises that a veterinary technician may be asked to teach a pet owner are included along with practical applications for the general hospital setting.

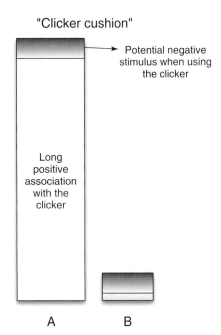

"Clicker cushion"

Potential negative
stimulus when using
the clicker

Long
positive
association
with the
clicker

A   B

Figure 8.21 (A) A long positive learning history with the clicker
should be in place before using the clicker in behavior modification. (B)Without this strong association the clicker may inadvertently become associated with or predictive of a negative stimulus
and become aversive.

Using a marker in the application of behavior modification

An event marker (clicker) is an invaluable tool in behavior modification. It can be used in behavior modification to simultaneously change the emotional response
of a stimulus or event, teach an alternate response, and
clearly mark subtle steps in a desensitization program.

It must be emphasized that before using the clicker for
behavior modification, the animal should have a long
and positive history with the clicker and associate a
positive emotional response to the clicker (Figure 8.21A
and B).

Without this strong association, the clicker may inadvertently become associated with or predictive of a negative stimulus and become aversive and will no longer
be a positive way to communicate with the animal.

A clicker must have a sufficiently positive association
before being used in the application of behavior modification.

- A clicker must have a sufficiently positive association
  before being used in the application of behavior
  modification.

A clicker will likely be ineffective if the animal is too
stressed (not taking treats) or if the animal is too stimulated to acknowledge the clicker. In both cases the stimulus should be decreased to a level at which the animal
is less emotional and can focus on training.

The clicker is a valuable tool to expedite behavior modification and should therefore be used appropriately and
accurately to keep its value and positive association.

Throughout this text we will use C/T (Click/Treat), CC
(Classical Counter Conditioning), RS (Response Substitution), and DS (Desensitization).

Generalization and behavior modification

As described in the section titled **Marker training techniques and skills**, generalization means to generalize a
behavior to different situations. With regard to behavior
modification, lack of generalization can be used to benefit the behavior modification process. When applying
any of the behavior modification techniques described,
the technician should attempt to create a situation that is
different from the past learning history. It is comparable
to trying to write on a blackboard that is already filled
with writing (previous learning history) versus starting
with a clean, unmarked blackboard. The goal should be
to create a fresh "clean" learning history whenever possible. For instance, if the animal has had a bad experience in an examination room, training should begin
in the waiting room. If a negative emotional experience
was created with one style of nail clippers, a different
style of nail clipper should be used in behavior modification.

Classical counter-conditioning

Whenever we interact with animals in training or otherwise, classical conditioning is taking place. The animal
will associate the situation and circumstances with a positive (pleasant), negative (unpleasant), or neutral (not
pleasant or unpleasant) experience. These associations
occur all of the time, whether we are conscious of them
or not.

Classical counter-conditioning is a technique used to
change a specific, previously created negative emotional
response to a stimulus to a positive emotional response.
In other words, a current situation that is frightening or
upsetting to the animal, for example, fear of large dogs,
is to be changed from the negative emotional response
of fear to tolerance or pleasantness; it is then taught an
alternate operant response (RS: see subsequent text).

When the animal's emotional state (i.e., fear) is
modified, the behaviors that often drive that emotion
(distance-increasing behaviors, over-reactivity) are also

decreased. This will make the application of RS and DS easier.

The positive emotional response should then quickly prompt subtle changes in the operant response of the animal. For example, if currently the sight of a large dog causes fear followed by the operant response of charging to the end of the leash to occur, when the driving emotion of fear is decreased, a change in the operant response of charging to the end of the leash also begins to be seen. Once the emotional state of the animal changes to a less reactive state, cognitive options and choices become more obvious to the animal. Charging at the end of the leash becomes slightly less intense, and/or the dog (the patient) is able to pause before reacting, which is the moment to incorporate RS by giving a cue for an alternate foundation behavior (sit, watch me, target, etc.). For example, operant behaviors like a slight pause before reacting or turning attention away from the stimulus will begin to occur. Those subtle changes can be reinforced with a clicker and therefore produce a change in the emotional response to the stimulus (if a strong positive association with the clicker is in place).

The previously fear-provoking stimulus becomes the cue for an alternate response and the animal begins to anticipate the introduction of the fear-provoking stimulus as an opportunity for reinforcement. The pet can then be cued by the presence of a stimulus to look at the pet owner (attention) or to target the pet owner's hand (note: hand targeting of the animals nose to the pet owner's hand should not be recommended initially for animals that are highly aroused and could redirect to the presented hand).

CC is also the easiest for owners to understand and apply. A pet owner can be told, "First, we will change how "Spot" feels about the situation (e.g., other dogs, veterinary clinic) so he will be less afraid. Once he is less fearful of _____ and even begins to LIKE _____, we will teach him other coping skills (rather than barking and lunging) that he can use in those situations."

As the improved emotional state should be seen relatively quickly if CC is applied properly, the pet owner is also reinforced therefore increasing pet owner's compliance and confidence.

Some mild issues may require only CC to change the behavior. For example: A rescued 4-year old sheltie, "Tag," nips at the pet owner's ankles (sometimes leaving marks) when the dishwasher makes a clicking sound. "Tag" is placed on leash (so the behavior cannot occur), a clicking sound is produced (it is helpful to find an easily producible clicking sound, other than the dishwasher, that triggers the response), immediately

followed by a treat or C/T. Beginning this process in a room or environment where the previous behavior of nipping ankles has NOT occurred (no past or little past learning history) will expedite the CC process.

Counter-conditioning is required when the criteria of DS to be successful cannot be met (see section titled **Systematic desensitization**). For example, if a sound intensity (e.g., thunder) and occurrence cannot be controlled or if the stimulus cannot be removed or avoided while the DS process occurs, CC will be key.

Classical counter-conditioning benefits:
– Is usually the easiest technique for pet owners to apply.
– Often a relatively quick emotional change is seen.
– Positive emotional response makes it easier for the pet to learn other coping skills (see section titled **Response substitution**)
– If the requirements for DS cannot be met, CC is critical.
– Makes the application of RS and DS easier or possibly not needed in mild cases.

Practical application of CC

To make a strong classical association the following should occur:
• The current stimulus that causes the negative emotional response must be at a low enough level that the patient does not react or reacts only very mildly.

   When applying CC, DS is usually also occurring because the stimulus (e.g., sight of large dog) is first introduced at a tolerable level. The stimulus should be noticed by the animal and acknowledged but not at a level at which the animal reacts strongly.

   Example: If the trigger is the presence of a large dog, the large dog must be far enough away so there is very little or no response from the patient.

   Example: If the stimulus is touching of the feet, touching a foot must occur at a level that does not elicit a significant response. Touch the foot = reinforcement. If touching of the foot is too high a stimulus, then touching the shoulder may need to occur first. This may mean touching of the shoulder is first marked (C/T).
• The presenting order must be correct.

   Example: large dog in sight, food is presented.

   Example: Touch the foot, give a treat, release the foot and the treat disappears.

   It is helpful to cue YOUR behavior first, for example, say "foot", technician touches foot, C/T. The cue "foot" begins to predict the foot touch (predictability is reinforcing, especially when working with fearful animals), food reinforcement, C/T.

- Outside environmental stimuli should be decreased; otherwise the animal may make an association with something in the environment other than large dogs.

   Example: Presentation of a basket muzzle containing food. Once the dog is enjoying eating out of the muzzle, put the muzzle away and ignore the dog for 5 min. NOTHING good happens to the dog until the muzzle reappears. The goal is for it to become very clear to the dog what is making the fun/food appear again (the muzzle).

- Once reactivity to the stimuli has decreased (large dog can be closer before there is any response from the patient or the intensity of the response is decreased) response substitution can be added.

   Example: Large dog in the distance, dog turns to pet owner anticipating a treat. Other responses, like looking at the pet owner and/or loose leashing walking away from stimulus, can now be incorporated into the treatment plan.

Fear and aggression cannot be reinforced or increased with food (Garcia and Koelling, 1966; Luescher and Martin, 2010; Martin, 2011).

- Fear and aggression cannot be reinforced or increased with food (Garcia and Koelling, 1966; Luescher and Martin, 2010; Martin, 2011).

More examples of CC:

- Counter-conditioning in a situation where a dog is fearful at the veterinary office

   Dog enters the veterinary clinic and receives treats.

- Counter-conditioning in a situation where a dog is fearful of thunderstorms.

   Thunderclap = peanut butter in mouth or other desired reinforcement.

- Counter-conditioning in a situation where a dog is aggressive to a new baby.

   When the baby is in the room, dog gets a stuffed food toy and attention. The toy is removed and the dog is ignored when the baby is not present.

- Counter-conditioning in the treatment of aggression between two dogs in the same household.

   Both dogs are tethered in the same room. Both dogs receive C/Ts while in the presence of the other dog.

- Counter-conditioning in a situation where a dog is fearful of a head halter

   Head halter is presented and the dog receives attention and treats. Head halter disappears and attention and treats cease until the head halter is produced again.

Response substitution

Response substitution is operant counter-conditioning. CC, as described earlier, is a classically associated response while RS is an operant-associated response.

The aim of RS is to replace undesirable behavior with desirable behavior in a given situation, the situation being the cue (discriminative stimulus) for the current undesirable behavior (Figure 8.22). Response substitution uses the situation in which undesirable behavior usually occurs (e.g., person at the door) as a discriminatory stimulus for the substituted desired behavior (i.e., go to a place - see section titled **Foundation behaviors**). The new, desired behavior should be incompatible with the undesirable behavior (i.e., go to crate or other place when person comes to the door is incompatible with charging the front door).

Response substitution is often used in conjunction with desensitization. For example, training relaxation or another foundation behavior, while gradually exposing a dog to increasingly intensive stimuli.

Response substitution can be explained to the pet owner as "teaching the pet a new, more appropriate coping skill" and explained further as, "Spot's current 'coping' skill when he is afraid is to charge the leash and try to make the scary thing go away, and it usually works, or so it seems to him. We are going to teach him a new coping skill and we will substitute that response for the current one. Over time, he will know that you will tell him what to do before he becomes upset and therefore the unpredictability of the situation will lessen and he will become calm. It will also help you because you will also know what to do and also become calm. It is response substitution for you too!"

If the dog's current "coping skill" is charging at the front door to "make people go away" the dog is taught an alternate coping skill of going to a bed or "place" for a reward when the doorbell rings. Both CC (stranger = food) and RS (go to a bed) occur simultaneously.

When the animal performs an unwanted behavior he should be distracted before cuing the alternate behavior to prevent chaining or linking of the unwanted behavior to the substituted behavior. For example, a dog barks at the window, the owner claps his hands to interrupt the behavior (not to frighten or scare the dog); dog turns attention toward pet owner, cue "go to your bed" is given; dog is rewarded for going to his bed. Interrupting the behavior with a hand clap prevents the behavior chain of the dog barking at window and then going to its bed for a reward.

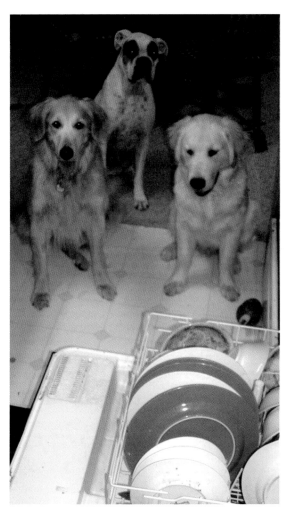

Figure 8.22 These dogs are cued to "sit" while the dishwasher is being loaded and then reinforced by getting to investigate the dishwasher.

RS is usually easier and more smoothly applied after some classical CC has already occurred.

> • RS is usually easier and more smoothly applied after some classical CC has already occurred.

It is important for owners to understand that the preferred behavior must be trained before attempting to use it in the desired situation. For example, it is not appropriate and much more difficult to begin initial training to sit to greet people the moment the dog is jumping on a visitor. Create calm training situations; then generalize the

situations before attempting to apply the newly trained behavior in a specifically needed situation (visitor at the door).

RS benefits:
– Gives the animal an "alternate coping skill" when unsure in a situation.
– The pet owner begins to focus on desired behavior rather than the undesired behavior.
– Response substitution also gives the pet owner an "alternate coping skill." For example, instead of tightening the leash in anticipation of barking and lunging, asking the dog to target away from the stimulus utilizing a fast-paced loose leash walking with turns and sits to increase distance from the stimulus.

Practical application of RS

• Choose an alternate and appropriate behavior to train that will not allow the unwanted behavior to occur.
   Shape or capture the behavior. Place it on a cue and train to fluency.
• Begin applying the new on cue and fluent behavior in a quiet environment. Training should be done in a situation unrelated to one in which the unwanted behavior occurs. Possibly begin "go to your bed" in a room away from the front door. Once the behavior has been learned in that situation, move "the bed" closer to the goal area (e.g., 20 feet from the front door).
• Once the dog is consistently responding fluently to the cue in a quiet environment, presentation of the stimulus that causes the unwanted behavior at a low intensity can be introduced. For example, if the dog barks every time someone comes to the door, have a friend walk up to the front door, and stand quietly without knocking. Before the dog reacts to the person, cue the dog to go to his bed. When he goes to his bed, immediately reward him. Often a remote reinforcement tool, like the Treat and Train (www.premier.com) is beneficial.
• Gradually increase the intensity of the eliciting stimulus – have people approach the door, ring the bell, and enter. If the dog fails to perform the behavior at any stage, return to the previous level and concentrate on training at the level of stimulus intensity until the dog is responding correctly, every time, before progressing to the next stage.
• Once training and behavior modification have begun, it is important to manage situations to prevent the dog from continuing to practice the undesirable behavior. Training will progress much more quickly if the dog's opportunity to perform the unwanted behavior is eliminated. When someone comes to your door unexpectedly, prevent the dog from barking

at the door by confining the dog in a room or crate when the guest first arrives. Bring the dog back out into the living area once everyone is settled.

More examples of RS:

Ask the pet owner what behavior he/she wants the dog to do: Instead of _____ I would like him to _____

– Instead of jumping on people I would like him to sit for greetings.
– Instead of begging at the table I would like him to go to his bed when we eat.
– Instead of jumping at the front door when the doorbell rings I would like him to go to his crate when he hears the doorbell.

Systematic desensitization

This is a technique used to reduce or eliminate a response (e.g., fear or aggression) to a stimulus (e.g., loud noise, strangers) through gradual and systematic exposure. The animal is trained to quiescence and relaxation before beginning the DS process. The stimulus is then introduced at a low intensity (i.e., recording of a noise at low intensity, stranger from a distance) and the animal is rewarded (CC) for relaxed behavior or performing an alternate behavior (RS). Once the animal has habituated to the stimulus at a low intensity, the intensity is systematically and gradually increased, and the procedure repeated.

Specific aspects of the stimulus are systematically added without causing a full or intense reaction in the animal.

This aspect of DS is often the most difficult because identifying the specific aspects of the stimulus and then placing them into a systematic hierarchy must be determined and extrapolated from watching the animal's body language and getting the pet owner's observations and input from past experiences.

Once the characteristics of the stimulus can be determined and are placed into a DS hierarchy, variables are added one at a time, decreasing one variable as another is added.

DS can be explained to pet owners by instructing them: "We are going to figure out, to the best of our ability, what characteristics of strangers bother "Spot" the most. Then we are going to create a plan to introduce those aspects gradually and one at a time."

Requirements for the systematic desensitization program

To utilize DS properly the following must occur:
• Identify the cause of the fear.
• Reproduce the cause of the fear.

• Identify a starting point where the animal is not afraid (relaxed and still taking treats).
• Control the intensity of the fear-provoking stimulus.
• Control exposure to the fear-provoking stimulus (it does not occur spontaneously or randomly).

If the above criteria cannot be met, DS cannot be effectively applied and behavior modification should focus around CC and RS. As other aspects of the treatment plan are successfully put into place, DS can be reconsidered (if still needed) at the follow-up appointment.

Creation of a systematic desensitization plan

The goal of DS is to increase tolerance to a stimulus. This is comparable to building a muscle; the patient may be slightly uncomfortable at times but learns that it can tolerate the stimulus at that specific level, even if slightly uncomfortable. At the next application of DS, the patient learns to tolerate a bit more as its tolerance "muscle" grows in size.

1. Identify characteristics and variables of the stimulus that influence the animal's anxiety level and response. This can increase your insight into the causes of the anxiety and make it easier to create an accurate anxiety hierarchy.

   Examples of possible variables:
   ◦ Distance away from the stimulus.
   ◦ Sound/loudness of the stimulus.
   ◦ Speed/movement of the stimulus.
   ◦ Specific characteristic of the stimulus.

   Example: "Spot" was diagnosed with fear-induced aggression toward unfamiliar men.

   Discuss with the pet owner the possible characteristics of unfamiliar men and ask the pet owner to rank the characteristics on a scale of 1–10, with 10 being a strong reaction.

2. Prioritize the characteristics into a graded (on a scale of 1–10, for example) anxiety hierarchy, and then break down those characteristics into manageable components. Place the characteristics that bother the animal the most at the end of the list.

   The anxiety hierarchy is a graded list of the situations related to the fear-provoking stimulus.

   Constructing an accurate anxiety hierarchy is very important as it provides the framework for approaching the problem. To create an accurate hierarchy, thought and discussion with the pet owner are critical.

   First analyze the problem with the pet owner into situational components. Ask the pet owner, "What situation is the most difficult for 'Spot'"? Constructing the anxiety hierarchy has its own therapeutic value by helping the pet owner analyze the pet's specific fears into an objective format, thereby increasing understanding of the problem and the specific triggers of that fear.

(a) Ask the pet owner to describe a situation in which "Spot" is least likely to respond aggressively to the stimulus (i.e., least scary), and to describe the worst case scenario the behavior would occur in (the most "scary").

For example, "Spot" would not react to a familiar, light skinned, nonbearded man in shorts and a shirt at a distance. "Spot" would be most upset by a bearded, dark skinned man, wearing a dark coat and carrying an umbrella, at the front door in the evening.

Grade the characteristics on a scale of 1–10 (10 being the most difficult or upsetting) and place the items in order from the least upsetting to the most upsetting by asking the pet owner to think about each situation and rate the difficulty of that situation for the pet.

Begin with items so mild that they are practically nonfrightening. The smaller the steps, the faster the DS process goes. Raising a characteristic too quickly or adding multiple characteristics at once without decreasing other characteristics will cause the problem to worsen (actually sensitizing rather than desensitizing).

This ranked list of anxiety-evoking items constitutes the hierarchy that you will use in your treatment. Modifications, additions, combining of items, and further breaking down of items on the hierarchy may be made at any time during the desensitization therapy (Table 8.10).

3. Determine a nonstressful starting point

Determine what contexts or interactions the animal can tolerate without a stress reaction. A good barometer that a characteristic has been increased too quickly is that the dog suddenly stops taking treats or starts roughly grabbing at the treat. Subtle body language signals, such as conflict and displacement behaviors (see Chapter 2), may also indicate the dog is starting to reach his threshold of tolerance for the situation. If a nonstressful starting point cannot be determined, DS cannot be properly applied and a nonstressful starting point may need to be created, using drug desensitization first.

4. Create "practice" situations

(a) Each characteristic should be increased individually, not simultaneously.

(b) As one characteristic is intensified, another characteristic may need to be temporarily lessened. For example, the patient may have learned to tolerate a

Table 8.10 Spot's anxiety hierarchy for fear of men.

Characteristic of stimulus	Anxiety rating
Women	2
Carrying an object (book)	2
Dark clothing	6
Volume of voice	7
Dark skin tone	8
Men with facial hair	9
Close proximity (3 feet)	10

In this DS plan for "Spots" fear aggression toward men, the first stimulus to be incorporated would be a woman at a distance. Other variables are added according to the anxiety hierarchy without adding multiple variables at the same time.

stationary man in close proximity but when introducing a moving man, the distance from the patient should be increased.

(c) The intensity of each characteristic should be increased gradually – always staying below the arousal threshold (see Figure 8.29).

(d) Progression to the next level of intensity should be accomplished without eliciting undesirable behavior (i.e., a look at the stimulus should be reinforced but a hard, tense stare is an indication the level has been increased too quickly).

(e) Clicker training can be a very valuable tool in the desensitization process to influence the emotional response of the animal.

A marker or clicker is extremely valuable in the desensitization process because it is possible to pinpoint the exact reinforceable moment, for example, the relaxation of a shoulder during desensitization of restraint. Probably the most important use of the clicker in behavior modification is in changing the animal's motivation before it becomes distressed. It is possible to influence the animal's reaction to the stimulus by clicking before it reaches its arousal threshold or by clicking just as it begins to reach the arousal threshold. In other words, click before the aggressive response occurs – the moment before it makes the decision to react can swing the animal away from previously learned behaviors (charging at the end of the leash, aggressing during restraint). At that point, the stimulus should not be increased but maintained at that level until the animal relaxes and then desensitization may continue.

Helpful hints:

– The smaller the steps, the faster the progress made.
– DS always "works" when applied properly. If progress is not being made, likely multiple variables are being

added simultaneously, variables are being raised too quickly, the characteristics of the stimulus were not prioritized properly, or a nonstressful starting point was not determined.

- Think about what you are about to do and decrease it by 50%.
- Implementing systematic desensitization inconsistently or too rapidly can cause the problem to worsen.

Conclusion

A combination of the behavior modification techniques is almost always occurring simultaneously but it is important for the veterinary technician to be able to tease aspects of the those techniques out of the treatment plan to properly understand and then be able to explain them to the pet owner.

For instance, a dog that has had an adverse emotional response to a nail trim in the past can quickly be taught to target its paw to a hand (RS) while being clicked and treated (CC), therefore changing the emotional response of the event (having the feet touched). The paw is gradually held for longer lengths of time in the hand. When pressure on the paw is added, the length of time the paw is held is decreased (DS).

Drug desensitization

The goal of drug desensitization is to address the suspected pathologic dysfunction of the neurotransmitter system leading to or worsening the problem behavior or behavior disorder.

Antianxiety drugs (not sedatives) are administered to the animal at a high enough level to prevent the fearful reaction to the stimuli. The intensity of the stimuli may stay the same, but there is a gradual reduction of the drug over time so that the animal becomes gradually more aware of the frightening stimuli.

Drug desensitization is used when the intensity of the stimulus cannot be controlled, or when there are too many frightening stimuli to use systematic desensitization.

Additionally, it can help to make behavior modification easier to apply, giving the owner a starting point for desensitization, and improving compliance and treatment success (see Chapter 9).

Systematic desensitization and drug desensitization may be used simultaneously.

Other
Interruption of behavior

Interrupting behavior is **not** meant to teach a specific behavior or to punish a behavior but is used to temporarily stop a behavior so an alternative cue can be given. If a behavior is not disrupted before giving another cue, the behaviors may be inadvertently chained together (i.e., stimulus outside becomes cue to bark and the barking becomes the cue to go to the mat). If behavior is interrupted, it is less likely behaviors will be chained.

Interruptions could include clapping hands, patting your leg, or picking up a dragline to get the dog's attention. Ideally the interruption should not elicit fear or panic in the animal. It should be performed in a nonconfrontational manner and be just enough to get the pet's attention and interrupt the thought process so another cue for an alternative behavior can be given.

Cease punishment

Pet owners should also stop all retrospective scolding or physical punishment. Punishment is likely to increase or cause fear. Fear produces unpredictable side effects and rarely the desired effects. Punishment is comparable to a bomb going off; unpredictable and unfocused damage is caused with collateral damage occurring in the process. Especially pet owner-applied punishment (i.e., scolding, physical punishment, dominance roles) is detrimental and counter-productive to any treatment plan.

As it is nearly impossible for pet owners to apply punishment correctly, such punishment becomes unpredictable, increasing stress. Instead of using punishment, pet owners should be taught to gently interrupt behavior and use response substitution to cue another behavior.

Remote punishment

Remote punishment involves the application of an aversive stimulus without the pet owner being present.

As discussed previously, punishment should not be associated with the pet owner (or another person or stimulus) and must occur when the behavior occurs and must occur every time the behavior occurs. The remote punishment should not be operated by the pet owner but instead only be activated by the pet's behavior (i.e., cans falling off counter when the pet investigates the counter).

Side effects for remote punishment remain the same as with other punishment. Inadvertent associations can be made, including fear of sounds or fear of entering the space where the punishment occurred.

The primary advantage of remote punishment is that it is less likely the pet owner will be associated with the punishment. Therefore, the pet should learn to cease the behavior even when the pet owner is absent (Landsberg *et al.*, 2013).

Euthanasia or rehoming

Euthanasia may be a responsible and appropriate decision when the quality of life for the pet, the pet owner, or other pets in the home is poor, or when animals and people are at risk for serious emotional and physical harm, and treatment is not a viable option. It is a complex decision that the veterinarian will make along with the pet owner after obtaining an extensive history and possible referral to a veterinary behavior specialist.

The veterinarian may recommend rehoming as an option if the pet's behavior problem or disorder is not likely to worsen in a new home or if the environment in the new home can be controlled in such a way that triggers are no longer an issue (i.e., a home without other pets or a home with no children).

If the pet owner is not at peace with the decision, then the owner should be given the option of a behavior consultation with a veterinary behaviorist.

Grief counseling of client

Chapter 5 detailed grief counseling to pet owners. Grief counseling is a primary responsibility of the veterinary technician. Grief will occur whether the pet owner is euthanizing or rehoming the pet. Grief is a process and veterinary technicians should assist the pet owner through the process, being aware of grief that is not progressing and be able to refer the pet owner to an appropriate mental health professional when needed.

The practical applications of behavior modification

Foundation behaviors

Foundation behaviors are trained behaviors that are likely to be required to successfully apply the prescribed behavior modification techniques. These behaviors and skills are useful to teach any animal (with species modifications) and should be included in all problem prevention plans (i.e., puppy classes)

Targeting

Targeting is a very useful behavior tool and can be used in many applications of behavior modification. How to shape targeting has been discussed earlier in this chapter.

Target to hand

Targeting to the handler's hand can be cued when a potential problem stimulus (i.e., unknown animal or person) is seen by the handler and used as a prompt to turn the dog away from the stimulus before it can react (emergency u-turn). Once turned, fast-paced loose leash walking with numerous sits and turns can be added to increase the distance from the stimulus. A hand target should not be used when the patient is overly aroused or has a history of redirecting bites.

> • A hand target should not be used when the patient is overly aroused or has a history of redirecting bites.

Targeting to a hand is also useful for teaching loose leash walking. The hand can be presented as a prompt to help show the dog the desired position of walking beside a person.

Hand target recall

Very frequently the pet owner's recall cue has been "poisoned" and associated with a negative emotional event. This can happen inadvertently. For example, a dog that shows signs of separation anxiety may begin to associate being called in from outside with the owner's departure. The owner lets the dog outside to eliminate just before leaving the home. The dog is called inside and then the owner leaves.

In instances where the recall cue has been "poisoned," the behavior must be retaught using a new cue. If targeting has a strong positive emotional response, it can be used to prompt the recall behavior. Later, should the handler so desire, the cue for the recall can be changed to a different cue, such as a whistle or novel verbal cue.

Attention

Attention is really another targeting skill, targeting of the eyes to the handler. Eye contact can be captured and shaped. The behavior of making eye contact may need to first be desensitized if in the past eye contact was discouraged or if the animal is not comfortable with looking directly at the owner. Initially, any eye contact is C/T. Once it is predictable it can be placed on cue. Distractions and duration can be added systematically to the behavior.

Offered eye contact (without a cue from the pet owner) to the owner on walks and during training is a behavior that should be highly reinforced throughout the life of the dog. When working with a dog that has over-reactivity to stimuli, the owner should be coached to mark and reinforce offered eye contact in a variety of contexts. The dog quickly learns offering calm attention to his owner results in good things. A verbal cue, such as "Eyes" or "Watch," should also be taught because this can be beneficial when playing a game of opposites; "Look" and "Watch" (see subsequent text).

Game of opposites: "look" and "watch"

Just as people notice changes in the environment, so do dogs. It is natural for all animals to notice a sudden change in the environment. This awareness is a natural survival mechanism and it keeps us safe. We notice it, assess the threat, and then usually recognize the stimulus as nothing to worry about. For example, you are sitting in a coffee shop and you see a person walk in the front door, you assess the situation and as long as the person appears to be of no threat, you return to your conversation. Some dogs are anxious and unsure about certain stimuli in the environment and assess what we would consider nonthreatening stimuli as a threat. Initially expecting a dog to just ignore and look away from such stimuli is impractical and perhaps impossible for the dog.

Teaching a game of opposites, "look" and "watch", can help change the dog's emotional response to stimuli. These cues will initially be taught in a nondistracting environment using capturing and shaping and should not be associated with the presence of triggers during the early stages of training. They are a pair off opposite behaviors. "look" will be used to mean look at something away from the handler and "watch" will mean look at the handler. A directional cue (finger point) may be useful with "look" in order to indicate what direction the dog is to look. *Control Unleashed* by Leslie McDevitt is a great resource for teaching the skills and adding in distractions systematically.

Initially the handler will use the cues "look" and "watch" in a variety of contexts within the house and yard and with inanimate objects such as a toy or chair. Once the dog has learned the cues and CC to the fear-provoking stimulus has already occurred on walks, the owner can ping pong back and forth between "look" and "watch" (and other known cues) in the context of previous triggers.

Default looking at stimuli and offered eye contact should still be rewarded as well but eventually they will be placed on a variable ratio of reinforcement.

Ultimately, if the owner is consistent with marking and rewarding for the sight of triggers, two things will start to happen. First, the dog will begin to anticipate earning a C/T for the presence or sound of a trigger and will begin to anticipate the stimuli as an opportunity for reinforcement. This moment often occurs when the click is delayed slightly. The dog looks at the stimulus and then turns toward the pet owner, curious as to why it was not clicked for seeing the stimulus. This turning away from the stimulus should be highly rewarded. The second side effect is that the dog will start to look for triggers not because he is worried or concerned, but because it has become a game; the motivation of the behavior has changed. This change in the emotional response will also be evident in the body language of the dog.

Basic cued behaviors – sit, down, come, loose leash walking

Cued behaviors are critical for applying and building on any behavior modification plan. When a patient has no available on-cue behaviors such as sit or down, the behavior technician must begin by teaching a cued behavior that can be used in later aspects of the treatment plan (i.e., RS and DS).

The ability to successfully cue a behavior that produces a reliable response will be necessary any time the pet owner needs to assist the pet when it is unsure what to do or before it reacts to a stimulus. Without cued behaviors it is difficult to communicate to the animal an alternative method for getting out of a situation.

For example, a frightening stimulus is approaching in the distance, the pet owner can cue other behaviors like "look" or "watch" and then cue fast-paced walking, while increasing distance from the stimulus with quick turns and sits (or a combination of behaviors). Initially the steady flow of information is a distraction from the frightening stimulus. Later, as the dog's anxiety decreases, the learning history becomes, "I can do this and get reinforced AND the scary things weren't so scary after all."

Practice tip: These cues and fast-paced walking should be practiced often without any triggers present. Otherwise the owners change in pace and quick cues will become a predictor of stimuli in the environment.

The veterinary technician often teaches the pet owner how to train the basic cued behaviors of targeting, watch, look, come, sit, down, and loose leash walking. Techniques for capturing and shaping, adding a cue and basic fluency should be covered and written materials should be provided for the owner to refer to. Cued behaviors will be used during CRR (cue → response → reward) interactions, RS, DS, and to guide the pet owner in focusing on what behavior he/she wants the pet to DO rather than undesirable behavior.

Only the behaviors that are required to apply the treatment plan should be taught at the initial consultation to keep from overwhelming the pet owner. Later, the veterinarian and veterinary technician should refer the pet owner to the veterinary hospital's qualified trainer for further training.

Before training foundation behaviors, the veterinary technician should determine by discussion with the pet owner and by assessing the animal's body language if a previous cue for any of these behaviors has been "poisoned" (see cueing). If so, a different type of cue should be used to reteach the behavior.

Place – go to a specific location

Teaching a dog to go to a specific location is useful as a preventive tool as discussed in Chapter 7 but settle on a mat will also be utilized during many behavior modification exercises. It should be noted that teaching an animal to go to a "place" is not the same as teaching relaxation, although "place" is frequently used in the shaping of relaxation (see below). Specifically, go to a place might be used in a desensitization program with a dog that displays signs of territorial aggression toward strangers at the front door.

NOTE: It is possible to teach the dog to go to a small piece of cloth on the floor. Once the "place" cue is reliable the cloth can be made smaller and smaller. Eventually it will be possible to carry a very small piece of cloth with you so a "place" is readily available when you travel with your dog.

Example:
- Shaping "place"
- Place a towel or mat on the floor as a target.
- Mark the dog for looking or turning its head toward the mat; toss the treat toward the mat.
- Mark the dog for any movement toward the mat; toss the treat past the mat.
- Mark as the dog turns from picking up the treat and turns toward the mat; toss the treat onto the mat.
- Mark for 2 ft on the mat, toss the treat off the mat.
- Mark for 3 or 4 ft on the mat, toss the treat off the mat.
- Once the dog is readily going to the mat cue a "down" (taught in a previous session), mark and toss the treat off the mat.
- Fade out the verbal cue "down" by waiting for the dog to offer the behavior before the C/T.
- Once the dog is readily offering the behavior of going to the mat and lying down, the cue "place" can be added.
- Fluency of the "down" on the mat can be gradually shaped by working on distractions, duration, and distance.

Applications of behavior modification

The following exercises are examples of behavior modification exercises that may be included in a prescribed treatment plan. The discussed techniques are only examples of how the behavior modification exercises could be applied. The veterinary technician may need to modify the exercises for each patient and situation and communicate any significant modifications to the veterinarian. Significant changes may indicate a change in the treatment plan is required (adding medications, etc.).

As the patient and pet owner progress through treatment, the techniques may be modified at follow-up appointments. All aspects of CC/RS/DS should be reviewed before applying these techniques.

CC/RS/DS behavior at the door

Foundation skills needed: sit or down, go to a mat or other location

Possible Training Tools needed: A remote reward system is very helpful for reinforcing at a distance from the door.

A head halter may be required for dogs that react very quickly and intensely at the door so the dog can be efficiently prompted and reinforced for another behavior.

Avoid practicing unwanted behavior with visitors during the treatment period. The following exercise should be controlled with the dog on leash and collar for safety. Alternatively, a tether or baby gate may prevent escapes from the home.

1. If the dog has been trained to go to a mat previously, the mat cue can be used at the door to expedite training. First, CC of the sound of the doorbell may be required. Doorbell = Treat. As the doorbell sound begins to mean treats, the sound of the doorbell can be transferred as the cue "go to your mat". Using a prerecorded doorbell that can easily be controlled, for instance on a smart phone, can be very helpful. Sound of doorbell → cue "go to your mat" → C/T

2. Teach the dog to sit on his mat at the door for a food treat without any visitors at the door. It may also be beneficial to do practice sessions at a back door where there has been less learning history.

3. Incorporate training sessions at the door. With the dog sitting at the door, jiggle the door knob or crack the door, and reward the dog for remaining seated. If the dog leaves the mat do not respond or reprimand him. With the next repetition, decrease the stimulus; touch or reach for the door handle rather than jiggling it.

4. Eventually, you should be able to open and close the door without visitors there and reward the dog for

sitting. Safety factors (dog leashed or behind a baby gate) should be in place to prevent escaping out the door.

5. Repeat the above, but add a light knock by the handler before you open and close the door.
6. Gradually, you can increase the intensity of the knock without the dog breaking the sit. This is adding more distraction to the training.
7. Add the doorbell sound back into the training and transfer as the cue for "go to your mat."
8. Next, start with someone familiar to the dog at a distance (20 ft) from the door. Repeat steps 3–7. When you open the door acknowledge the person's presence. Say "Hello," the visitor should respond accordingly. Close the door and reward the dog for staying on the mat.
9. Gradually the familiar person's distance to the door may be reduced. Start with the person about 20 ft away, and gradually reduce the distance to 19 ft, 18 ft, and so on while repeating the above exercise.
10. Eventually, the person should be standing 6 ft away from the door while the dog maintains the sit position. The owner and the familiar "visitor" should reward the dog for sitting by tossing a food treat to him.
11. Once the dog is comfortable and successful with several familiar people, repeat the above exercise with less familiar people.

CC/RS/DS of muzzle or head halter

Training a dog to wear a basket muzzle or head halter utilizes the same techniques and will be used interchangeably in the following text.

A pet owner may be instructed to desensitize his/her dog to wearing a muzzle or head halter if the dog has a well-established bite history, or if the owner is in doubt of his/her ability to manipulate the environment so that the dog can remain below his threshold consistently.

A basket muzzle can be used to reduce the risk of injury. A head halter can be used to redirect a dog that is reactive to a stimulus. The basket muzzle and head halter are not a treatment for aggressive behavior because they do not change the underlying motivation. They are used as a management and safety tool while implementing behavior modification. They serve to minimize injury if an incident should occur and can be used as a step in many DS processes. For example, when the dog has been DS to a stimulus while behind a gate but the next step of the DS plan requires the dog to be able to move freely, having a basket muzzle on the dog allows for increased safety. It is comparable to the dog wearing a "moving" gate. Once the dog is successful

using a basket muzzle in a specific situation, the next step could be using a head halter in the same situation. Steps to classical (counter) condition and desensitize the dog to a basket muzzle or head halter:

1. Short training sessions that last 5 min or less are best.
2. Take the basket muzzle out and put cheese or peanut butter inside the basket so the dog is prompted to reach his nose in to lick the treat out. This is classical conditioning.
3. Lower the muzzle down to your side and allow the dog to approach and stick his nose in on his own. Keep your hand still and allow the dog to approach. NEVER reach forward with the muzzle (or head halter nose loop); instead let the dog push his nose into the muzzle. Reaching forward toward the dog is likely to make the dog back away.
4. If the dog is wary and will not approach the muzzle, place the muzzle on the floor and step on the strap so he cannot pick it up and run away with it. Begin targeting the muzzle on the floor, C/T for any interaction. Once interacting with the muzzle has become an opportunity for reinforcement, begin again at step 3.
5. The muzzle or head halter should disappear suddenly along with all attention and interaction. Ignore the dog for 1 min. Bring the muzzle/head halter out; the dog should become excited when he sees the basket muzzle or head halter, indicating CC has occurred.
6. After the dog is showing excitement when you get the muzzle out and readily pushing his nose in the muzzle to eat the treats, you may start placing the strap around the back of his head.
7. An alternate step is to mark and reward the dog for putting his nose in the muzzle or head halter nose loop as an offered behavior (without food to prompt him). This step can be incorporated once the classical conditioning component has occurred.
8. Once you have attached the muzzle, you will need to adjust it so it fits well and the dog is not able to pull it off.
9. After attaching the neck strap, it is important to give the dog treats through the muzzle. Canned cheese is ideal for this.
10. The muzzle and head halter should be incorporated into a variety of activities to prevent them from becoming a predictor of potential stressful situations. If the muzzle or head halter are only used when visitors come to the home or the dog goes to the veterinarian, the positive association will be diminished.

CC/RS/DS to a person, animal, or other stimulus

The requirements to apply behavior modification are the same regardless of the stimulus (review CC, RS, DS). For this example, we will use presence of a stranger as the stimulus.

Foundation skills: watch, look, target, sit or down, go to a mat, relaxation, fast-paced heeling, and emergency U-turns.

Possible training tools needed: Clicker and treats, a well-fitted collar or harness, and a 4 to 6-ft leash, possibly a head halter and/or basket muzzle.

Note: Each step will involve several repetitions. With the reset for another repetition, start again at the same starting point. With successive repetitions the ending point will be gradually closer to the goal behavior. Varying the difficulty level is beneficial to incorporate some very easy repetitions. Thus, the exercise does not seem to always be getting more and more difficult.

1. Begin classical counter conditioning and response substitution (operant counter conditioning) to the presence of the person at a distance. If a nonstressful starting point from the stimulus cannot be found, a calming cap may be required and/or medications may be needed. Give small but highly desirable food treats (or other high level reinforcement) while the stimulus is in view. Start with the least threatening stimulus (perhaps a woman if the dog is more reactive to men). The dog should be below a level of reactivity. He may orient toward the stimulus but should readily take treats and be able to look away from the stimulus. Remove the stimulus and ignore the dog for a minute. When the stimulus reappears, look for signs of less attentiveness toward the stimulus and either C/T for looking at the stimulus or for turning attention back to the handler (operant offered behaviors).

2. Response substitution (operant counter conditioning): Add cues "look" (look at the stimulus) and "watch" (attention toward pet owner) which have been taught previously. Offered (uncued) looks and watches should also continue to be reinforced.

3. With the stimulus present but stationary, utilize desensitization and response substitution. This step may be explained to the owner with the analogy – "If you were afraid of spiders would it be easier for you to approach the spider or have the spider approach you?" It is usually less stressful to approach the stimulus then to have the stimulus approach you. Gradually decrease the dog's distance from the stimulus while performing fast-paced walking, turns, look, watch, and sit. Simultaneously reward the dog with high-value reinforcements (classical counter-conditioning) frequently after each behavior (Figure 8.23).

4. Once the dog is comfortable working around the stationary person from a distance of 8-10 feet, increase the distance from the stimulus and now incorporate some slow movement by the stimulus. The (distraction) person still stays in place but shifts his/her weight or walks in place, while the dog works closer to him/her. After success at this step with the dog remaining calm, non-reactive, and able to easily respond to known cues at a distance of 8-10 feet, progress to step 5.

5. This step incorporates the stimulus and the dog/handler simultaneously walking parallel with each other and at a distance that the dog is relaxed. Gradually the distance from each other can be reduced but it should be done at a pace that allows the dog to remain calm. Each time the handler cues the dog to perform a stationary behavior, the distraction person should also slow down or stop moving.

6. Variations of the same exercises, adding in other stimuli, may be repeated as needed, before progressing to the final step.

7. The final step is when the patient remains stationary with the handler and the stimulus gradually approaches. This usually is much more difficult for the dog.

Have the patient in a sit or down position by the pet owner and directly facing the stimulus. Sit is usually easier at this point but if the down position is associated with previously taught relaxation it may be the behavior of choice. Ideally, relaxation has been previously taught and can then be used during this step. The distraction person or stimulus is at a nonstressful starting point.

a. The handler cues "sit" which cues the distraction person to begin slowly walking in a zig zag (parallel to the dog and gradually decrease the distance) pattern toward the patient. At any point if the dog glances toward the stimulus, C/T. C/T any attention toward the handler and for responding to the look and watch cues. A high rate of reinforcement is ideal. While the dog is still relaxed but may be showing subtle indicators of increased distraction, for example, he is slower to respond to cues or is having difficulty looking away from the stimulus, the handler will cue the dog to sit again (even if he is still sitting) and reward him. This is also the cue for the distraction person to stop walking, pause briefly, and then walk away and return to the original starting point. This reset acts as a functional reward for the dog and is a

CHAPTER 8

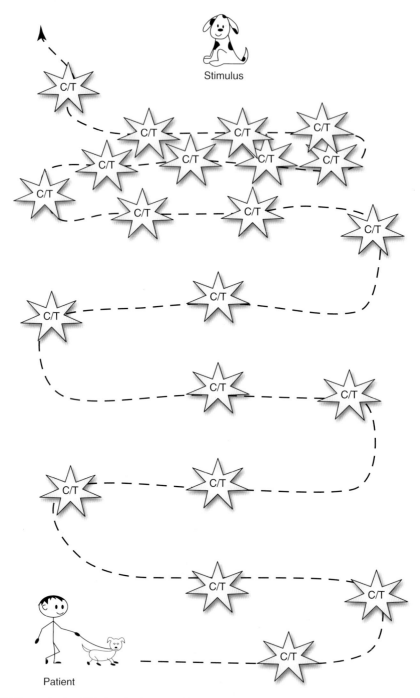

Figure 8.23 DS/CC/RS to a stimulus: With the stimulus present but stationary, utilize DS, CC and RS to the stimulus. Gradually decrease the dogs distance from the stimulus while performing fast paced walking, turns, look, watch, and sit and C/Ting at each response. A higher rate of reinforcement may be required as the distance to the stimulus is decreased.

form of negative reinforcement; the intensity of the stimulus is decreased (social pressure is removed). Ideally this reset should happen before the dog begins to show conflict or displacement behaviors, such as prolonged staring, taking treats roughly, or trying to avoid the stimulus. It is beneficial to increase and then decrease the criteria (distance the stimulus approaches) with repetitions on this exercise rather than making each repetition more difficult.

b. Incorporate the stimulus walking in a curved path toward the patient, then walking at an angle, and finally straight toward the patient. Add other variables but always decrease one characteristic before adding another characteristic (see section titled **Systematic desensitization**) (Figure 8.24).

Implementation tip: Alternate between these exercises during the training session. Going back to easier versions (while working on Step 7a take a break and go back to Step 3 for a few repetitions) may help to rejuvenate the DS process and allow for faster progress.

CC/RS/DS thunderstorms/sounds

Foundation skills: relaxation and other foundation behaviors

Possible training tools needed: clicker and treats, mat, sound CD

Goals: This exercise has two goals. The first is to promote relaxation and CC to the sounds that have previously induced fear or anxiety. The second is to teach the animal a "safe" place to go when it hears these sounds. For thunderstorm anxiety, it is beneficial for the safe place to be located in an interior room, such as a walk-in closet that is void of windows (decreasing lightening) where the sound of thunder is muffled (Figure 8.25).

1. Refer to training relaxation. The mat that cues relaxation and has a previously positive association should be used. Before a training session a DS hierarchy must be created. Determine what sounds the dog reacts to and at what volume levels before beginning the process.

2. Begin the training session with no sound. During the training session, play a recording of thunderstorms/sounds at a volume that do not induce fear. Always begin a new training session at the lowest volume. Cue for relaxation or if too difficult, cue for an alternate response. Just as the "look" cue was taught as a game for the animal, a "listen" cue can also be taught, thus changing the emotional response associated with the sound.

3. Add the sound at a level the dog notices but does not otherwise react. C/T (or just toss a treat) at the

moment he acknowledges the sound. Cue another foundation behavior.

4. Gradually increase the volume (one level at a time) during the training session. The dog should not show signs of fear or anxiety because the volume is increased gradually and kept at a subarousal threshold. If the dog begins to show signs of fear, cannot respond to a cue, or stops consuming treats, the volume has been increased too rapidly. Progress more slowly.

5. Eventually, you will be able to play the recording at a high volume without the dog reacting fearfully. Once you have achieved this goal, the mat may be used during actual storms.

CC/RS on a walk

Foundation skills: watch, look, target, sit, or down.

Possible training tools needed – Head halter, in some cases also a basket muzzle, calming cap in extreme cases, double leash, citronella spray to deter leash animals from approaching.

Frequently the pet owner may need to use CC and RS on walks, especially if the dog is over-reactive to people/other dogs. In such a situation DS would be difficult because the stimuli cannot be controlled. Therefore the pet owner should be instructed to CC and do RS if stimuli are suddenly presented and before intervention is needed.

1. If the stimulus is seen at a distance that the dog will easily tolerate, the owner should give the dog high-value treats while the stimulus is present (CC). If the stimulus is approaching or too close for the dog to tolerate, the pet owner should give another cue, like "let's go" and possibly use a hand target to target away from the stimulus (RS). NOTE: initially a head halter may be required to prompt the behavior of turning away. Turning away from the stimulus and increasing distance at the moment the dog acknowledges the stimuli is often reinforcing in itself to a fearful dog. Pet owners should be encouraged to use yards and driveways to turn their pet away from the stimulus while it passes. Visual barriers such as cars, trees, and bushes can also help the dog to be successful with RS while the stimulus passes.

2. The patient must be kept busy with fast-paced walking and turns and sits. Other cued behaviors can be added, such as targeting and "watch." The key mistake pet owners make is that they require the pet to sit while watching the stimulus approach. In reality, RS should be fast paced – almost an aerobic workout. Over time, as the pet begins to be less concerned with

stimuli, the handler will find it is not necessary to move as quickly or as far away from the stimulus.

Relinquishment exercises

Foundation skills needed: Sit

Possible training tools needed: The dog should initially be tethered to a stable point for this exercise.

Food bowl exercises

A common situation in which dogs show aggression is over their food. Management by feeding the dog in a location away from people and animals will need to be implemented. Some owners may decide that management rather than treatment is their preferred option. In treating severe food bowl aggression, the following protocol is recommended:

1. Feed the dog in a new place and use a different food bowl (preferably an old saucepan with a long handle) so that the dog does not associate feeding with past learning experiences (Figure 8.26).
2. Tether the dog securely with a leash and a buckle collar.

3. Measure out the amount of food to be fed in a different container that is out of reach of the dog. Cue the dog to "sit," place three kibbles in the saucepan, lower the pan to the dog so that he can eat the food out of the pan. The owner should continue to hold the sauce pan and be turned sideways and avoid direct eye contact while the dog is eating.
4. Prior to pulling the empty pan away, cue the dog to sit again. This adds predictability. When the dog sits, move the pan away and add a few more kibbles into the pan.
5. Continue in this manner until all the food is fed.
6. If the dog shows any aggression at any time, (which would be unusual due to the gradual nature of the exercise), leave the area for a few minutes until the dog is no longer aroused. Return and continue as before but with less kibble or kibble of lower value. The exercise may need to be discontinued if aggression reoccurs.
7. Once the dog is comfortable with being fed in this manner, gradually start adding more food into the bowl with each repetition.

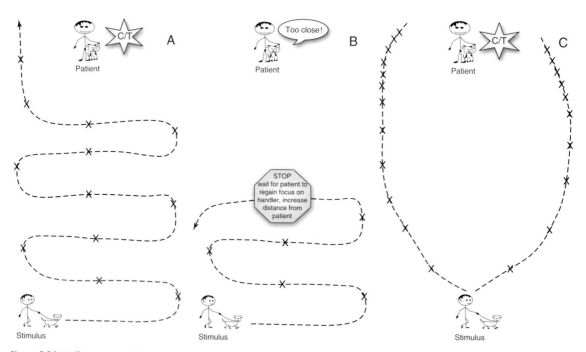

Figure 8.24 Walking patterns for DS. a) Stimulus approaches in a zigzag pattern while the patient is reinforced for an alternative behavior. X's note potential reinforcement opportunity for the patient, just as the stimulus turns toward or passes in front of the patient. b) If at any point the patient is unable to respond to a cue, starts to show conflict or displacement behaviors, or becomes too focused on the stimulus, a cue should be given to the person approaching to stop, when the patient calms and can again focus on the handler the stimulus increases distance from the patient and approaches at a more gradual pace. c) Incorporate the stimulus walking in a curved path toward the patient, d) Incorporate the stimulus walking at an angle toward the patient, e) Incorporate the stimulus walking straight toward the patient.

Figure 8.24 (*Continued*)

Figure 8.25 "Iris" in her safe place during a storm.

8. The next step involves gradually lowering the bowl to the floor. Go back to only 3 kibbles at a time in the bowl. With each repetition the bowl will be closer and closer to the ground until it is resting on the ground.

9. At this point, let go of the saucepan handle for a short period of time, and gradually increase the time. The dog will be cued to sit prior to removing the empty pan to add more food to it.
10. Gradually increase the amount of food being added to the pan each time.
11. Once you place 1/3 of the ration into the saucepan at once, using a ladle, start adding the remaining food into the saucepan as the dog eats.
12. Finally, all the food is placed into the saucepan at once and while the dog is eating, add or toss special treats such as cheese and hotdogs from a distance that does not elicit aggression.
13. Do not pet the dog while he/she is eating.
14. Progress should be gradual; do not be tempted to move forward too quickly or you could destroy any progress that has been made.
15. In the future, C/T when walking past the food bowl and toss a high-value treat into the bowl.

Exchange DS exercise

Dogs are natural resource guarders. Edible objects such as bones or rawhides, as well as inedible objects such

Figure 8.26 An adapted food bowl to begin the desensitization process for food bowl guarding.

as socks, Kleenex, or plastic wrappers may be guarded. These objects become much more valuable as the owner tries to get the stolen item away from the dog. Often the dog has been conditioned to run with the item as the pet owner chases. A behavior chain is created; obtaining a valuable object cues the pet owner to give chase (conflict situation created), which prompts the dog to defensively guard the object. During treatment, the goal is to change the dog's emotional response from one of fear to one of anticipation of reinforcement for relinquishment. The initial circumstance of having a valuable object must be changed to a positive emotional response of anticipating an opportunity for reinforcement and a "drop it" cue taught. This can be accomplished by teaching a release cue, such as "drop it," using positive reinforcement. While teaching "drop it," further conflict should be avoided. This may require using management by picking up or making unavailable any items which may be guarded by the dog.

1. The pet owner should be encouraged to capture "drop it" anytime the dog drops an object (toy) throughout the day by C/T at the moment the object is dropped. The dog should begin to associate dropping objects with the C/T and begin to offer the behavior. The cue "drop it" can be added.
2. Create a DS hierarchy listing the dog's least valued items to the most valued items. Start with low valued items. For safety tether the dog to a stable point with a leash attached to its buckle collar.
3. Start by showing the dog an object that has no value, such as a large rock at the end of the dogs reach on the tether.
4. Place the object about 3 ft away from the dog and cue "drop it." As you pick up the object C/T, tossing

the treat to the dog. Next place the object 2.5 ft away. Give the "drop it" cue, pick the object up, C/T. As the exercise progresses and the dog begins anticipating a reward, chain "sit" and "drop it" together. Cue "sit" → dog sits → cue "drop it" → pick up the object, C/T. Repeat the exercise while continuing to place the object closer and closer to the dog. Note: even though the dog is not releasing the object in response to the "drop it" cue, the cue is providing information about what the owner is about to do (pick up the object then give the dog a treat).
5. If at any time the dog tries to grab the object, cue "sit." And continue as long as the dog is not anxious or aggressive.
6. Set up exchanges in the same manner with slightly more coveted objects.
7. Gradually move up the previously prepared DS hierarchy, moving to more valuable objects.
8. Do exchanges with objects the dog has spontaneously taken possession of. Use special food rewards for releasing the object. When safe to do so, return the object to the dog or offer an alternative appropriate chew toy.
9. Do exchanges with "hot" objects the dog has spontaneously taken possession of. Use special food rewards for releasing the object. When safe to do so, return the object to the dog or offer an alternative appropriate chew toy.
10. Generalize the above exercises in different environments with different people.

Independence training
Foundation skills needed: Sit, down, place, relaxation
  Possible training tools needed: Video camera

  Independence training is often used when it has been determined that the pet has an unhealthy overattachment to the owner. Any behaviors that can be performed without being in direct or visual contact can be used to shape independence.

  For example, going to a place or mat can be trained initially next to the pet owner. Gradually the distance between the mat and the owner is increased. Later, sending the dog to a mat out of the pet owner's vision can be included. A tethered interactive food storage toy can be used when he is resting on the mat away from the pet owner. Tethering the food storage toy makes it impossible for the dog to carry the toy while following the owner.

  Sit-stay and down-stay should be trained to fluency as described below:

The 3-Ds of fluency are focused upon when teaching duration behaviors such as sit-stay or down-stay and should be added separately and in sequence.

1. **D**uration
2. **D**istance
3. **D**istractions

1. Initially, cue "sit" and then pause before giving a C/T. The dog in essence has to hold the position longer before receiving the reward.
2. Some people choose to make the "sit" or "down" cue the only cue used and duration is gradually taught with the single stationary cue. Others prefer to have a separate cue to signal to the dog to continue doing what they are doing, such as a verbal cue, "stay," or a hand signal (hand out in front as if motioning to stop). While teaching duration avoid repeating the cue or continue to hold your hand out.
3. Train duration first without moving away. Be aware that staring at the dog to hold him in place could quickly become part of the cue. Then when the handler looks away from the dog, the dog gets up. Vary the time. Do not always make it longer. End on a good note and set the dog up to succeed. If you see the dog getting ready to break the stay, it is best to avoid clicking and treating. Otherwise you are likely to reinforce the early movement of breaking the stay and inadvertently teach the dog to break the stay. Instead, reset the dog and make the next repetition easier, so that the dog is successful.
4. Once you have worked up to a 30-s stay without moving away from the dog, start adding the next variable – distance. You will need to make the duration shorter when adding the new variable.
5. Cue the dog (Sit, Stay). Take a half step or one step away from your dog, click, return immediately, and treat.
6. Continue in this fashion. When you start to add distractions, decrease the other variables. Distractions could be the handler doing something (jumping jacks, turning around, singing, etc.), other people, dogs, or toys. Always set the criteria at a level at which the dog has a realistic chance at being successful. If you are not progressing, most likely it is because multiple criteria are being raised at once. Reassess.
7. It is important to time the click when the pet owner is away from the pet and has not begun to return to the pet. This will encourage a positive emotional response to the pet owner leaving. Dog thinks, "Move away from me so I can get clicked!"

DS to departure cues and planned departures

Pet owners often have a predeparture pattern that predicts to the pet that the owner is preparing to leave. The pet suffering from separation anxiety often gets more anxious as it recognizes that the owner is preparing to depart. The goal with DS to departure cues is for these cues to lose their predictive value as a signal the owner is going to leave the pet and thus minimize the pet's anxiety associated with predeparture routines.

The owner should make a list of things to do prior to a routine departure. An example of a predeparture list might include turn off the TV, turn on the radio, take phone off the charger, let the dog outside, put on shoes, brush teeth, confine the dog to the bedroom, pick up keys, open the garage, set the alarm and exit the garage door.

Several times throughout the day when the owner is not leaving, some of these behaviors should be performed. For example, the owner may put on her shoes, brush her teeth, then sit down and watch a movie. The owner should not attempt to agitate the dog or get the dog's attention. In fact the owner should just ignore the dog during this time and be nonchalant. Ideally the owner should attempt to avoid the dog seeing these departure cues when she does actually have to leave the dog. The owner might exit out a different doorway or put things in the car at night.

Once DS to departure cues has been accomplished, the next step may be to desensitize the dog to planned departures. The early stage of this is combining a relaxed down stay with the departure cues as a distraction. A remote treat dispenser, such as the Treat and Train®, can be helpful in this process to disassociate the treat from the owner. Another alternative is to give the dog a long lasting food storage toy tethered by his bed.

The owner cues the dog to settle on his bed and performs departure cues randomly without leaving the dog or going out of sight. The dog is rewarded for calm behavior with either the food storage toy or remote treat dispenser, or the owner clicks and tosses a treat to the dog. Eventually the goal is for the owner to progress through the departure routine and then leave for short periods of time. Gradually the time the owner is gone is increased but should be variable (some short and some longer). At this point it would be important to be utilizing a long lasting food storage toy. Upon return of the owner, the dog should initially be ignored to avoid overexcitement with return.

This process can be very time consuming and difficult to perform without sensitizing the dog. If the dog becomes anxious during the process, the frequent departures and leaving of the dog may actually create more anxiety with departure. Video can be helpful to allow the owner to assess the dog's behavior while the owner is out of sight. While working on DS to planned departures, it is important to avoid leaving the dog or have a different routine that signals an actual departure versus the training session (i.e., the dog is confined to a specific room for actual departures and is loose in the house during training). DS to departure cues and planned departures should be used in conjunction with a complete treatment plan for separation anxiety, which may include medication options.

Handling issues

Foundation skills needed: Previous conditioning to the clicker is useful.

Possible training tools needed: Basket muzzle if there is a previous bite history while being handled or there is concern that the dog may bite.

The first goal of desensitization to handling exercises is to teach the pet to tolerate and enjoy all types of handling from familiar people. The second goal is to teach the pet to tolerate more intensive, firm, or unfamiliar forms of handling that might be necessary for restraint, grooming (including nail trimming, ear cleaning, and combing), teeth brushing, and veterinary care. The goal is to change the emotional response associated with being handled from fear or agitation to one of relaxation or contentment.

Step 1: Teaching tolerance

The goal of handling exercises is to accustom the pet to accept and enjoy all types of handling from familiar people. Before beginning, a DS hierarchy should be created; the areas where the pet is most likely to react should be placed at the end of the hierarchy.

1. Begin by working with the pet only when it is calm and in a relaxed environment.

2. Gently but very briefly touch a body part that is the least likely to cause anxiety (ears, mouth, paws, belly, and hair coat), C/T (see Figure 8.27a and b).

3. Anticipate the pet's mood and reaction and always stop before the pet displays uneasiness or undesirable behavior. The goal is to C/T for tolerance of the touch without getting a reaction.

4. When the animal begins to eagerly anticipate the touch, a cue can be given, "hug" and the body part touched, C/T. Repeat the exercises, gradually lengthening the duration and firmness of the touch (do not increase both duration and firmness at the same time).

Step 2: More Intensive Handling

The goal of step 2 is to accustom the pet to accept mildly unpleasant types of handling, including venipuncture, from familiar and unfamiliar people.

1. If the dog has had a previously bad experience with handling (such as at the veterinary hospital), DS should first occur in an environment as dissimilar as possible from where the bad experience occurred.

Figure 8.27 a) and b) Gently but very briefly touch a body part that is the least likely to cause anxiety and then click and treat.

2. If the body cues have been taught as described previously, they may be used. Cue "hug" and gently touch, pet, stroke, or massage various areas of the body and collar and C/T.

3. Gradually increase the intensity of touching, pushing, patting, and grasping different areas of the body (e.g., face, feet, muzzle, ears) as the pet earns clicks and treats for it. For example, when preparing for venipuncture, rub the cephalic vein, C/T; gently pinch over the vein, C/T; gently scratch the vein with a fingernail, C/T; insert the needle, draw blood, C/T.

CC/RS/DS to the veterinary hospital

Unfortunately, patients often develop a negative emotional response to the veterinary hospital. In these cases, a nonstressful starting point must be found before behavior modification can commence. Where will the dog take a highly valued reinforcement? Initially it may be in the car in the parking lot. CC should occur first, taking the dog to the hospital and only give treats and then leave. The next step may be taking treats in the waiting room and doing training – then leaving.

When entering an examination room, it should not be a room in which the dog has had a previous bad experience. The dog is anticipating being restrained and instead should be given treats and then leave the examination room. Handling exercises should be trained previously and can later be instituted and applied by a technician while the dog is still in the parking lot, then waiting room, and finally the examination room.

Relaxation

Foundation skills needed: "Down", "Go to your Mat"
  Training tools needed:
– A portable mat, different from a favorite bed or a place previously used to teach "place". The new mat will initially be the cue for relaxation. Later the cue will be transferred to the verbal cue "relax" (or whatever cue is chosen).
– Leash.

Considerations:

Teaching relaxation can be added to "place" but is different in that the focus is on shaping relaxation rather than going to a specific location. "Relax" can then be generalized to multiple environments, even when the mat or "place" is not available; for example, on a walk or during thunderstorms.

Because the clicker can cause a strong emotional response of excitement, the clicker may not be effective in shaping relaxation with all dogs.

Teaching to relax on cue is a behavior that can be included in many aspects of behavior modification and should be considered a foundation skill. Relaxation can become a default offered behavior when the dog is unsure of what to do and should become a problem prevention tool taught early in the dog's life. The following protocol was modified from Chill Out Fido by Nan Arthur.

1. Ask the pet owner what the dog looks like when it is most relaxed. That will be the behavior that is shaped. The position described by the pet owner can also be captured by C/T when the dog assumes the position but the following shaping should occur to teach deep relaxation in many situations and environments.

2. With the dog out of the room, scatter 5–10 treats on the mat, ensuring a positive response to the mat.

3. Bring the dog into the room on leash and passively allow him to investigate the treats on the mat. Begin every relaxation training session in the same manner. The leash may be held or dropped and stepped on. The leash restriction is used to associate relaxation with the leash and also keeps the dog from wandering during the training session.

4. As the dog eats the treats off the mat, drop a few more treats onto the mat; as the dog begins to eat those treats, drop one treat at a time between the dog's front paws, also on the mat. Quietly dropping the treats rather than treating from the hand should occur because being given a treat from the hand overly excites some dogs. Dropping the treat also prompts the dog to lower its head.

5. It was noted previously that a clicker is not usually recommended when training relaxation because excitement is often an emotional response to the clicker. Instead, use a quietly spoken word as the marker, a quiet verbally spoken "good" could be the marker, for example. Begin by first assuming a relaxed position yourself. Do not interact with the dog; become completely disengaged from the dog. Pretend the dog is invisible.

6. Once the dog begins interacting with the mat do not reinforce the dog for staring at you. Reward instead when he diverts his attention away from you. Begin reinforcing for sniffing the mat or otherwise disengaging from you.

7. Once the dog begins to understand that less activity is being reinforced, begin shaping for less intense behavior such as less intense sniffing, sitting, lying down, or lowering head, and marking the behavior with the verbal "good" and treat. It should also be noted that a treat lower on the reinforcement

hierarchy may be the best treat of choice, creating less excitement. Excitement is counter-productive to shaping relaxation.

8. Next begin shaping for more obvious signs of relaxation. A yawn or deep breath can be captured. Reinforce as close and quietly to the dog's front feet as possible, reinforcing lowering of the head.

9. Practice with the leash on the dog with you standing, which teaches the dog to relax on leash while you are standing. Place the behavior on a cue ("chill", "relax", etc.)

10. Transfer the cue of the sight of the mat to the verbal cue. Practice the exercise with the dog on leash but without the mat present. Give the new verbal cue, pause, present the mat, and continue transferring the cue as previously described.

11. Generalize and train to fluency.

Staying safe

When a pet is being seen for a behavioral disorder, it is likely that the pet is fearful and may or may not have exhibited aggression. Before interacting with the pet, the veterinary technician should have minimally obtained the following information:

1. Age of the animal. The age will give insight into the length of learning history of the animal, in other words, how much time the animal has had to practice the coping skill it has utilized to control the environment in the past. The "coping" behavior may be actively avoiding the situation (leaving), aggressing to make the stimulus increase distance, or some other behavior like a stereotypic stress relieving behavior. A dog that has had a lengthy history of conflict-induced aggression may no longer demonstrate conflict behaviors before a bite.

2. Past bite history. Past behavior will be the best predictor of future behavior. How many times has the animal bitten? Does it give warning signals (i.e. conflict behaviors)? How easily is the behavior triggered? Has the pet inhibited its bite in the past and does the animal bite multiple times or leave after the first bite?

3. Known and identifiable triggers. Usually the pet owner can identify triggers of aggression when the veterinary technician asks, "What would you tell me not to do with 'Fluffy' because it might upset her and trigger the response?" If the owners cannot identify triggers, the veterinary technician should continue to listen to the history being obtained by the veterinarian before moving forward. The triggers will likely be identified as a more detailed history

of prior episodes is obtained. Use extreme caution when working with an older aggressive patient that does not inhibit its bite or bites multiple times and triggers are unknown. Such cases should be referred to a veterinary behaviorist.

Safety techniques for the behavior consultation room

When working with an aggressive or fearful animal during a behavior consultation, the following suggestions can help decrease the chances of an aggressive episode:

- Keep interruptions to a minimum – Any change of environment, including knocks on the door or people entering and leaving the consultation room can incrementally push the patient toward the bite threshold. Keep all interruptions, noises, or other "surprises" to a minimum during the consultation.

- Keep movement and variables low during the consultation. Although having all members of the family present is important for obtaining the behavioral history and it is important to have all members present to discuss the prescribed treatment plan implementation, it is also important to keep distractions and uncontrolled stimuli to a minimum. Very young children may not be appropriate for the consultation.

- Tethers: A wall or floor tether can be used if the bite threshold and bite history are unclear. Identify triggers as quickly as possible so they can be avoided or applied systematically and not accidentally (see Figure 8.28).

- Mobile chair: A rolling desk-type chair can be used by the technician to move out of the tethered space if needed. The chair can also be used to turn away from

Figure 8.28 Wall tethers can be utilized when working with an animal with a bite history or unknown bite history

the dog if conflict behaviors are seen or if an aggressive situation occurs. Use a chair that can turn and be pushed away if needed.

Understand the animal's arousal and bite thresholds

All dogs have a level at which they will bite. They also have thresholds for other levels of threat, such as growling, snarling, and snapping. The first step is to determine potential risk factors. Typical risk factors include categories of people to whom the dog was not socialized, certain ways of being touched, pain, presence of food, and other dogs. Presentation of any one of these risk factors by itself may elicit threat or biting, depending on the dog's particular threshold level.

A combination of more than one risk factor at the same time usually evokes a higher level of threat. In many situations, a dog that has bitten "for no reason" may have been exposed to a novel combination of risk factors at once, pushing him over his "Bite Threshold" (Figure 8.29).

For example, Stanley, an 8-year-old poodle, was not socialized to children, is uncomfortable around loud noises and is arthritic. Stanley has never bitten anyone before. One day the neighbor's 3-year-old child comes over blowing a whistle and falls on Stanley. Stanley bites the child. The pet owners say Stanley was unprovoked. Stanley was pushed over his bite threshold. Helping pet owners understand their dog's bite threshold will help them to realize the bite was not unprovoked and they can then learn to recognize when they are reaching the dog's bite threshold and change the environment before a bite can occur.

Greeting a fearful patient

If the patient has been known to be fearful in the examination room in the past, the following suggestions should be incorporated for his next visit.

Control as many antecedents as possible

Make sure the pet does not have to wait in the reception area but can enter the examination room immediately. Have the pet owner keep the animal in the car until the examination room is ready. This will keep arousal and anxiety related to anticipation from rising. Be in the exam room before the patient enters. Many dogs will almost immediately begin guarding the space in the examination room unless the technician is in the room first. As said previously, best predictor of behavior is past behavior. If the dog has had issues in the past, ask the owners not to feed him on the day of his appointment. Have a range of food reinforcements available but also

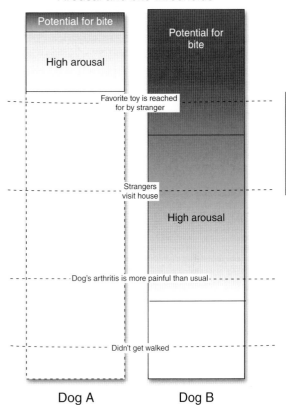

Figure 8.29 Arousal and bite threshold. Dog A has a high threshold for arousal and biting. Dog B is frequently in a high arousal state and is therefore more easily reaches its bite threshold.

ask the pet owner to bring the pet's favorite treat. Ignore the patient when they enter the room and explain to the owner that you are trying to be nonthreatening toward his/her pet.

CC and DS to your presence

As the medical history is obtained, ignore the dog but toss the very best treats possible (i.e., chicken) (see Figure 8.30). Every veterinary examination room should have a can of "canned cheese," canned dog food, hot dogs, or cooked chicken chunks in the freezer. If the client is concerned that you are giving "table food" – something you have recommended the owner not to do, explain that this is specifically why it is important that they do not give table food at home, otherwise it would not be a "treat" and "special" to the pet.

Figure 8.30 Veterinary technician tossing treats to a patient. Alicea Schaeffer RVT, VTS (Behavior), KPA-CTP, CPDT-KA.

If the fearful patient will not take the treats you have tossed, ask the owner to offer the treats to his/her dog. Frequently, it only takes an offered "safe" treat from the owner for the dog to sample what you have tossed.

If the pet remains hidden behind the owner, ask the owner to walk across the room away from the pet (Figure 8.31). At this point the patient will decide whether it is "safer" to hide alone or to follow the owner. By getting the dog to walk across the room you are creating an opportunity for him to gain confidence when nothing "bad" occurs when he walks across the room. An area of safety has been created. If the dog does not follow the owner, have the owner kneel and offer or toss a treat across the room to the pet.

Figure 8.31 Pet owner walking to opposite side of the examination room with the patient following. Alicea Schaeffer RVT, VTS (Behavior), KPA-CTP, CPDT-KA.

Figure 8.32 Technician sitting sideways and where the pet owner and patient were sitting previously. Alicea Schaeffer RVT, VTS (Behavior), KPA-CTP, CPDT-KA.

Once the pet and owner have left the "safe" area, the technician can sit where the dog was previously hiding (Figure 8.32). The technician should turn sideways, avert his eyes from the pet and nonchalantly toss treats to the pet creating a "bread crumb trail" leading to the technician. DO NOT TALK TO THE PET OR LOOK DIRECTLY AT IT. Continue calmly talking to the pet owner in a relaxed fashion, regardless of what the pet does. Pet owners often feel ashamed of the way their pet behaves at the veterinary clinic. It is important that you assist the client in relaxing by telling him/her the pet is only afraid and it is ok, you are hoping to calm its fears.

As the pet begins to take treats closer to you, offer a treat from your upturned hand. Make sure not to remove your hand until the pet has turned to walk away (Figure 8.33). The movement of your hand can cause a fearful dog to become aggressive. If the dog is "stretching" or "snatching" the treat from your hand, be very still and do not increase any aspect of the interaction until the dog chooses to move away on its own.

Once the dog is comfortable and not showing signs of fear when taking treats out of your flat hand, hold the treat closer to your body for the dog to take it from you. Continue until eventually your hand with the treat is next to your body. At this point the dog may not leave once it has eaten the treat. This is the point where you can offer another treat while you scratch the dog's chest (Figure 8.34). Always allow the dog to retreat whenever it feels the need, allow the dog to be in control of the interaction. Eventually the dog will begin not leaving you and may even lean against you. Even at this point,

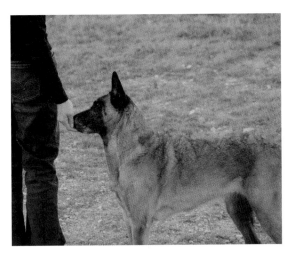

Figure 8.33 Hand offering treat with palm up and avoiding reaching into the dog's space. The hand may be moved once the patient has moved away or initiated further contact.

Figure 8.34 Dog beginning to relax as the technician scratches chest, still sitting sideways and avoiding eye contact. Alicea Schaeffer RVT, VTS (Behavior), KPA-CTP, CPDT-KA.

do not stand or change your posture until the pet leaves on its own. You can toss treats across the room to move the dog away from you if needed.

Next, stand and toss treats again. The pet should now trust you enough to begin seeking your attention. Quietly ask for a "sit" and then reward. It is likely at this point you have just won a permanent friend.

If the dog will not take any treat at any point in the appointment, a "nonstressful" starting point has not been found. If the dog is truly hungry (the owner has restricted food before the appointment) and you are using a treat "that cannot be refused" then this patient is in extreme distress. The next step is to determine

when the patient stopped taking treats. Would he take treats in the owner's car in the parking lot? Then that is the place to begin the process. This may also be a case in which anxiolytic medications are required to create a nonstressful starting point.

Conclusion

Veterinary technicians are an instrumental tool in the positive resolution of behavior problems and behavior disorders that threaten the human–animal bond. By understanding the motivations that drive behavior, potential diagnosis and treatments that may be prescribed, and with practiced applications, they can become the pet's behavior case manager, working with the veterinarian, the qualified trainer and pet owner to successfully apply prescribed techniques.

References

Ahn, H. and Picard, R. (2006) Affective cognitive learning and decision making: The role of emotions, in *Proceedings of the 18th European Meeting on Cybernetics and Systems Research (EMCSR 2006)*.

Behavior, A. V. S. A. B (2007) AVSAB Position Statement: The use of Punishment for Behavior Modification in Animals.

Coppinger, R. and Coppinger, L. (2001) *Dogs: A Startling New Understanding of Canine Origin, Behavior & Evolution*, Scribner, New York City, New York, USA.

Depue, R.A. and Iacono, W.G. (1989) Neurobehavioral aspects of affective disorders. *Annual Review of Psychology*, **40**, 457–492.

Friedman, S. (2009a) Behavior Fundamentals: Filling the Behavior-Change Toolbox Behavior Fundamentals: Filling the Behavior-Change Toolbox North American Veterinary Conference, Orlando, FL.

Friedman, S.G. (2009b) *Functional assessment: hypothesizing the predictors and purposes of problem behavior*, North American Veterinary Conference, Orlando, FL.

Garcia, J.K. and Koelling, R.A. (1966) Relation of cue to consequence in avoidance learning. *Psychomic Science*, **4**, 123–124.

Gershoff, E.T. (2002) Physical punishment by parents and associated child behaviors and experiences: A meta-analytic and theoretical review. *Psychological Bulletin*, **128**, 539–579.

Gray, J. (1990) Brain systems that mediate both emotion and cognition. *Cognition & Emotion*, **4** (3), 269–288.

Guy, N.C., Luescher, U.A., Dohoo, S.E. *et al.* (2001) Risk factors for dog bites to owners in a general veterinary caseload. *Applied Animal Behaviour Science*, **74** (1), 29–42.

Horwitz, D., Mills, D.S. and British Small Animal Veterinary Association (2009) *BSAVA Manual of Canine and Feline Behavioural Medicine*, British Small Animal Veterinary Association, Quedgeley, Gloucester England.

Horwitz, D. and Neilson, J.C. (2007) *Blackwell's Five-Minute Veterinary Consult Clinical Companion : Canine And Feline Behavior*, Ames, Iowa, Blackwell Pub.

Hunsberger, J.G., Newton, S.S., Bennett, A.H. *et al.* (2007) Antidepressant actions of the exercise-regulated gene VGF. *Nature Medicine*, **13** (12), 1476–1482.

Ksenych, E. and Liu, D. (1992) *Conflict, order, and action : readings in sociology*, Canadian Scholars' Press, Toronto.

Landsberg, G.M., Hunthausen, W.L. and Ackerman, L.J. (2013) *Behavior Problems of the Dog and Cat*, Edinburgh, Saunders/Elsevier.

LeDoux, J.E. (1996) *The Emotional Brain : The Mysterious Underpinnings of Emotional Life*, Simon & Schuster, New York.

Luescher, A., Martin, K.M. (2010) Dogs! & Cats: Diagnosis and Treatment of Behavior Problems, Purdue University.

Luescher, A. and Shaw, J. (2007) DOGS! Principles and Techniques of Behavior Modification Notes, Purdue University, West Lafayette, IN.

Martin, K.M. (2011) *Puppy Start Right: Foundation Training for the Companion Dog*, Sunshine Books, Inc, Waltham, MA.

Milgram, S. (1963) Behavioral study of obedience. *Journal of Abnormal Psychology*, **67**, 371–378.

Mulvaney, M.K. and Mebert, C.J. (2007) Parental corporal punishment predicts behavior problems in early childhood. *Journal of Family Psychology*, **21** (3), 389–397.

Panksepp, J. (1998) *Affective Neuroscience : The Foundations of Human and Animal Emotions*, Oxford University Press, New York.

Pryor, K. (6/25/2002) "The Poisoned Cue: Positive and Negative Discriminative Stimuli." http://www.clickertraining.com/node/164 2013 (accessed 22 May 2014).

Pryor, K. (2009) *Reaching the Animal Mind: What the Clicker Training Method Teaches Us About Animals*, Scribner, New York.

Psychology, A. f. A. S. (2007–2012) Psychological Benefits of Exercise from http://www.appliedsportpsych.org/resource-center/health-fitness-resources/psychological-benefits-of-exercise/ (accessed 22 May 2014).

Ramirez, K. and John G. Shedd Aquarium (1999) *Animal Training: Successful Animal Management through Positive Reinforcement*, Shedd Aquarium, Chicago, IL.

Salman, M.D., Hutchinson, J.M., Ruch-Gallie, R. *et al.* (2000) Behavioral reasons for relinquishment of dogs and cats to 12 shelters. *Journal of Applied Animal Welfare Science*, **3** (2), 93–106.

Strassberg, Z., Dodge, K., Pettit, G. and Bates, J. (1994) Spanking in the home and children's subsequent aggression toward kindergarten peers. *Development and Psychopathology*, **6**, 445–445.

Straus, M.A.M. and Paschall, M.J.M. (2009) Corporal punishment by mothers and development of children's cognitive ability: a longitudinal study of two nationally representative age cohorts. *Journal of Aggression, Maltreatment & Trauma*, **18** (5), 459–483.

Wood, L. (2008) *Clicker Bridging Stimulus Efficacy*, Hunter College, New York.

9 Introductory neurophysiology and psychopharmacology

Sara L. Bennett[1] and Carissa D. Sparks[2]

[1] VCA Berwyn Animal Hospital, Berwyn, IL, USA

[2] Purdue University Veterinary Teaching Hospital, West Lafayette, IN, USA

CHAPTER MENU

Introduction

This chapter explores the most important cells of the nervous system – neurons. The nervous system is the information highway of the body. This multicellular system is directly responsible for the vast communication that is occurring every second of every day. The brain is the supervisory center of the nervous system and is the most complex organ in the body. The anatomy and physiology of the brain are discussed; however, owing to its intricacies, information will focus on the functional anatomy pertaining to behavior. Because the brain is such a convoluted organ, it has mechanisms protecting it from the general circulation. The blood–brain barrier (BBB) is described, and the basic anatomy and physiology underlying drug effects are considered. Neurotransmitters in the brain producing behavioral effects are elaborated on, and pharmacokinetics and psychopharmacology are discussed.

- The nervous system is the information highway of the body.

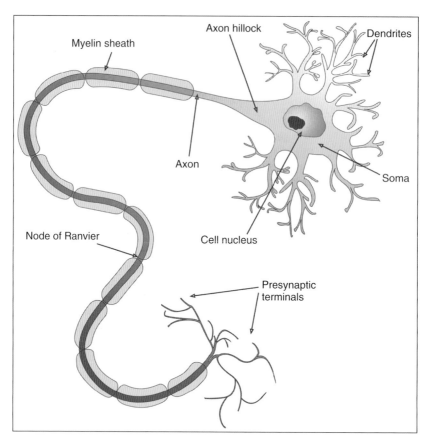

Figure 9.1 Neuron. (Illustration by: Carol Bain, DVM).

Basic neurophysiology

The nerve cell is the functional unit of the nervous system. There are four main structures to every neuron; the soma, dendrites, axon, and presynaptic terminals. Each neuron has a specific purpose: to transmit messages through electrical impulses to adjacent neurons until this information reaches the brain.

The soma is also referred to as *the cell body*. It contains the nucleus and the organelles necessary for cellular life and communication (Meyer and Quenzer, 2005).

Dendrites branch out from the soma and are the major receiving apparatus responsible for taking signals from other neurons and transmitting them into the soma. Dendrites branch out similarly to a tree and are covered with spines. These specialized dendritic spines vary in morphology and receive excitatory input from other neurons. It is hypothesized that the abrupt changes occurring with these structures are involved with learning and memory (Hedges and Burchfield, 2006).

Axons are much longer than dendrites, often extending several feet in length in some animals. Axons act as the conduction unit of the neuron. They are covered with a fatty layer called *the myelin sheath*, which serves as an insulator. The myelin sheath wraps around the tubular axon and is interrupted at regular intervals called *nodes of Ranvier*. These interruptions accelerate the conduction down the axon. Electrical impulses are carried through the axon to presynaptic terminals (Cunningham and Klein, 2007; Figure 9.1).

Presynaptic terminals branch out from the end of the axon and contain presynaptic vesicles that secrete neurotransmitters to other cells. The axon fires and these neurotransmitters are released into the synaptic cleft. Neurochemicals cross the synaptic cleft and attach to specialized receptors on adjacent nerve or muscle cells specific for that chemical (Figure 9.2). Depending on the neurotransmitter released and the receptor site bound to, excitement, inhibition, or initiation of enzymatic reactions will occur. It is here where most psychotropic

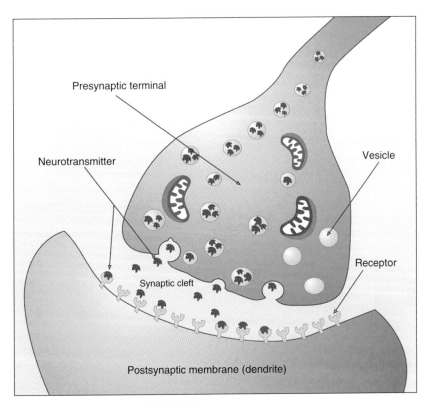

Figure 9.2 Neurotransmission. (Illustration by: Carol Bain, DVM).

medications initiate their effects (Hedges and Burchfield, 2006). Impulse communication is about a third of a millisecond at which time the neurotransmitter must be deactivated. Neurotransmitters are deactivated from the receptors by diffusion into the extracellular fluid, enzymatic metabolism, or reuptake into the presynaptic terminal to be used again (Grilly, 2006).

An average neuron forms thousands of synapses with other neurons. These interactions between neurons are responsible for all perceptions, memories, thoughts, and behavior. Learning is the process in which specific experiences alter our nervous system and influence our behavior. The Hebb rule states that learning involves strengthening of a synapse that is repeatedly active when the postsynaptic neuron fires (Carlson, 2002).

- These interactions between neurons are responsible for all perceptions, memories, thoughts, and behavior.
- Learning is the process in which specific experiences alter our nervous system and influence our behavior.

The central nervous system (CNS) consists of the brain and the spinal cord. The brain is divided into several major parts, the hindbrain, the midbrain, the forebrain, the basal ganglia, and the olfactory bulb (Meyer and Quenzer, 2005; Figure 9.3).

Hindbrain

The hindbrain consists of the brainstem, connecting the brain to the spinal cord, and the cerebellum. The brainstem is made up of the medulla oblongata and the pons (Figure 9.4). These structures are primarily responsible for respiratory and cardiac function. Cranial nerves pass through the medulla to transmit information from the head and the neck to the spinal cord. Therefore, damage to this area can result in a wide range of neurologic deficits (Hedges and Burchfield, 2006). The pons incorporates a portion of the reticular formation, a collection of nuclei forming a network responsible for attention and arousal (Carlson, 2002). The cerebellum is primarily involved with coordination but has also been implicated in attention and cognition (Hedges and Burchfield, 2006).

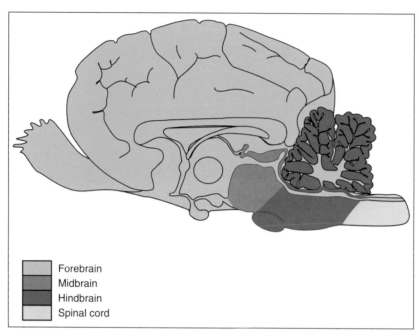

Figure 9.3 Color-coded brain structures (forebrain, midbrain, hindbrain, and spinal cord). (Illustration by: Carol Bain, DVM).

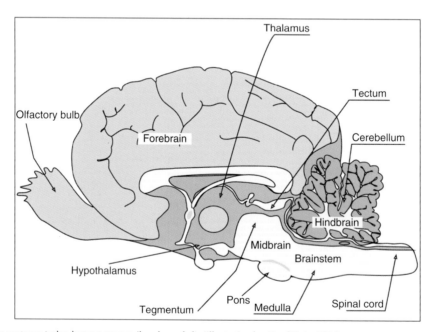

Figure 9.4 Brain anatomy (color, but not necessarily color coded). (Illustration by: Carol Bain, DVM).

Midbrain

The midbrain is located dorsal to the brainstem and envelops the tectum and tegmentum (refer to Figure 9.4). These structures play a role in visual reflexes and reactions to moving stimuli. They are also involved in arousal, attention, and behaviors modulated by rewards (Carlson, 2002; Hedges and Burchfield, 2006). Within the tegmentum are several other structures, some of which are important for organizing behaviors such as predation and defensive rage (Meyer and Quenzer, 2005).

Forebrain

The forebrain is the largest portion of the brain and contains a wide array of structures involved with learning. The forebrain is predominantly comprised of gray matter and is covered by the cerebral cortex. The cortex is divided into two hemispheres that are connected by millions of axons. The largest of these axon pathways is called *the corpus callosum* (Meyer and Quenzer, 2005). The cerebral cortex is further divided into four lobes in each hemisphere: the frontal, the parietal, the temporal, and the occipital lobes (Figure 9.5). Other structures of the forebrain that are not necessarily associated with a specific lobe include the thalamus/hypothalamus, basal ganglia, and olfactory bulb (refer to Figure 9.4). Each lobe of the cortex consists of several structures responsible for specific functions. Each lobe transmits electrochemical impulses to other areas of the brain in which the information is further analyzed and perceived. This vast and intricate communication coordinated within the brain is how memories and perceptions are formed (Meyer and Quenzer, 2005).

Parietal lobe

The parietal lobe lies caudal to the frontal lobe and dorsal to the temporal lobe (refer to Figure 9.5). The rostral portion of the parietal lobe consists of the somatosensory association cortex. It receives electrical impulses from the body and the head relative to pain, temperature, touch pressure, and position of the limbs and sense of joint movement. The caudal portion is responsible for cognition and selective attention.

Occipital lobe

The occipital lobe is considered the visual cortex and interprets sensory information from the eye. With regards to behavior, the occipital lobe functions in conjunction with the parietal lobe to form the cognitive association area (King, 1987).

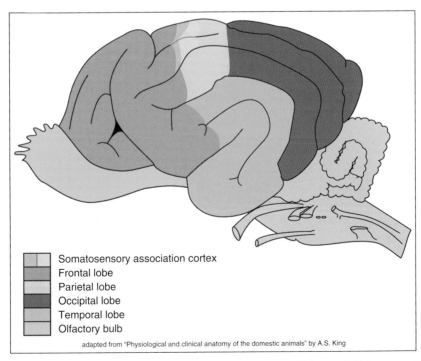

Somatosensory association cortex
Frontal lobe
Parietal lobe
Occipital lobe
Temporal lobe
Olfactory bulb

adapted from "Physiological and clinical anatomy of the domestic animals" by A.S. King

Figure 9.5 Color-coded brain lobes (somatosensory association cortex, frontal lobe, parietal lobe, occipital lobe, temporal lobe, and olfactory bulb). (Illustration by: Carol Bain, DVM).

CHAPTER 9

Temporal lobe

The temporal lobe is considered the interpretative association area and is concerned with learning and memory. The temporal lobe harbors the limbic system, which is comprised of the hippocampus and the amygdala (Figure 9.6). The limbic system is important in behavior because it is considered the emotional center of the brain. It is involved with fear, aggression, affection, initiative, imagination, and anxiety. All of these emotions contribute to individual personality. Specifically, the amygdala interprets facial expressions, processes stressful stimuli, and modulates fear and aggressive responses. The hippocampal formation is involved with learning and spatial memory rather than emotion, but it is also implicated with the stress response (Hedges and Burchfield, 2006; King, 1987).

Basal ganglia

The basal ganglia are a group of nuclei that lie deep within the brain and encompass a variety of complex structures. This area of the brain is not as well understood as other areas but is known to receive signals from the cerebral cortex and project these signals to other regions (Cunningham and Klein, 2007). They are most often associated with movement regulation but appear to possess functions associated with obsessive compulsive disorder, depression, and dementia (Hedges and Burchfield, 2006).

Frontal lobe

Although the frontal lobe is not as developed in dogs as it is in humans, it has many responsibilities pertaining to behavior. The frontal association area contributes to general alertness, intelligence, and temperament of each individual (King, 1987; refer to Figure 9.5).

Hypothalamus/thalamus

The hypothalamus and the thalamus are a major division of the forebrain (refer to Figure 9.4). The hypothalamus is most commonly known for its role in homeostasis. Specific to behavior, the hypothalamus works in conjunction with the hippocampus and amygdala to control the emotions of rage and aggression. The thalamus is a distribution center taking information from one region of the brain and projecting it to the appropriate portion of the cerebral cortex (Carlson, 2002; Meyer and Quenzer, 2005).

Olfactory bulb

The olfactory bulb is located in the most rostral part of the brain in most animals (refer to Figures 9.4 and 9.5). Axons from the olfactory bulb project to the amygdala, limbic cortex, and the piriform lobe. All of these structures are important in reproductive behavior (Carlson, 2002).

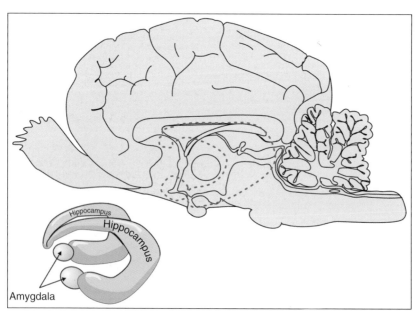

Figure 9.6 Amygdala and hippocampus. (Illustration by: Carol Bain, DVM).

Figure 9.7 Synthesis of acetylcholine.

Blood–brain barrier

The brain and the spinal cord are bathed in the cerebrospinal fluid (CSF), which acts as a cushion for the brain, nourishment for cells, and a conduit for hormones. Cells in the brain form tight junctions around the capillaries, preventing extracellular fluid from entering the CNS. This semi-permeable barrier is considered the BBB. The BBB is directly responsible for protecting the CNS from toxins and fluctuations of extracellular fluid. It also prevents neurotransmitters from leaking into general circulation. Because of this protective barrier, only specialized medications can penetrate into the CNS. Solubility, ionization, and polarity are a few of the important characteristics of every medication that directly affect the absorptive quality of the drug. Only lipid-soluble, unionized, and nonpolar medications can cross the BBB (Cunningham and Klein, 2007; Bill, 2006).

Neurotransmitters

Neurotransmitters are the chemicals released from presynaptic vesicles under specific stimulation and used in the brain to transmit information from one neuron to another. Hundreds of chemicals have been identified in the nervous system as being, or having the potential of being, a neurotransmitter. This section focuses on the most common neurotransmitters pertaining to behavior (Grilly, 2006).

> • Neurotransmitters are the chemicals released from presynaptic vesicles under specific stimulation and used in the brain to transmit information from one neuron to another.

Acetylcholine

Acetylcholine (ACh) is synthesized in nerve terminals from a vitamin, called *choline*, and acetyl-CoA (Figure 9.7). This neurotransmitter is primarily excitatory and is distributed throughout the CNS and the peripheral nervous system (PNS). The functions of ACh on the CNS are not well understood but are implicated in chemosensory associations and are responsible for triggering rapid eye movement (REM) sleep. ACh is also involved in facilitating perceptual learning and controls functions of the hippocampus, including the formation of memories (Carlson, 2002; Table 9.1). In the PNS, ACh activates muscles and is the major neurotransmitter in the autonomic nervous system. ACh will bind to two receptor types referred to as *nicotinic and muscarinic*. Nicotinic receptors are located in both the CNS and the PNS and are considered the "fast" receptors. Evidence suggests that when they are activated, other neurotransmitters are released, resulting in a myriad of effects (Grilly, 2006). Muscarinic receptors are considered the "slow" receptors and are involved with the formation of memory, learning, and movement (Hedges and Burchfield, 2006). An enzyme called *acetylcholinestrase* (AChE) located in the synaptic gap degrades ACh by hydrolyzing it into acetate and choline. This degradation is different from other neurotransmitters in which postsynaptic activity is regulated via reuptake. Choline is then actively taken back into the cell and reused for more ACh synthesis (Grilly, 2006).

Monoamines

There are four neurotransmitters that belong to the monoamine family. These include dopamine (DA), norepinephrine (NE), epinephrine, and serotonin (5-HT). The first three are further classified as catecholamines, whereas 5-HT is considered an idolamine (Carlson, 2002).

Dopamine

DA is synthesized through a series of interactions of various enzymes. Two amino acids, called *phenylalanine*

Table 9.1 Neurotransmitters, functions and primary locations.

Neurotransmitter	Function	Location
Acetylcholine	Perceptual learning	Throughout CNS and PNS
	Formation of memories	Hippocampus
Dopamine	Attention	CNS
	Cognition	Basal ganglia
	Sociability	Limbic system
	Motivation	
	Reward	
Norepinephrine	Arousal	Throughout CNS and PNS
	Dreaming	Pons
	Anxiety	Hypothalamus
	Fear	Frontal cortex
	Mood	Hippocampus
	Attention	
	Processing information	
Serotonin	Regulates mood	CNS and PNS
	Anxiety	Brainstem
GABA	Reduces anxiety	Throughout CNS
	Promotes sleep	
	Muscle relaxation	
Glutamate	Learning/memory	Throughout CNS
	Cognition	
	Psychosis	
	Anxiety	

and tyrosine, are directly involved with the synthesis of L-dopa. The final product of these reactions is DA (Cunningham and Klein, 2007; Figure 9.8).

This neurotransmitter is found exclusively in the CNS because L-dopa does not cross the BBB. It is found in the basal ganglia and limbic system as well as other areas of the brain. Depending on the receptor site, it can be both excitatory and inhibitory. DA is responsible for autonomic functions, posture, fine motor movements, attention, cognition, sociability, motivation, and reward (Hedges and Burchfield, 2006; refer to Table 9.1).

There have been five receptor sites identified for DA, but only two of them are commonly used. DA is degraded by two different enzymes, monoamine oxidase (MAO-B) and catechol-O-methyltransferase (COMT). Both of these enzymes are found in the synaptic gap and deactivate DA. The majority of DA is reabsorbed by active transport back into the vesicles to be reused (Grilly, 2006).

Norepinephrine/epinephrine

NE and epinephrine are also called *noradrenaline and adrenaline*, respectively. They are synthesized in a similar manner as DA because DA is a precursor of NE and epinephrine (Cunningham and Klein, 2007; Figure 9.9).

These catacholamines are produced throughout the CNS and PNS, including the pons, hypothalamus, frontal cortex, hippocampus, and adrenal gland (Hedges and Burchfield, 2006). NE and epinephrine are responsible for arousal, dreaming, anxiety, fear, mood, hunger, thirst, attention, and the processing of information (Meyer and Quenzer, 2005). These neurotransmitters have been implicated in attention-deficit hyperactivity disorder as well as depression (Hedges and Burchfield, 2006; refer to Table 9.1).

There are two catecholamine receptors that differ in shape and affinity. These receptors are referred to as *alpha and beta*. Each of these receptor types is responsible for specific physiological effects. Similarly to DA, MAO-B and COMT can degrade NE and epinephrine,

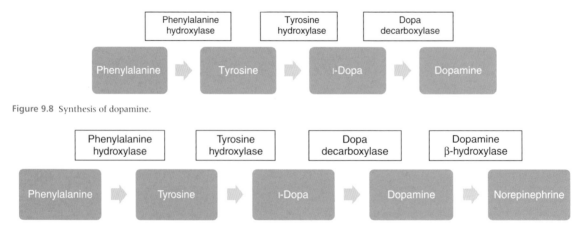

Figure 9.8 Synthesis of dopamine.

Figure 9.9 Synthesis of norepinephrine.

Figure 9.10 Synthesis of serotonin.

but the primary mechanism is reuptake into the vesicles (Meyer and Quenzer, 2005).

Serotonin

The synthesis of 5-HT occurs in two steps and involves the essential amino acid tryptophan (Figure 9.10; Carlson, 2002).

5-HT is found in both the CNS and the PNS and is involved in a wide array of physiological processes. In the CNS, 5-HT is synthesized in cell bodies found in the brainstem (Hedges and Burchfield, 2006). 5-HT regulates mood, anxiety, appetite, sleep, arousal, metabolism, the regulation of pain, and, to some degree, aggression (refer to Table 9.1).

Nine receptors have been identified and mediate the effects of 5-HT. The receptors most commonly associated with behavior are the type 1A and 2A receptors. The primary mode of termination is by reuptake through active transport (Carlson, 2002; Grilly, 2006).

Gamma-Aminobutyric acid

Gamma-Aminobutyric acid (GABA) is a product of glucose and glutamic acid and is widely distributed throughout the CNS. GABA is the primary inhibitory neurotransmitter in the brain and is responsible for reducing anxiety, promoting sleep, reducing seizure activity, and producing muscle relaxation (Carlson, 2002; refer to Table 9.1).

GABA receptors are complex and involve five binding sites. Each binding site has an affinity for a different drug. The first site is for GABA itself, the second is for a class of drugs commonly used in behavior modification called *the benzodiazepines*, the third is for barbiturates, the fourth for steroids, and the fifth for a poison found in an East Indian shrub (Carlson, 2002; Grilly, 2006).

Glutamate

Glutamate is the primary excitatory neurotransmitter and is widely distributed throughout the CNS. It is involved in sensory and motor function, learning, memory, and cognition (refer to Table 9.1). Glutamate interacts with other neurotransmitters to achieve numerous functions (Hedges and Burchfield, 2006).

Glutamate has three main receptors: kainate, metabotropic, and N-methyl-D-aspartate (NMDA). The kainate receptor is involved with epilepsy, the metabotropic receptor is implicated with anxiety, and the NMDA receptor plays an important role in learning, memory, and in the development of psychosis. The NMDA receptor is complicated and is continually under investigation for its potential involvement in learning and a variety of mental disorders.

Pharmacokinetics

Pharmacokinetics is defined as the movement of drugs into, through, and out of the body and includes the processes of absorption, distribution, metabolism, and excretion (Bill, 2006).

The most common methods of medication administration include intravenous injection (IV), intramuscular injection (IM), subcutaneous injection (SC), oral administration (PO), and transdermal absorption. Once drugs have been administered, they are absorbed from the site of administration into systemic circulation and distributed to the site of action (McCurnin and Bassert, 2006). Drugs interact with biologic tissues and vary in their effectiveness based on the binding affinity and specificity with receptors at the site of action. In the case of psychoactive medications, these sites of action are generally receptors in the CNS. However, most drugs have more than one site of action and can produce undesirable side effects. The goal of drug therapy is to administer a dose that maximizes the intended effect and minimizes side effects (Bill, 2006; Grilly, 2006).

> • The goal of drug therapy is to administer a dose that maximizes the intended effect and minimizes side effects.

Drugs may be either metabolized and excreted or excreted without being metabolized. Although enzymes in the brain destroy certain drugs, most metabolism of drugs occurs in the liver. Drugs or their metabolites are

CHAPTER 9

primarily excreted by the renal and hepatic systems. Other routes of elimination include skin, lungs, saliva, and through breast milk (Hedges and Burchfield, 2006; McCurnin and Bassert, 2006).

The half-life of a drug is the measurement of time that it takes for the maximum blood concentration to decrease to half after equilibrium. Therefore, the half-life is the amount of time for half of the drug to be eliminated from the system (Bill, 2006; McCurnin and Bassert, 2006).

Steady state is attained when serum concentrations from repeated administrations reach a state of equilibrium between doses administered and the amount of drug eliminated in a given time interval. The steady state can be calculated by multiplying the half-life by five (McCurnin and Bassert, 2006). The therapeutic window is the ideal range of a drug concentration. Drug concentrations below the range of the therapeutic window generally do not produce therapeutic effects. Alternately, drug concentrations above the range of the therapeutic window may show signs of toxicity. The goal of drug therapy is to reach steady state within the therapeutic window (Bill, 2006).

> • The goal of drug therapy is to reach steady state within the therapeutic window.

Drugs act through receptors. Drugs that bind to a receptor and block a natural neurotransmitter are called *antagonists* and inhibit the effects of a neurotransmitter. Drugs that bind to a receptor and activate the receptor to stimulate the cell are called *agonists* and facilitate or imitate the effects of a neurotransmitter (Bill, 2006). Psychoactive drugs work primarily through their variable agonist or antagonist roles, resulting in a shift in the balance of neurotransmitters or other active nervous system chemicals.

> • Psychoactive drugs work primarily through their variable agonist or antagonist roles, resulting in a shift in the balance of neurotransmitters or other active nervous system chemicals.

Drug categories

Drugs are used as an adjunct therapy to behavior and environmental modification to treat a behavioral problem. With a multifaceted approach to treatment, therapy is more likely to be successful than if either drugs or behavior modification is used alone (Overall, 2001; Horwitz and Mills, 2002).

> • With a multifaceted approach to treatment, therapy is more likely to be successful than if either drugs or behavior modification is used alone (Overall, 2001; Horwitz and Mills, 2002).

Giving an animal a behavioral drug with the intent to sedate it or slow down its reaction in order to address its behavioral problem is an inappropriate use of medication (Overall, 2004).

Before adding a medication as part of a treatment plan to address a behavioral problem, certain requirements should be met. First, it is imperative that a veterinarian–client–patient relationship has been established before prescribing psychoactive medications. The pet should undergo a thorough medical and behavioral history, as well as a physical examination and complete laboratory evaluation, including a complete blood count (CBC), chemistry profile, urinalysis, and thyroid panel. The clinician overseeing the case should have determined a working behavior diagnosis or diagnoses. In addition, he or she should be aware of side effects, drug interactions, and contraindications associated with the drug of choice (Overall, 2004). It is imperative that a diagnosis is made so an appropriate drug can be chosen; this prevents just treating behavioral signs (symptoms). These drugs are intended to address the specific underlying neurochemical mechanisms associated with the behavioral diagnosis and to help make implementation of the behavioral treatment plan easier to accomplish for the owner (Overall, 2004).

Most psychoactive medications are used off label for animals. Only a few have been approved for veterinary use by the Food and Drug Administration (FDA) in dogs to treat specific behavioral problems. Whenever possible, FDA-approved medications should be used before an alternative or generic medication. When an FDA-approved medication is not available for the diagnosis or for the species of intent, the owner should be counseled on the off label use of the chosen medication.

There are several different indications for the use of medications in a behavioral treatment plan. General indications include drug desensitization, failure of a treatment plan that initially comprised a behavior modification plan alone, or to address a behavioral problem that has a medical component.

The goal of drug desensitization is to address the suspected pathologic dysfunction of the neurotransmitter system, leading to or worsening the behavioral disorder? In addition, it can help to make behavior modification easier to apply, giving the owner a starting point for desensitization, and improving compliance and treatment success.

Specific indications include anxieties, such as separation anxiety, generalized anxiety, fears, and phobias; compulsive disorders, cognitive dysfunction syndrome, hyperkinesis, which is a rare pathologic hyperexcitability disorder, and aggression. When addressing a problem that includes aggression as a symptom, it is important to keep in mind some critical points. Firstly, there are no FDA-approved drugs for use in aggression. Secondly, there is always a degree of risk of disinhibition (loss of conscious control of the aggressive response), although this risk varies with the drug class chosen. Understanding the mechanism of action as well as label indications and contraindications of all drugs is imperative before prescribing or administering them. There is also a significant liability risk when treating aggression. The use of liability release forms for aggression as well as off label drug use is encouraged.

> • Understanding the mechanism of action as well as label indications and contraindications of all drugs is imperative before prescribing or administering them.

Several drug classes are discussed in this section. They include the tranquilizers/neuroleptics/antipsychotics, the anxiolytics, the antidepressants, including the tricyclic antidepressants (TCAs), selective serotonin reuptake inhibitors (SSRIs), and the monoamine oxidase inhibitors (MAOIs), the mood stabilizers, the atypical antidepressants, CNS stimulants, and a few other miscellaneous drugs (Table 9.2).

Tranquilizers/neuroleptics/antipsychotics

In this category, phenothiazines have historically been the most commonly used for behavioral reasons. In people, they are used for tranquilization and for the treatment of psychosis and behavioral arousal.

The mechanism of action mainly centers on the blocking of DA (D2) receptors, which leads to a decrease in spontaneous activity. In people, this is called *ataraxia* or a blunting of both normal and abnormal responses. While in this state, the ability to learn is often impaired.

Side effect presentation and severity typically depend on whether a high-potency or low-potency phenothazine is administered. The most common presentation seen in dogs and cats is tranquilization, hypotension, and some concern of decreased seizure threshold (Plumb, 2002, although Tobias *et al.*, 2006). Additional side effects may be seen with longer term use or the use of high-potency medications. These may include neuroleptic malignant syndrome, extrapyramidal signs, and tardive dyskinesia. Neuroleptic malignant syndrome is a rare and idiosyncratic syndrome mainly seen in people. It is expressed as autonomic system instability manifested by muscle rigidity, altered levels of consciousness, hyperthermia, and tachycardia (Simpson and Simpson, 1996). Extrapyramidal signs include resting tremors or stiffness or decreased movement of the facial muscles. Akathisia, identified by motor restlessness, agitation, and pacing, has been noted in some animals (Simpson and Simpson, 1996). Acute dystonia, described as abrupt onset facial and neck muscle spasms, has also been noted (Simpson and Papich, 2003). Tardive dyskinesia, described as facial contortions, abnormal movements of the tongue and mouth, or twisting postures that can affect the face, limbs, and trunk, is mainly seen in people after long-term administration of antipsychotics (Simpson and Simpson, 1996; Simpson and Papich, 2003).

Acepromazine is a low-potency phenothiazine and historically has been one of the most frequently used drugs to decrease mobility and reactivity in veterinary patients in an attempt to address undesirable behaviors. It has a wide variety of uses, including a preanesthetic agent, an antiemetic (Plumb, 2002), and for "aid in controlling intractable animals" (PromAce®–package insert. Fort Dodge). A state of profound sedation with a poor anxiolytic effect is typically seen. This, along with the antiemetic effect, makes it an appropriate choice for preanesthesia but can leave the animal more reactive to noises potentially resulting in a startle response, so caution should be taken with handling an animal under the influence of acepromazine. Unfortunately, its effect merely slows down the pet's physical reaction, whereas the mental anxiety the pet is experiencing remains minimally affected. This makes acepromazine an inappropriate choice for use alone in animals with noise phobias or other anxieties, as it has been historically used.

> • This makes acepromazine an inappropriate choice for use alone in animals with noise phobias or other anxieties.

Table 9.2 Common veterinary behavior medications.

Class	Drug family	Drug	Indications	Time to effect	Side effects	Contraindications
Tranquilizers/ neuroleptics/ antipsychotic	Phenothiazine	Acepromazine PromAce	Chemical restrain, tranquilization, preanesthetic	Oral: 1–2 h Injectable: 15 min	Hypotension, decreased seizure threshold (?), tranquilization, behavioral disinhibition, decreased learning, paradoxical excitation	Not beneficial for anxiolysis, noise phobia, separation anxiety. Caution with aggression
Anxiolytic	Azapirone – serotonin 1A receptor agonist	Buspirone, Buspar	Anxiety, fear, mild phobias	4–6 weeks for maximal effect	Behavioral changes in cats	Do not use in conjunction with MAOIs
	Benzodiazepine – GABA receptor potentiation	Diazepam, Valium	Fear response, panic	Oral: 1–2 h	Sedation, muscle relaxation, polyphagia, behavioral disinhibition, paradoxical excitation, acute hepatic necrosis (cats)	Caution with aggression
	Benzodiazepine	Alprazolam, Xanex	Fear response, panic	Oral: 1–2 h	Same as diazepam, thought to be less sedating	Caution with aggression
	Benzodiazepine	Clonazepam, Klonopin	Fear response, panic	Oral: 1–2 h	Same as diazepam; thought to produce less sedation and less polyphagia	Caution with aggression
	Benzodiazepine	Lorazepam, Ativan	Fear response, panic	Oral: 1–2 h	Same as diazepam; possibly safer on the liver in cats	Caution with aggression
Antidepressant	Selective serotonin reuptake inhibitor (SSRI)	Fluoxetine, Prozac, Reconcile* *Reconcile is FDA approved for treating Separation anxiety in dogs	Anxiety, chronic fear, compulsive disorder, aggression	4–6 weeks for maximal effect	Mild lethargy, anorexia Nausea, vomiting, diarrhea, constipation, insomnia, increased agitation, tremors, increased anxiety, increased aggression	Do not use in conjunction with MAOIs, TCAs, other SSRIs; Caution with tramadol, other serotoninergic drugs
		Paroxetine, Paxil	Same as fluoxetine	4–6 weeks for maximal effect	Same as fluoxetine plus: Urinary retention, constipation	Same as fluoxetine
		Sertraline, Zoloft	Same as fluoxetine	4–6 weeks for maximal effect	Same as fluoxetine	Same as fluoxetine
		Citalopram,Celexa	Same as fluoxetine	4–6 weeks for maximal effect	Same as fluoxetine plus: Increased cardiac sensitivity in dogs	Same as fluoxetine
	Tricyclic antidepressant (TCA)	Clomipramine, Clomicalm* *Clomicalm is FDA approved to treat separation anxiety in dogs	Anxiety, chronic fear, compulsive disorder	3–4 weeks for maximal effect	Sedation, anticholinergic effects: dry mouth, dry eye, mydriasis, urine retention, constipation, tachycardia or other arrhythmia; antihistaminic effect; aggression	Do not use in conjunction with MAOIs, SSRIs, other TCAs; Glaucoma, keratoconjunctivitis sicca (KCS- dry eye), cardiac arrhythmias, seizures, urinary retention, or thyroid disease

Class	Mechanism/Description	Drug	Indication	Onset	Side effects	Contraindications
		Amitriptyline, Elavil	Same as clomipramine	3–4 weeks for maximal effect	Same as clomipramine	Same as clomipramine
		Imipramine, Tofranil	Same as clomipramine	3–4 weeks for maximal effect	Same as clomipramine	Same as clomipramine
		Doxepin, Sinequan	Same as clomipramine	3–4 weeks for maximal effect	Same as clomipramine plus: Strong antihistaminic effect	Same as clomipramine
	Monoamine oxidase inhibitor (MAOI)	Selegiline, L-deprenyl, Anipryl* *Anipryl is FDA approved for treating cognitive dysfunction syndrome in dogs	Cognitive dysfunction syndrome, anxiety, pituitary dependent hyperadrenocorticism (HAC) in dogs	4–8 weeks for maximal effect	Increased motor activity, vomiting, diarrhea, agitation, restlessness, disorientation, stereotypic behavior with high doses, "Cheese effect"	Do not use in conjunction with other MAOIs (including amitraz), SSRIs, or TCAs. Tramadol, St. John's Wort, Griffonia seed extract, other opioids, alpha-2 agonists, phenylpropanolamine
Mood stabilizer	Antiepileptic drug, tricyclic compound	Carbamazepine	Impulsive, explosive aggression	Unknown in animals	Nausea, dizziness, elevated liver values, blood dyscrasias, dermatologic lesions, aggression	Do not use in conjunction with MAOIs
Atypical antidepressant	Mixed serotonin agonist/antagonist	Trazodone	Anxiety, fear, phobias	1–2 h	Vomiting, diarrhea, sedation, increased anxiety, irritability or aggression	Do not use in conjunction with MAOIs
	Tetracyclic antidepressant/serotonin and norepinephrine reuptake inhibitor	Mirtazapine	Anxiety, chronic fear, appetite stimulation	1 h	Polyphagia, agitation, tremors, muscle twitching, tachycardia, decrease seizure threshold, antinausea, antiemetic effects, and antilibidic effects	Do not use in conjunction with MAOIs
CNS stimulant		Methylphenidate, Ritalin	Hyperkinesis, narcolepsy	Unknown in animals	Hyperactivity, agitation, aggression, hypertension, lower seizure threshold	Do not use in conjunction with MAOIs
		Dextroamphetamine (injectable)	Hyperkinesis, narcolepsy	30 min to 2 h	Same as methylphenidate plus: tremors, GI upset, dry mouth	
Miscellaneous	Alpha-2 agonist	Clonidine	Anxiety, fear, panic	1–2 h	Vomiting, diarrhea, sedation, hypotension, bradycardia, increased anxiety, irritability	Do not use in conjunction with MAOIs

Additional side effects that can be seen with the use of acepromazine include inhibition of learning, making the implementation of behavior modification challenging; and paradoxical excitation, primarily in horses and cats, but can include increased aggressive response and/or the loss of bite inhibition in any species. Therefore, extreme caution should be used, and safety measures such as basket muzzles should be implemented when used in animals with a history of aggression.

> • Therefore, extreme caution should be used, and safety measures such as basket muzzles should be implemented when used in animals with a history of aggression.

Anxiolytics

Anxioytics are a group made up of the benzodiazepines, azapirones, antihistamines, and barbiturates.

Benzodiazepines work by potentiating the inhibitory effect of GABA. This occurs by binding to the GABA A receptor and strengthening the binding of GABA to this receptor. The effects seen include sedation, decreased anxiety, muscle relaxation, seizure control, although these effects tend to be dose dependent. Behaviorally, these medications are used to help treat events connected to intense anxiety or panic, such as thunderstorm or other noise phobias, separation anxiety, or to decrease the fear response in "pariah" or the victim cat in cases of intercat aggression (Lindell *et al.*, 1997). For the maximal anxiolytic effect to be seen, one must administer these medications at least 1 h, sometimes as early as 2 h, before initiation of anxiety-producing stimuli.

Some additional effects may also be seen with the use of benzodiazepines. Increased appetite, sometimes profound, can be noted; this may be beneficial in counteracting the anorexia seen secondary to the use of some antidepressants. Similar to acepromazine, memory deficits can be identified as well. These can be recognized by difficulty in learning new material, or the animal may seem to forget what has been previously taught. Decreasing the ability to learn may be a useful side effect if used during fearful situations, such as a visit to the veterinarian's office when a stressful procedure must be performed on the pet.

Paradoxical reactions, such as idiosyncratic excitation, agitation, and restlessness can also be seen in dogs and cats.

In addition, disinhibition of behaviors can also occur. In people, a loss of conscious inhibition of hostility,

aggression, or rage has been documented. In animals, these medications should be used with extreme caution in aggression, as they can decrease bite inhibition, similar to what can be seen with acepromazine.

Acute hepatic necrosis in cats is a rare, but often fatal, potential side effect of benzodiazepines. It has been documented with diazepam, but the risk is present with the other benzodiazepines as well. There have been cases reported with almost every drug in this class. It is recommended to evaluate liver values before and within 5 days of starting medication when benzodiazepines are used in cats (Center *et al.*, 1996).

> • It is recommended to evaluate liver values before and within 5 days of starting medication when benzodiazepines are used in cats (Center *et al.*, 1996).

These are also class IV controlled substances and do carry a risk of abuse by owners; therefore, additional monitoring and recording of prescriptions is necessary.

These medications can be used as needed for event treatment, such as fireworks associated with holidays. If they are administered chronically, as may be done with separation anxiety, they should be weaned gradually before being discontinued. The general rule is to decrease the administration by 25–30% per week or slower (Schwartz, 2005). This helps prevent recurrence of behavioral signs and withdrawal, such as nervousness, tremors, or seizures.

Several different drugs in this class have been used for anxiety control in dogs and cats. Some more commonly used ones include diazepam (Valium®), alprazolam (Xanax®), clonazepam (Klonopin®), and lorazepam (Ativan®). Each has a relatively short half-life, much shorter than is seen in people, making frequent dosing important. Variation does occur with the half-life, frequency, and intensity of side effects with each drug in the class. All benzodiazepines are metabolized in the liver and excreted through the kidneys, although intermediate metabolites and their effect on the liver vary.

Diazepam may have duration as short as 4 h, leading to a frequent dosing requirement. In addition, some individual pets may experience significant sedation with less anxiolysis. This medication can be quite effective in some individuals. Some experts believe clonazepam may be less sedating and have less of a polyphagic effect relative to other benzodiazepines. Individual responses and variation to dose and effects do occur. Alprazolam has also been considered to have less sedative effect compared to other benzodiazepines.

Some veterinary behaviorists believe that lorazepam may be safer for the liver, as it does not have any intermediate metabolites that must be processed by the liver, although there have been a few cases of acute hepatic necrosis in cats seen with this medication.

The azapirones are another drug class that can be classified as anxiolytic but also have antidepressant effects. Buspirone (Buspar®) is the drug most commonly used in veterinary behavior medicine from this class. It is classified as a 5-HT 1A receptor agonist, as it has very specific affinity for the 5-HT 1A receptors. Its mechanism of action is interesting in that it initially activates autoreceptors, which actually potentiate negative feedback. Over time, however, these receptors will become progressively desensitized as with SSRIs. This leads to enhanced activation of postsynaptic 5-HT 1A receptors (Blier and de Montigny, 1998).

The degree of anxiety control is mild, making buspirone inappropriate for profound panic states. The late receptor reregulation effects results in a delayed anxiolytic response compared to the benzodiazepines. It may take until 4–6 weeks to see the full effect of this medication. The degree of specificity for the 5-HT 1A receptor makes side effects associated with activity at other 5-HT receptor minimal and makes this a relatively safer medication. It can have a bitter taste, making it more difficult to disguise for cats.

> - The degree of anxiety control is mild, making buspirone inappropriate for profound panic states.

Antidepressants

The antidepressant classes that will be discussed include the TCAs, SSRIs, and the MAOIs.

Tricyclic antidepressants

The TCAs are structurally similar to phenothiazines (central three-ring structure) and work by inhibiting the reuptake of NE and 5-HT by the presynaptic plasma membrane transporters. Commonly used drugs in this class include clomipramine (Clomicalm®), amitriptyline (Elavil®), imipramine (Tofranil®), and doxepin (Sinequan®). These are used to treat a variety of anxiety and compulsive disorders, as well as some forms of aggression in dogs and cats. Specific diagnoses applicable to this drug class include separation anxiety, generalized anxiety, compulsive disorders, such as lick granulomas or psychogenic alopecia, and anxiety-related urine

marking. Additional effects include adrenergic effects, such as sedation or syncope; anticholinergic effects, such as dry mouth, dry eye, mydriasis, urine retention, constipation, tachycardia, or other arrhythmias; and antihistaminic effects. Clomipramine and doxepin show the most antihistaminic effects in this drug class. Clomipramine administration has been associated with changes in measured thyroid levels. Although it is not thought to cause clinical hypothyroidism in dogs, it can complicate monitoring maintenance levels in dogs currently being treated for hypothyroid disease (Crowell-Davis and Murray, 2006).

These drugs have a narrower therapeutic window than the SSRIs. An overdose of a tricyclic antidepressant near 15 mg/kg can lead to death by fatal cardiac arrhythmia within hours (Johnson, 1990, Simpson and Papich, 2003). Cats tend to be more sensitive to TCAs than dogs. This is most likely because these drugs are metabolized by glucuronidation.

TCAs may take 3–4 weeks for maximal effect. TCAs should be weaned gradually if they are to be discontinued after 3–4 weeks of use. TCA are contraindicated in patients with glaucoma, keratoconjunctivitis sicca (KCS-dry eye), cardiac arrhythmias, seizures, urinary retention, or thyroid disease. They should not be used with MAOIs, as this greatly increases the risk of serotonin syndrome. After discontinuing a TCA, a minimum of 14 days should elapse before starting a MAOI. Clomipramine is more specific for 5-HT than other TCAs. Dogs metabolize clomipramine faster than people do. The half-life in dogs is approximately 5 h compared to 24 h in people. The label dose for clomipramine formulated as Clomicalm® is 2–4 mg/kg q 24 h; however, many experts agree that it may be more efficacious when administered every 12 h rather than every 24 h in dogs (Landsburg *et al.*, 2003; Crowell-Davis and Murray 2006).

Clomicalm®, manufactured by Novartis, is a chewable flavored tablet formulation of clomipramine that is labeled for separation anxiety in dogs. It is not recommended for use in aggressive dogs per the label.

Selective serotonin reuptake inhibitors

SSRIs are derivatives of TCAs. Their mechanism of action is by inhibiting the reuptake of 5-HT by the presynaptic plasma membrane transporters. They also desensitize the 5-HT1A autoreceptors over time.

Commonly used drugs in this class include fluoxetine (Reconcile® and Prozac®), paroxetine (Paxil®), sertraline (Zoloft®), and citalopram (Celexa®). They are used to treat various anxieties, fears, aggressions, and compulsive disorders in dogs and cats. They tend to have fewer side effects than TCAs and a safer therapeutic window. Owing to the reregulation of some of the receptors, expect 4–6 weeks to see the full therapeutic effect. As with many of the other medications already discussed, SSRIs should be weaned off gradually when dosing chronically.

Additional effects include mild lethargy or anorexia, although these are usually mild and resolve within 1–2 weeks. More concerning side effects include nausea, vomiting, diarrhea, constipation, insomnia, increased agitation, tremors, increased anxiety, and rarely, increased aggression. Individual variation within the spectrum of side effects can be seen.

As with TCAs, SSRIs should not be used in combination with MAOIs because of the risk of serotonin syndrome. When changing from fluoxetine to a MAOI, it is recommended to wait 5 weeks after discontinuing the fluoxetine before starting the MAOI. Fourteen days should elapse after discontinuance of a MAOI and beginning a SSRI. SSRIs should be used cautiously when the patient is concurrently administered with tramadol, as this synthetic opiate analgesic also has 5-HT and NE reuptake activity, and this combination can lead to serotonin syndrome. It has been documented that dogs have an increased cardiac sensitivity to citalopram (Celexa®); therefore, use with caution in this species (Celexa Product information, 2013).

Fluoxetine

A common human trade name for fluoxetine is Prozac®, and the veterinary trade name is Reconcile®. Fluoxetine is considered to be less likely to disinhibit aggression than other behavior modifying drugs commonly used.

The generic, tablet, and capsule form of fluoxetine is inexpensive. Transdermal formulations of fluoxetine have been used in cats to ease daily administration. Unfortunately, there is no evidence at this time that transdermal formulations result in consistent and therapeutic blood levels; therefore, rendering this formulation type ineffective and potentially harmful in cats (Ciribassi et al., 2003).

Lilly/ Elanco's product, Reconcile®, is a flavored chewable tablet that is labeled for separation anxiety in conjunction with a behavior modification plan in dogs. This formulation is not recommended for use in aggression per the label.

Paroxetine

Paroxetine (Paxil®) is another SSRI related to fluoxetine. It may be more likely to have anticholinergic side effects, such as urine retention or constipation, and these may be more apparent in cats. Slowly titrating the dose over the first week can help to avoid or alleviate side effects, and the patient should be monitored closely. Paroxetine, in some opinions, may be less likely to cause agitation that is sometimes seen with fluoxetine. It also has a shorter half-life than fluoxetine.

Monoamine oxidase inhibitors

MAOIs work by blocking oxidative deamination or breakdown of intracellular monoamine neurotransmitters (5-HT, NE, and DA) by the enzyme, monoamine oxidase, found within the mitochondria. There are two types of MAOs and MAOIs, types A and B. Type A breaks down mainly 5-HT, NE, DA, and tyramine, whereas type B preferentially destroys phenylethylamine and DA. The drugs that inhibit MAO-A are considered less selective and not routinely used in veterinary medicine. It is interesting to note that the degree of inhibition of each neurotransmitter is species specific, and individual variation can be seen within any species.

Selegiline

Selegiline, also known as L-deprenyl or Anipryl®, is the only MAOI currently used in veterinary behavior medicine. Selegiline is used primarily for Parkinson's and Alzheimer's diseases in people but used for cognitive dysfunction syndrome (CDS) in dogs and cats. Anipryl® is labeled for pituitary-dependent hyperadrenocorticism (HAC) in dogs and for cognitive dysfunction syndrome in dogs.

Selegiline has additional mechanisms of action beyond inhibiting the breakdown of neurotransmitters by monoamine in the mitochondria. It also inhibits the presynaptic reuptake of DA, NE, and 5-HT. In addition, it modulates DA levels by inhibiting some autoreceptors, preventing degradation, and increasing turnover. It decreases oxidative stress secondary to the DA degradation and may also enhance the action of superoxide dismutase and catalase, two free radical scavengers that help to increase the elimination of free radicals. It also increases levels of phenylethylamine, which is a neuromodulator of DA responses. It helps to increase the release and decrease the reuptake of DA (Campbell et al., 2001, Crowell-Davis and Murray, 2006, Pfizer, Inc., 1998).

The many different actions of selegiline lead to a variety of effects seen in the patient. These include elevated mood or decreased anxiety. Anxiolysis is one of the main uses of this drug for veterinary behavioral therapy in Europe.

Selegiline has also been shown to decrease oxidative damage (Campbell et al., 2001; Crowell-Davis and Murray, 2006; Pfizer, Inc., 1998). This is important because oxidative damage of DA pathways is considered a significant mechanism in the pathogenesis of Parkinson's disease, and free radicals also contribute to Alzheimer's disease in people and CDS in animals.

High doses may cause stereotypic behaviors because of the increase in DA. Motor activity may be increased as a result of selegiline's metabolic products, including amphetamine and methamphetamine, as well as phenylethylamine, which also has amphetamine effects. It is therefore recommended to administer this medication in the morning so the pet does not keep the owner up at night. In addition, vomiting, diarrhea, agitation, restlessness, or disorientation may be occasionally seen. Because of the metabolic products, this drug does have the potential for abuse by people, so monitoring and recording of prescriptions are recommended.

Before administering an MAOI, it is important to be aware of all medications, including parasiticides and herbal remedies that the pet is taking. MAOIs should not be used concurrently with other TCAs, SSRIs, or MAOIs, as there is a significant risk of developing serotonin syndrome or toxicity with these combinations. Serotonin syndrome occurs when the concentration of 5-HT in the brain becomes too high, reaching toxic levels. Clinical signs that can be seen include nausea, confusion, agitation, muscle rigidity, tremors, salivation, hyperthermia and may lead to seizures, coma, and death. This is most commonly the result of an MAOI combined with another antidepressant (usually a TCA or SSRI), and the inhibition of neurotransmitter degradation from the MAOI is coupled with reuptake inhibition from the antidepressant but can occur with other combinations as well. Multiple MAOIs should not be combined. Amitraz, a topical parasiticide is also an MAOI. It is found in Mitaban®, Preventic® collars, and the spot on flea and tick treatment, CERTIFECT™. Other combinations can potentially lead to serotonin syndrome. Diets high in tryptophan could also create this because the amino acid tryptophan is the precursor to 5-HT. Some over-the-counter herbal supplements can have this unintended effect also. St. John's Wort can act as MAOI or broad spectrum reuptake inhibitor (Schwartz, 2005), and Griffonia seed extract is comprised of 5-hydroxytryptophan, another part of the synthesis of 5-HT (Crowell-Davis and Murray, 2006). Other medications commonly used to manage concurrent disease processes in older patients can also negatively interact with selegiline. The synthetic opiate analgesic, tramadol, has 5-HT and NE reuptake actions. There have been case reports of agitation, stupor, and death when selegiline was combined with other opioids. Caution should be used when these medications are

combined or used concurrently (Plumb, 2002). Extreme fluctuations in blood pressure can occur when selegiline is combined with phenylpropanolamine (PPA), a drug commonly used for urinary incontinence, or alpha-2 agonists.

- Before administering an MAOI, it is important to be aware of all medications, including parasiticides and herbal remedies that the pet is taking.

There is also an interaction called *the cheese effect* that occurs more commonly in people, but there have been a few cases reported in individual animals. It occurs when larger amounts of certain cheeses or wine are ingested while taking an MAOI, and the level of tyramine in the gut increases because MAOIs prevent inactivation of tyramine, which leads to increased NE. This can create a phenomenon in which vasoconstriction and an increase in blood pressure occur simultaneously, leading to a hypertensive crisis. This is more likely to occur with nonselective MAOIs (MAOA-Is) but could potentially occur in sensitive individuals. Therefore, it may be prudent to limit the pet's cheese intake with concurrent use of selegiline (selegiline FDA professional monograph).

Mood stabilizers

Mood stabilizers are used to mediate extreme changes in mood and help treat mania and depression in people, particularly lithium. Many have historically been used to facilitate seizure control, particularly valproic acid and carbamazepine. Their behavioral effects aim to decrease impulsivity, emotional reactivity, and aggression. They are uncommonly used in veterinary behavior medicine.

Carbamazepine has a similar structure to TCAs and acts on ion channels to decrease high-frequency repetitive firing. This was the mechanism implicated for seizure control, although its short half-life makes it less effective in this regard. It also has other nonspecific actions on many neurotransmitters, and its psychotropic mode of action is unknown. Carbamazepine is generally used for impulsive, explosive aggression but almost always in conjunction with other behavior modifying drugs. Side effects to be aware of and to monitor for include nausea, dizziness, elevated liver values, blood dyscrasias, and dermatologic lesions. At minimum, a CBC and chemistry panel should be checked before starting therapy and again 1 month after treatment or after a dose increase.

Atypical antidepressants

There are several atypical antidepressants that are becoming more frequently used as adjuncts to behavior treatment plans. These include nefazodone (Serzone®), bupropion (Welbutrin®), trazodone (Desyrel®), and mirtazapine (Remeron®), but the list is expanding rapidly (Simpson and Simpson, 1996). Trazodone and mirtazapine are discussed in the following sections.

Trazodone

Trazodone is a mixed 5-HT agonist/antagonist. It works as a weak inhibitor of 5-HT reuptake at presynaptic 5-HT receptors and as an antagonist at postsynaptic 5-HT receptors. The active metabolite, *m*-chlorophenylpiperazine, also has some agonistic effect at 5-HT 1 receptors, which may also increase 5-HT by mediating inhibitory effect of GABA (Simpson and Simpson, 1996). Trazodone is commonly used in people as an antidepressant, anxiolytic, sleep aid, and anti-obsessional.

The synergistic effect of trazodone in combination with an SSRI or TCA can be helpful when additional anxiety control is needed, but the risks or side effects of benzodiazepines are too severe (Gruen and Sherman, 2008). Trazodone has also been used alone or as needed for specific events (e.g., fireworks, thunderstorms). It has also been used to facilitate postsurgical crate confinement.

Trazodone typically has minimal anticholinergic effects, but vomiting, diarrhea, or sedation can be noted. These are less likely if the dose is started low and titrated up. Uncommonly, increased anxiety, irritability, or aggression can be seen, and the pet should be monitored for these side effects. This medication has also been reported to have the lowest seizure risk of the drugs in the antidepressant class (Gruen and Sherman, 2008).

Mirtazapine

Mirtazapine is considered a second generation or tetracyclic antidepressant that works through presynaptic alpha-2 adrenergic receptor antagonist activity and increases 5-HT and NE activity (Quimby *et al.*, 2011). Traditionally, mirtazapine was used as an antidepressant in human medicine but has also been commonly used as an appetite stimulant in cats. It does have anxiety decreasing effects in dogs and cats. Additional effects to note include antinausea, antiemetic effects, and antilibidic effects (Quimby *et al.*, 2011; Coskun *et al.*, 2009). As typical for drugs in behavior medicine, there is a potential risk for increased irritability and serotonin syndrome. Owing to the lack of glucuronidation capabilities in the cat, it is administered typically every 72 h rather than daily as in the dog.

CNS stimulants

CNS stimulants are uncommonly used in veterinary behavior medicine and are indicated for a few behavioral disorders, mainly for narcolepsy or hyperkinesis (pathologic hyperactivity) in dogs. There are several side effects associated with this class of medication because of the stimulant nature of these drugs. They are contraindicated in patients with glaucoma, heart disease, or an animal that has taken MAOIs in the last 14 days (Crowell-Davis and Murray, 2006).

Dextroamphetamine is an injectable formulation, which can be used in the clinic to attempt to diagnose hyperkinesis, as its effect occurs rapidly but has short duration. It is rarely used.

Methylphenidate (Ritalin) works by enhancing DA release and inhibiting DA and NE reuptake. This leads to a paradoxical calming effect in some overactivity disorders, learning deficits, or some types of aggression in people. Methylphenidate is indicated for narcolepsy and hyperkinesis in dogs but is contraindicated in dogs showing hyperactivity from other causes, such as conditioned behaviors. True hyperkinesis is rare. Diagnosis confirmation with a drug trial using methylphenidate should only be undertaken if behavior modification treatment for the other differentials for hyperactivity has failed and the clinician has a strong suspicion for hyperkinesis as a differential diagnosis. The medication is typically started at a low dose and incrementally increased every 1–2 days. If at any point, the hyperactivity worsens, the drug trial is discontinued. The dose titration is important because the effect on the patient's activity level usually falls in a reverse bell curve effect. A lower dose may be ineffective, seen as no change in the degree of hyperactivity, but as the dose is incrementally increased, a point in which the activity level drops dramatically will be found. This will be considered near the therapeutic dose for that individual dog. If the dose increase is continued, the dog's activity will increase back to baseline and potentially even higher.

Miscellaneous drugs

Clonidine is a centrally acting alpha-2 agonist used to control blood pressure in people but is also thought to have some analgesic and anxiolytic effects because it can decrease NE release in the brain (Schweimer *et al.*, 2005). Clonidine can be administered as needed for fear-inducing situations up to every 12 h. It may take up to 2 h for the anxiolytic effect and is expected to have a duration of 4–6 h (Ogata and Dodman, 2011). Starting with a low dose and titrating up to effect is recommended. In people, it is mainly metabolized in the liver and excreted in urine. Potential side effects to monitor

Table 9.3 Possible indications for drug therapy.

Behavior disorder or other considerations	
Fear and/or anxieties	Multiple stimuli
	Stimuli cannot be avoided
	Intensity of stimuli cannot be controlled
	Cannot determine a nonstressful starting point for desensitization to begin
	Self injurious behavior
Aggression	Multiple triggers
	Triggers cannot be identified
	Triggers cannot be managed or avoided
	Threshold for aggression very low
	Little warning before aggressive response
	Nongraduated response
Compulsive disorder	Decrease frequency/intensity of behavior so behavior modification possible
	Decrease frequency/intensity of conflict behaviors that have the potential for developing into a compulsive behavior (usually from frustration)
Cognitive dysfunction	Slow progression of cognitive dysfunction
	Adjunct symptomatic therapy if new fears and anxieties, insomnia develop
Condition of the human–animal bond	Broken or severely damaged human–animal bond
	Owner is afraid of the pet
	Owner contemplating euthanasia or rehoming, seeking help as a "last resort"

for include vomiting, diarrhea, hypotension, tachycardia or bradycardia, sedation, increased irritability or anxiety, or anticholinergic effects. In order to monitor cardiovascular side effects, it may be prudent to measure heart rate in animals taking this medication and compare it to the individual's baseline. Additional research with this medication in veterinary behavior is ongoing.

Conclusion

The nervous system is a complexity of neurons and neurotransmitters communicating important information at specific moments. The brain is the most intricate of all the organs in the body. The various structures in the brain work in conjunction to attain life and personality. There are over 50 neurotransmitters in the body, but the neurotransmitters most commonly associated with behavior are the monoamines and GABA. There are many different drugs and drug classes that can be useful tools in the comprehensive treatment plan for behavioral disorders. Whether the main diagnosis centers around fear and anxiety, compulsive disorder, aggression, cognitive dysfunction, or hyperkinesis, the same basic plan should be followed for every patient to make an educated decision on whether drugs are indicated (see Table 9.3), and if so, which is the most appropriate drug for that case. A thorough behavior and medical

history should be obtained, and a working diagnosis should be made by a licensed doctor of veterinary medicine after a doctor–client–patient relationship has been established. Potential drug interactions or concurrent illnesses should be identified prior to medication being prescribed. The client should be educated about side effects, contraindications, and length of time to effect for the medication prescribed for his or her pet. Adequate follow-up with the client and patient is imperative to monitor treatment success and to make adjustments as needed.

By obtaining a thorough understanding of neurophysiology, pharmacokinetics, and psychopharmacology, a veterinary technician can be prepared to assist and educate clients regarding the treatment of their pet's behavioral disorders, thus helping to preserve the human–animal bond.

References

Bill, R.L. (2006) *Clinical Pharmacology and Therapeutics for the Veterinary Technician*, 3rd edn, Mosby Inc., St. Louis, MO.

Blier, P. and de Montigny, C. (1998) Possible Serotonergic mechanisms underlying the antidepressant and anti-obsessive–compulsive disorder responses. *Biological Psychiatry*, **53**, 193–203.

Campbell, S., Trettien, A. and Kozan, B. (2001) A noncomparative open-label study evaluating the effect of selegiline hydrochloride in a clinical setting. *Veterinary Therapeutics*, **2** (1), 24–39.

Carlson, N.R. (2002) *Foundations of Physiological Psychology*, 5th edn, A Pearson Education, Inc., Boston, MA.

Celexa Product information 2013, Forest Pharmaceuticals; Warner-Lambert Company, St. Louis, MO.

Center, S.A., Elston, T.H. and Rowland, P.H. (1996) Fulminant hepatic failure associated with oral administration of diazepam in 11 cats. *Journal of the American Veterinary Medical Association*, **209**, 618–625.

Ciribassi, J., Luescher, A. and Pasloske, K.S. (2003) Comparative bioavailability of fluoxetine after transdermal and oral administration to healthy cats. *American Journal of Veterinary Research*, **64** (8), 994–998.

Coskun, M., Karakoc, S., Kircelli, F. and Mukaddes, N.M. (2009) Effectiveness of mirtazapine in the treatment of inappropriate sexual behaviors in individuals with autistic disorder. *Journal of Child and Adolescent Psychopharmacology*, **19** (2), 203–206.

Crowell-Davis, S. and Murray, T. (2006) *Veterinary Psychopharmacology*, Blackwell Publishing Company, Ames.

Cunningham, J.G. and Klein, B.G. (2007) *Textbook of Veterinary Physiology*, 4th edn, Elsevier, Philadelphia, PA.

Grilly, D.M. (2006) *Drugs and Human Behavior*, 5th edn, Pearson Education, Inc., Boston, MA.

Gruen, M. and Sherman, B. (2008) Use of trazodone as an adjunctive agent in the treatment of canine anxiety disorders: 56 cases (1995–2007). *Journal of American Veterinary Medical Association*, **233**, 1902–1907.

Hedges, D. and Burchfield, C. (2006) *Mind, Brain and Drug: An Introduction to Psychopharmacology*, Pearson Education, Inc., Boston, MA.

Horwitz, D. and Mills, D.S. (2002) *BSAVA Manual of Canine and Feline Behavioural Medicine*, British Small Animal Veterinary Association, Quedgeley, Gloucester.

Johnson, L.R. (1990) Tricyclic antidepressant toxicosis. *Veterinary Clinics of North America, Small Animal Practice*, **20**, 393–403.

King, A.S. (1987) *Physiological and Clinical Anatomy of the Domestic Mammals*, Oxford University Press, Oxford.

Landsburg, G., Hunthausen, W. and Ackerman, L. (2003) *Handbook of Behavior Problems of the Dog and Cat*, 2nd edn, Saunders, Edinburgh.

Lindell, E.M., Erb, H.N. and Houpt, K.A. (1997) Intercat aggression: a retrospective study examining types of aggression, sexes of fighting pairs, and effectiveness of treatment. *Applied Animal Behaviour Science*, **55**, 153–162.

McCurnin, D.M. and Bassert, J.M. (2006) *Clinical Textbook for Veterinary Technicians*, 6th edn, Elsevier Saunders, St. Louis, MO.

Meyer, J.S. and Quenzer, L.F. (2005) *Psychopharmacology Drugs, The Brain, and Behavior*, Sinauer Associates Inc., Sunderland, MA.

Ogata, N. and Dodman, N. (2011) The use of clonidine in the treatment of fear-based behavior problems in dogs: an open trial. *Journal of Veterinary Behavior.*, **6**, 130–137.

Overall, K. (2001) Pharmacologic treatment in behavioral medicine: the importance of neurochemistry, molecular biology and mechanistic hypotheses. *The Veterinary Journal*, **162**, 9–23.

Overall, K. (2004) Paradigms for pharmacologic use as a treatment component in feline behavioral medicine. *Journal of Feline Medicine and Surgery*, **6**, 29–42.

Pfizer, Inc. (1998) *Freedom of Informations Summary: Anipryl® (selegiline hydrochloride) tablets for use in dogs*, Pfizer Inc., Groton, CT.

Plumb, D.C. (2002) *Veterinary Drug Handbook*, 4th edn, Iowa State Press, Ames.

PromAce®–Package insert. Fort Dodge 2000. Fort Dodge Animal Health Fort Dodge, Iowa 50501 USA by Fort Dodge Animal Health Fort Dodge, Iowa 50501 USA (Injection) Ayerst Laboratories, Inc. Rouses Point, NY 12979 (Tablets) I 02300 Rev. Aug. 2000 02wc.

Quimby, J.M., Gustafson, D.L., Samber, B.J. and Lunn, K.F. (2011) Studies on the pharmacokinetics and pharmacodynamics of mirtazapine in healthy young cats. *Journal of Veterinary Pharmacology and Therapeutics*, **34** (4), 388–396.

Schwartz, S. (2005) *Psychoactive Herbs in Veterinary Behavior Medicine*, Blackwell Publishing Company, Ames.

Schweimer, J., Fendt, M. and Schnitzler, H.U. (2005) Effects of clonidine injections into the bed nucleus of the stria terminalis on fear and anxiety behavior in rats. *European Journal of Pharmacology*, **507**, 117–124.

Simpson, B. and Simpson, D. (1996) Behavioral pharmacotherapy. Part I. Antipsychotics and Antidepressants. *Compendium on Continuing Education for the Practicing Veterinarian*, **18** (10), 1067–1081.

Simpson, B.S. and Papich, M.G. (2003) Pharmacologic management in veterinary behavioral medicine. *The Veterinary Clinics of North America: Small Animal Practice*, **33**, 365–404.

Tobias, K., Marioni-Henry, K. and Wagner, R. (2006) A retrospective study on the use of acepromazine maleate in dogs with seizures. *Journal of the American Animal Hospital Association.*, **42**, 283–289.

Further reading

Dodman, N. and Shuster, L. (1998) *Psychopharmacology of Animal Behavior Disorders*, Blackwell Science, Malden.

Caspi, A., Sugden, K. and Moffitt, T.E. (2003) Influence of life stress on depression: moderation by a polymorphism in the 5-HTT gene. *Science*, **301** (291–293), 386–389.

Hariri, A.R., Mattay, V.S., Tessitore, A. *et al.* (2002) Serotonin transporter genetic variation and the response of the human amygdala. *Science*, **297**, 400–403.

Wanamaker, B.P. and Massey, K.L. (2009) *Applied Pharmacology for Veterinary Technicians*, Saunders Elsevier, St. Louis, MO.

Appendix Section 1
Forms and questionnaires

The appendices can be downloaded and printed at www.wiley.com/go/shaw/behavior

Appendix 1
Canine behavior history form part 1

Name_____ Phone_____

Address_____ City_____ State_____ Zip_____

Email:_____ Alternate phone_____

Household: #adults (>18 years):_____ #children:_____ ages:_____

#dogs (including patient):_____ #cats:_____ #other animals:_____

Who is the primary caretaker of the dog?

❏ Husband   ❏ Child _____   ❏ N/A

❏ Wife   ❏ Other _____

Name	Breed	Sex	Age (years)
Patient			
Dog 2			
Dog 3			
Dog 4			

Patient Information:

Weight (kg): _____   Body condition: Thin 1 2 3 4 5 Obese

Age neutered: _____years _____months ❏ Unknown

Current medical problems: _____

Current medications: _____ Dose rate (mg/kg q..): _____

_____ Dose rate (mg/kg q..): _____

Origin:

❏ Own breeding   ❏ Pet shop   ❏ Other_____
❏ Breeder   ❏ Humane society   ❏ Don't know
❏ Private home   ❏ Stray

Age removed from litter: _____   ❏ Unknown

Age obtained by owner: _____   ❏ Unknown

Canine and Feline Behavior for Veterinary Technicians and Nurses, First Edition. Edited by Julie K. Shaw and Debbie Martin.
© 2015 John Wiley & Sons, Inc. Published 2015 by John Wiley & Sons, Inc.
Companion Website: www.wiley.com/go/shaw/behavior

If obtained as a puppy, how was the puppy raised?

- ❏ In house
- ❏ In kennel/garage
- ❏ Loose outside
- ❏ Puppy mill
- ❏ Other
- ❏ Don't know
- ❏ N/A

If obtained as a puppy, how did you select that particular puppy from the litter?

- ❏ Breeder selected
- ❏ No choice
- ❏ Most outgoing
- ❏ Most timid
- ❏ Biggest
- ❏ Smallest
- ❏ Looks
- ❏ Other_____
- ❏ N/A

If previously owned, for what primary purpose was the dog kept?

- ❏ Adult's pet
- ❏ Family pet
- ❏ Children's pet
- ❏ Show dog
- ❏ Breeding
- ❏ Guard dog
- ❏ Farm/outside dog
- ❏ Obedience
- ❏ Service/working dog
- ❏ Hunting dog
- ❏ Research/teaching
- ❏ Other_____
- ❏ Don't know
- ❏ N/A

Primary purpose for which dog was obtained?

- ❏ Adult's pet
- ❏ Family pet
- ❏ Children's pet
- ❏ Show dog
- ❏ Breeding
- ❏ Watch/guard dog
- ❏ Farm/outside dog
- ❏ Obedience
- ❏ Service/working dog
- ❏ Hunting dog
- ❏ Other_____

Average number of hours dog is left alone per week-day?_____

Schedule on weekdays

- ❏ Is consistent
- ❏ varies

Where is the dog when left alone?

- ❏ Cage
- ❏ Confined in a room
- ❏ Loose in living area
- ❏ Basement
- ❏ Garage
- ❏ Outside kennel
- ❏ Outside tied
- ❏ Loose in yard
- ❏ Other_____
- ❏ N/A

Where is the dog at night?

- ❏ Cage
- ❏ Confined in a room
- ❏ Loose in living area
- ❏ Basement
- ❏ Garage
- ❏ Bedroom
- ❏ On person's bed
- ❏ Outside
- ❏ Other_____

Exercise (walks):

- ❏ <1/week
- ❏ several/wk
- ❏ once/day
- ❏ twice/day
- ❏ 3x/day
- ❏ >3x/day

Exercise schedule

- ❏ Is consistent
- ❏ varies during week

Average hours of walking exercise per day: _____

Dog is walked on:

- ❏ Off leash
- ❏ Harness
- ❏ Flat collar
- ❏ Head Halter
- ❏ Choke chain
- ❏ Pinch collar

Reason walked with that specific training tool:

_____

Training:

- ❏ Dog has been trained to go into a crate readily
- ❏ Attended puppy classes (<4months)
- ❏ Dog has been trained with a clicker
- ❏ Dog is a trained service dog
- ❏ Attended classes over 4 months of age
- ❏ Dog has been shown in trials
- ❏ Dog is trained for other work

At what age did puppy/obedience classes start? _____years _____months   don't know

Level of training:

- ❏ Basic (come, sit, down, heel on leash)
- ❏ Average (Basic plus: heel off leash, stay)
- ❏ Advanced

Performance of dog in class/training situation:

- ❏ Poor
- ❏ Fair
- ❏ Good
- ❏ Excellent
- ❏ Don't know/N/A

Performance elsewhere:

- ❏ Poor
- ❏ Fair
- ❏ Good
- ❏ Excellent
- ❏ Don't know/N/A

Training aids used:

- ❏ Off leash
- ❏ Head halter
- ❏ Choke collar
- ❏ Pinch collar
- ❏ Flat collar
- ❏ Harness
- ❏ Front clip harness
- ❏ Don't know/N/A

Reason:

_____

Types of discipline:

❑ None ever	❑ Startling	❑ "Dominance" roll
❑ Response substitution	❑ Physical	❑ Water spray
❑ Verbal reprimand	❑ Shock	❑ Other_____
❑ Distracting	❑ Time out	❑ _____

Feeding:

Diet	%	Brand
Dry		
Canned		
Table food		
Other		

Feeding schedule:

❑ 1/day   ❑ 2 times/day   ❑ >2 times/day   ❑ ad lib

Feeding schedule:

❑ is regular   ❑ Feeding schedule varies

Food treats   Type:_____ Contingent on behavior ❑ yes ❑ no

Temperament:

How would you generally describe your dog's temperament (check all that apply):

❑ Friendly to owner	❑ Aggressive to strangers	❑ Hyperexcitable
❑ Aloof	❑ Shy of strangers	❑ Super "submissive"
❑ Aggressive to owner	❑ Happy, outgoing	❑ Fearful (environment)
❑ Friendly to strangers	❑ Inhibited	❑ Fear of noises
❑ Aloof to strangers	❑ Anxious	❑ Don't know

Comments:_____

_____

What was the temperament of the dog as a puppy:

❑ Friendly to owner	❑ Aggressive to strangers	❑ Hyperexcitable
❑ Aloof	❑ Shy of strangers	❑ Super "submissive"
❑ Aggressive to owner	❑ Happy, outgoing	❑ Fearful (environment)
❑ Friendly to strangers	❑ Inhibited	❑ Fear of noises
❑ Aloof to strangers	❑ Anxious	❑ Don't know

Comments:_____

_____

Presenting problems (in order of importance to owner):

1 _____

2 _____

3 _____

4 _____

What have you tried so far to treat the problem(s)?

_____

_____

_____

_____

_____

Comments and status of the human animal bond?

_____

_____

_____

_____

_____

_____

_____

_____

_____

Appendix 2
Canine behavior history form part 2

Dog's name _____ Owner's name _____

	Neutral	Friendly	Hyper	Fearful	Anxious	Defensive Aggression	Offensive Aggression	Don't know
General behavioral profile How does your dog react to the following (if the dog has experienced the situation in the past)?								
Unfamiliar people at door								
Unfamiliar people in home								
Unfamiliar people, neutral Territory, on leash								
Same, off leash								
Same approaching/try to pet, on leash								
Children, bikes, skateboards								
Joggers (adults)								
On leash whiles cars, trucks go by								
Children 1–6 years								
Children 7–11								
Children 12–18								
Unfamiliar dogs on property								
Unfamiliar dogs off property on leash								
Same off leash								
Owners leaving								
Owners returning								

Canine and Feline Behavior for Veterinary Technicians and Nurses, First Edition. Edited by Julie K. Shaw and Debbie Martin.
© 2015 John Wiley & Sons, Inc. Published 2015 by John Wiley & Sons, Inc.
Companion Website: www.wiley.com/go/shaw/behavior

Nail trimming								
Grooming								
Bathing								
Wiping feet								
Owner reaching over head or Touching on head								
Owner touching other places								
Owner lifting dog up								
Grasping collar, restraining dog								
Roughhousing								
Approach or take food dish while dog is eating								
Taking away bone/toy/stolen object								
Approach dog on his bed								
Disturbing sleeping dog								
Stepping over lying dog								
Verbal reprimand								
Physical punishment								
Putting on/taking off collar								
Staring at dog								
Car rides								
Stranger approaching car								
Vacuum cleaner								
Broom								
Thunder								
Loud noises (other than thunder)								

Comments on behavior during consultation:

_____

_____

_____

_____

_____

_____

_____

_____

_____

_____

_____

_____

_____

_____

_____

_____

_____

_____

_____

Problem history: **Problem #**

General description: What happens? Where does it happen? Who is present? What are the triggers?

How does the dog behave (including body language before and afterwards) and how do people react?

_____

_____

_____

_____

_____

_____

Most recent incident:

_____

_____

_____

_____

_____

Second most recent:

_____

_____

_____

_____

_____

The earliest incident:

_____

_____

_____

_____

_____

Age problem started:_____ months_____ years

Any changes at that time?_____

_____

_____

Progression:

❑ same   ❑ increasing   ❑ decreasing

Frequency:

❑ >10 times/day   ❑ 1-10 times/day   ❑ 1-6 times/week   ❑ <1 times/week

PRELIMINARY DIAGNOSIS:

1. _____   3. _____

2. _____   4. _____

Medication: _____   Dosage: _____

TREATMENT PLAN:

_____

_____

_____

_____

_____

_____

_____

_____

_____

_____

_____

_____

_____

_____

_____

_____

_____

_____

_____

_____

_____

Appendix 3
Feline behavior history form part 1

Name_____ Phone_____

Address_____ City_____ State_____ Zip_____

Email:_____ Alternate phone_____

Household: #adults (>18 years):_____ #children:_____ ages:_____

#cats (including patient):_____ #dogs:_____ #other animals:_____

Who is the primary caretaker of the cat?

❑ Husband   ❑ Child   ❑ N/A

❑ Wife   ❑ Other _____

Name	Breed	Sex	Age (years)
Patient			
Cat 2			
Cat 3			
Cat 4			

Patient Information:

Weight (kg):_____   Body condition: Thin 1 2 3 4 5 Obese

Age neutered:_____ years_____ months_____❑ Unknown

Current medical problems: _____

Current medications:_____ Dose rate (mg/kg q..):_____

_____ Dose rate (mg/kg q..):_____

Origin:

❑ Own breeding   ❑ Pet shop   ❑ Other_____

❑ Breeder   ❑ Humane society   ❑ Don't know

❑ Private home   ❑ Stray

Canine and Feline Behavior for Veterinary Technicians and Nurses, First Edition. Edited by Julie K. Shaw and Debbie Martin.
© 2015 John Wiley & Sons, Inc. Published 2015 by John Wiley & Sons, Inc.
Companion Website: www.wiley.com/go/shaw/behavior

Age obtained:_____(years)_____(months)_____ ❑ Unknown

If obtained as a kitten, how was the kitten raised?

❑   In house   ❑   Loose outside   ❑   Don't know

❑   Kennel/garage   ❑   Other   ❑   N/A

If obtained as kitten, how did you select that particular kitten from the litter?

❑   Breeder selected   ❑   Most timid   ❑   Prettiest

❑   No choice   ❑   Biggest   ❑   Other_____

❑   Most outgoing   ❑   Smallest   ❑   N/A

Age removed from litter: _____   ❑   Unknown

Age obtained by owner: _____   ❑   Unknown

If previously owned, for what primary purpose was the cat kept?

❑   Adult's pet   ❑   Breeding   ❑   Don't know

❑   Family pet   ❑   Farm/outside cat   ❑   N/A

❑   Children's pet   ❑   Research/teaching

❑   Show   ❑   Other_____

Is the cat declawed?

❑   no   ❑   front only   ❑   front and back

Age at declawing:_____years_____months_____ ❑   Unknown

Primary purpose for which cat was obtained:

❑   Adult's pet   ❑   Show   ❑   Other_____

❑   Family pet   ❑   Breeding

❑   Children's pet   ❑   Farm/outside cat

Average number of hours the cat is left alone per weekday: _____

Schedule on weekdays

❑   Is consistent   ❑   Varies

Where is the cat when left alone?

❑   Cage   ❑   Outside   ❑   N/A

❑   Confined in a room   ❑   Basement

❑   Loose in living area   ❑   Garage

Where is the cat at night?

- ❏ Cage
- ❏ Confined in a room
- ❏ Loose in living area
- ❏ Bedroom
- ❏ On person's bed
- ❏ Outside
- ❏ Basement
- ❏ Garage

Average hours of being outside per day: _____

Schedule

- ❏ Is consistent
- ❏ Varies

Types of discipline used:

- ❏ none ever
- ❏ response substitution
- ❏ verbal reprimand
- ❏ startling
- ❏ physical
- ❏ time-out
- ❏ water
- ❏ other_____

Feeding and Litter boxes:

Diet	%	Brand
Dry		
Canned		
Table food		
Other		

Feeding schedule:

- ❏ <1/day
- ❏ 2x/day
- ❏ 2x/day
- ❏ ad lib

Feeding schedule:

- ❏ is regular
- ❏ Feeding schedule varies

Food treats   Type: _____Contingent on behavior ❏ yes ❏ no

Fresh water provided:

- ❏ 1/day
- ❏ 1/day
- ❏ >2x/day
- ❏ >2x/day

Watering schedule:

- ❏ Is regular
- ❏ Varies during week

Number of dishes with feed: _____

Number of dishes with water: _____

Number of litter boxes: _____

Location of litter boxes (check all that apply):

❏ Living area	❏ Spare room	❏ Basement
❏ Kitchen	❏ Laundry room	❏ Hallway
❏ Bathroom	❏ Closet	❏ Other

Type of litter box:

❏ Open	❏ Covered	❏ Varies

Type of litter:

❏ Clumping	❏ Shavings	❏ Sand
❏ Clay	❏ Newspaper	❏ Other

Is litter

❏ Deodorized/scented	❏ No odor control	❏ Don't know

Type of litter

❏ is consistent	❏ varies	❏ N/A

Liners used:

❏ No	❏ Always	❏ Varies

Litter boxes scooped:

❏ <1x/week	❏ several x/wk	❏ >1x/day
❏ weekly	❏ daily	❏ N/A

Litter boxes washed:

❏ <1/month	❏ weekly	❏ >daily
❏ monthly	❏ several x/wk	❏ N/A

Cleaner used:

❏ Strong disinfectant	❏ Bleach	❏ Other_____
❏ Pine cleaner	❏ Mild soap	❏ N/A
❏ Lemon cleaner	❏ Water only	

Temperament:

How would you generally rate the cat's temperament?

❏ Friendly	❏ Hyperexcitable	❏ Offensive aggressive
❏ Aloof	❏ Shy of people	❏ Don't know
❏ Inhibited	❏ Fearful (environment)	
❏ Anxious	❏ Fear aggressive	

Comments:_____

What was the temperament of the cat as a kitten?

❏ Friendly   ❏ Hyperexcitable   ❏ Offensive aggressive

❏ Aloof   ❏ Shy of people   ❏ Don't know

❏ Inhibited   ❏ Fearful (environment)

❏ Anxious   ❏ Fear aggressive

Presenting problems (in order of importance to owner):

1 _____

2 _____

3 _____

4 _____

What have you tried so far to treat the problem(s)?

_____

_____

_____

_____

Comments and status of the human–animal bond?

_____

_____

_____

_____

_____

_____

_____

Appendix 4
Feline behavior history form part 2

Cat's name_____ Owner's name_____

<table>
<tr><td colspan="9" style="text-align:center">General behavioral profile
How does your cat react to the following (if the cat has experienced the situation in the past):</td></tr>
<tr><th></th><th>Calm</th><th>Friendly</th><th>Hyper</th><th>Neutral</th><th>Fearful</th><th>Anxious</th><th>Aggressive</th><th>Don't know</th></tr>
<tr><td>Unfamiliar people in home</td><td></td><td></td><td></td><td></td><td></td><td></td><td></td><td></td></tr>
<tr><td>Same approaching, wanting to pet</td><td></td><td></td><td></td><td></td><td></td><td></td><td></td><td></td></tr>
<tr><td>Babies</td><td></td><td></td><td></td><td></td><td></td><td></td><td></td><td></td></tr>
<tr><td>Children</td><td></td><td></td><td></td><td></td><td></td><td></td><td></td><td></td></tr>
<tr><td>Unfamiliar cats on property</td><td></td><td></td><td></td><td></td><td></td><td></td><td></td><td></td></tr>
<tr><td>Nail trimming</td><td></td><td></td><td></td><td></td><td></td><td></td><td></td><td></td></tr>
<tr><td>Giving medication</td><td></td><td></td><td></td><td></td><td></td><td></td><td></td><td></td></tr>
<tr><td>Grooming</td><td></td><td></td><td></td><td></td><td></td><td></td><td></td><td></td></tr>
<tr><td>Petting</td><td></td><td></td><td></td><td></td><td></td><td></td><td></td><td></td></tr>
<tr><td>Lifting cat up</td><td></td><td></td><td></td><td></td><td></td><td></td><td></td><td></td></tr>
<tr><td>Restraining cat</td><td></td><td></td><td></td><td></td><td></td><td></td><td></td><td></td></tr>
<tr><td>Putting cat in carrier</td><td></td><td></td><td></td><td></td><td></td><td></td><td></td><td></td></tr>
<tr><td>Roughhousing</td><td></td><td></td><td></td><td></td><td></td><td></td><td></td><td></td></tr>
<tr><td>Disturbing sleeping cat</td><td></td><td></td><td></td><td></td><td></td><td></td><td></td><td></td></tr>
<tr><td>Stepping over lying cat</td><td></td><td></td><td></td><td></td><td></td><td></td><td></td><td></td></tr>
<tr><td>Cat same household approaching</td><td></td><td></td><td></td><td></td><td></td><td></td><td></td><td></td></tr>
<tr><td>Other cat outside</td><td></td><td></td><td></td><td></td><td></td><td></td><td></td><td></td></tr>
</table>

Canine and Feline Behavior for Veterinary Technicians and Nurses, First Edition. Edited by Julie K. Shaw and Debbie Martin.
© 2015 John Wiley & Sons, Inc. Published 2015 by John Wiley & Sons, Inc.
Companion Website: www.wiley.com/go/shaw/behavior

Dog same household approaching								
Strange dog outside								

Comments on behavior during consul:

_____

_____

_____

_____

_____

_____

_____

_____

_____

Problem history: **Problem #**

_____

General Description: What happens? Where does it happen? Who is present? What are the triggers?

How does the cat behave (including body language before and afterwards) and how do people react?

_____

_____

_____

_____

_____

_____

_____

Most recent incident:

_____

_____

_____

_____

_____

_____

Second most recent:

_____

_____

_____

_____

_____

The earliest incident:

_____

_____

_____

_____

Age problem started:_____ months_____ years

Any changes at that time? _____

_____

_____

_____

_____

Progression:

❑ same   ❑ increasing   ❑ decreasing

Frequency:

❑ >10 times/day   ❑ 1-10 times/day   ❑ 1-6 times/week   ❑ <1 times/week

PRELIMINARY DIAGNOSIS:

1. _____   3. _____

2. _____   4. _____

Medication: _____   Dosage: _____

TREATMENT PLAN:

_____

_____

_____

_____

_____

_____

_____

_____

_____

_____

_____

_____

_____

_____

_____

_____

_____

_____

_____

_____

_____

_____

_____

_____

_____

_____

_____

_____

_____

_____

Appendix 5
Trainer assessment form

Assessment criteria	Notes	0–5 (5 is excellent)
Welcomes potential clients to observe a class prior to making a decision to enroll		
Explains a skill and gives examples of how the skill is useful in everyday life		
Demonstrates the skill		
Utilizes handouts and other instructional guides		
Circulates though the students giving assistance and guidance when needed		
Remains conscious of the emotional and motivational state of all animals in the classroom setting and acts appropriately		
Arranges the classroom to optimize the success of each handler and animal		
Does not become focused on one student		
Keeps the class moving at an appropriate pace		
Can adjust their teaching plan as needed for individual student's needs		
Is professional and respectful at all times to owners/handlers		
Is appropriate and liberal with positive reinforcement to both the owners and animals.		
Is familiar with TAG Teach and utilizes it frequently and appropriately to instruct clients		

Canine and Feline Behavior for Veterinary Technicians and Nurses, First Edition. Edited by Julie K. Shaw and Debbie Martin.
© 2015 John Wiley & Sons, Inc. Published 2015 by John Wiley & Sons, Inc.
Companion Website: www.wiley.com/go/shaw/behavior

Uses appropriate management tools to decrease unwanted behaviors while teaching the desired behaviors		
Utilizes only humane training methods which promote and protect the human–animal bond and are not harmful to the handler or dog in any way		
Does not recommend or utilize choke collars, pinch collars, electronic shock collars or physical punishments		
Does not coach or advocate the outdated "dominance hierarchy theory" and the subsequent confrontational training and relationship that follows from it		
Recommends and utilizes training tools such as head collars and no pull harnesses on an individual basis or as recommended and prescribed by the veterinarian		
Understands the value of education and attends continuing education seminars regularly		
Is a certified member of a standardized and policed credentialing program		
Because of variables in dog breeding, temperament, owner commitment and experience, a trainer cannot and should not guarantee the results of his/her training, although should ensure client satisfaction		
Builds and maintains a mutually communicative, respectful and professional relationship with veterinary professionals		
Understands their role on the veterinary behavior team and does not diagnose behavior disorders or change the prescribed treatment plan.		
Total points		

Appendix 6
Determining pet owner strain

Life area	Manifestation of strain
Mental and emotional	❒ Stress and a feeling of being "used up" ❒ Worry or anxiety ❒ Anger toward your pet ❒ Fear your pet may hurt you or a loved one ❒ "Aloneness" and alienation ❒ Feelings of "hopelessness" when it comes to your pet ❒ Feelings of "not being able to go on" if your pet were to die
Health	❒ Health issues due to stress (weight loss or gain, headaches, etc.) ❒ Declined self-care ❒ Decreased energy ❒ Injury from you pet
Social	❒ Embarrassment ❒ Shame or guilt ❒ Fear of stigma / social disapproval ❒ Alienation ❒ Limit or cease having house guests ❒ Guilt when socializing outside the home ❒ Neglected relationships or giving up relationships that make you happy to tend to your pet's psychological and emotional needs ❒ Fear of being away from your pet ❒ Giving up hobbies ❒ Fear of injury to strangers
Financial	❒ Distraction during work day ❒ Financial liability / lawsuits ❒ Property damage and destruction ❒ Cost for treatment, medication, training, etc.
Family environment	❒ Fear for safety of family members ❒ Discord with significant other ❒ Strained relationship with extended family members ❒ Alienation by extended family

Canine and Feline Behavior for Veterinary Technicians and Nurses, First Edition. Edited by Julie K. Shaw and Debbie Martin.
© 2015 John Wiley & Sons, Inc. Published 2015 by John Wiley & Sons, Inc.
Companion Website: www.wiley.com/go/shaw/behavior

Appendix 7
Canine behavior plan of care

Consultation Date:_____

Client's Name:_____ Phone:_____ Email:_____

Address:_____ City:_____ State:_____ Zip:_____

Dog's Name:_____ Age:_____ Breed:_____ M ☐ Mx ☐ F ☐ Fx ☐

Canine Behavioral Diagnosis		
Aggression	**Target of Aggression**	☐
☐ Conflict-induced	☐	☐
☐ Possessive	☐	**Ingestive**
☐ Disease/Pain induced	☐	☐ Coprophagia
☐ Fear/Defensive induced	☐	☐ Pica
☐ Idiopathic	**Anxiety Disorders**	☐ Predatory Behavior
☐ IDA + Motivation	☐ Generalized Anxiety	**Eliminative**
☐ IDA-H + Motivation	☐ Global fear	☐ Housesoiling
☐ Alliance induced	☐ Separation Anxiety	☐ Urine marking
☐ Status induced	☐ Sound/Thunderstorm phobia	☐ Excitement urination
☐ Learned	☐ Specific fear or phobia	☐ Extreme fear/appeasement urination
☐ Maternal/hormonal induced	☐ Acute conflict behaviors/stereotypy	**Other**
☐ Play induced	☐ Compulsive disorder	☐ Cognitive dysfunction
☐ Redirected	Specific fear(s) or phobia (s) noted:	☐ Hyperexcitability
☐ Territorial	☐	☐ Conditioned unwanted behavior
☐	☐	☐

Prescribed Treatment Plan (see back for details and further information)		
Management	**Training**	☐ Shape relaxation
☐ Avoid triggers	☐ Marker training	☐ Leave it/ drop it
☐ Ignore attention seeking behaviors	☐ Lure reward training	☐
☐ Ignore at specific times	☐ Other training	☐
☐ Cue►response►reward interactions	☐ Agility training	☐
☐ Environmental modifications	☐ Concept training	☐
☐	☐ K9 Nose work® training	☐
	☐ Crate/confinement training	**Behavior Modification** (see back)
☐ Crate confinement	☐	☐ Counter-Conditioning
☐ Other confinement	☐	☐
☐	**Training Tools**	☐
☐ Umbilical cord	☐ Head halter	☐
☐ Change primary caregiver	☐ Basket muzzle	☐
☐ Increase mental stimulation	☐ Other muzzle	☐
☐ Walk off property	☐ Body harness	☐ Response Substitution
☐ Aerobic exercise	☐ No pull harness	☐
☐ Regular schedule	☐ Anxiety clothing	☐
☐ Dietary change	☐ Calming cap	☐
☐ Meal feed twice daily	☐ Drag line	☐
☐	☐ Tether	☐
☐	☐ Interactive toys/puzzles	☐ Systematic Desensitization
Other	☐ Pheromones	☐
☐ Interruption of behavior	☐ Remote Reward	☐
☐ Cease punishment	**Specific Behaviors to Train**	☐
☐ Remote punishment	☐ Targeting	☐
☐ Grief counseling	☐ Attention	☐
☐ Rehoming patient	☐ "Look" and "Watch"	☐ Other
☐	☐ Sit ☐ Down ☐ Recall	☐
☐	☐ Loose leash walking	☐
☐	☐ Go to a place	☐

Canine and Feline Behavior for Veterinary Technicians and Nurses, First Edition. Edited by Julie K. Shaw and Debbie Martin.
© 2015 John Wiley & Sons, Inc. Published 2015 by John Wiley & Sons, Inc.
Companion Website: www.wiley.com/go/shaw/behavior

Bite History
Has the dog bitten?   yes ☐   no ☐   Does the dog redirect aggression? ☐ yes   ☐ no
How severe were the bites?   Did not make contact ☐   Did not break skin ☐   Puncture ☐   Medical care needed ☐
Does the dog give warning before biting? ☐ yes   ☐ no   ☐ unknown
Note known triggers and other significant bite history:

Medical Conditions and Medications

Comments and Treatment Details

Veterinarian Signature: Date:

Appendix 8
Behavior problem list

Eliminative	Social	Ingestive
❑ Incontinence	❑ Barking/howling/whining	❑ Anorexia
❑ Diarrhea/vomiting	❑ Rolling in unsavory items	❑ Chewing objects
❑ House soiling	❑ Jumps up on people	❑ Coprophagia
❑ Urine Marking	❑ Demands attention	❑ Compulsive eating
❑ Urination on pheromones	❑ Demands touch	❑ Compulsive drinking
❑ Other _____	❑ Aggressive to owners	❑ Eating Grass/Plants
	❑ Aggressive to strangers	❑ Eating garbage
Grooming	❑ Aggr. to dogs/same household	❑ Pica
	❑ Aggr. to strange dogs	❑ Prey catching
❑ Licking self	❑ Aggr. to other animals	❑ Car etc. chasing
❑ Sucking on self	❑ Other _____	❑ Light/shadow chasing
❑ Chewing on self		❑ Stealing food
❑ Scratching self		❑ Fly snapping
❑ Checking hind end		❑ Air/mouth licking
❑ Other _____		❑ Other _____

Temperament related	Reproduction	Locomotory
❑ Depressed in appetent	❑ Cannibalism	❑ Circling/whirling
❑ Hyperexcitable/active	❑ False pregnancy	❑ Tail biting
❑ Hyper reactive	❑ Masturbation	❑ Pacing, figure 8s
❑ Nervous/anxious	❑ Mounting people	❑ Digging
❑ Fear of thunder	❑ Mounting animals	❑ Lameness/cond.
❑ Fear of loud noises exc. thunder	❑ Self nursing	❑ Roaming
❑ Fear of people	❑ Other _____	❑ Scratching objects
❑ Fear of situations		❑ Freezing
❑ Fear of objects/animals		❑ Other _____
❑ Other _____		

Comments:

Canine and Feline Behavior for Veterinary Technicians and Nurses, First Edition. Edited by Julie K. Shaw and Debbie Martin.
© 2015 John Wiley & Sons, Inc. Published 2015 by John Wiley & Sons, Inc.
Companion Website: www.wiley.com/go/shaw/behavior

Appendix 9
Technician observation

Date:_____   Client name_____   Pet name_____

	Start of Appointment	5 Minutes	15 min	30 min	End of appointment
Treats					
Treat proximity					
Interactions					
Trainability (1–10)					
General behavior					
Restrictions					
Significant events during appointment					

Canine and Feline Behavior for Veterinary Technicians and Nurses, First Edition. Edited by Julie K. Shaw and Debbie Martin.
© 2015 John Wiley & Sons, Inc. Published 2015 by John Wiley & Sons, Inc.
Companion Website: www.wiley.com/go/shaw/behavior

Appendix 10
Follow-up communation form

Client:		Date:	Patient Name:	

Problem List:

Problem #1				
Status of problem (cured 1 - 10 severe):				

Cured	Much Improved	Moderately Improved	Worse
Same	Slightly Improved	No Improvement	Considering euthanasia

Problem #2				
Status of problem (cured 1 - 10 severe):				

Cured	Much Improved	Moderately Improved	Worse
Same	Slightly Improved	No Improvement	Considering euthanasia

Problem #3				
Status of problem (cured 1 - 10 severe):				

Cured	Much Improved	Moderately Improved	Worse
Same	Slightly Improved	No Improvement	Considering euthanasia

Current Medications and Dose:	Comments:	

Current Treatment Plan and Application:	Comments:	Client Compliance (poor 1 - 10 excellent)

Canine and Feline Behavior for Veterinary Technicians and Nurses, First Edition. Edited by Julie K. Shaw and Debbie Martin.
© 2015 John Wiley & Sons, Inc. Published 2015 by John Wiley & Sons, Inc.
Companion Website: www.wiley.com/go/shaw/behavior

Specific Concerns, Discussion and Suggestions

Next Contact Scheduled for :

Signature: | Printed Name:

Appendix 11
Behavior diary

Month: _____

Behavior	1	2	3	4	5	6	7	8	9	10	11	12	13	14	15	16	17	18	19	20	21	22	23	24	25	26	27	28	29	30	31
10 (Excellent)																															
9																															
8																															
7																															
6																															
5																															
4																															
3																															
2																															
1 (poor)																															
Day of month	1	2	3	4	5	6	7	8	9	10	11	12	13	14	15	16	17	18	19	20	21	22	23	24	25	26	27	28	29	30	31

Canine and Feline Behavior for Veterinary Technicians and Nurses, First Edition. Edited by Julie K. Shaw and Debbie Martin.
© 2015 John Wiley & Sons, Inc. Published 2015 by John Wiley & Sons, Inc.
Companion Website: www.wiley.com/go/shaw/behavior

Notes/signficant events/ medication

1	
2	
3	
4	
5	
6	
7	
8	
9	
10	
11	
12	
13	
14	
15	
16	
17	
18	
19	
20	
21	
22	
23	
24	
25	
26	
27	
28	
29	
30	
31	

Appendix 12
Adult cat (3 months to ~12 years) questionnaire

Owners name:_____ Today's date:_____

Cat's name:_____ Cat's age (DOB):_____

1. How would you describe your cat's litter box training?
   - ❑ Great, not having any accidents
   - ❑ OK, a few accidents (less than once a month)
   - ❑ Could be better, several accidents a week
   - ❑ Not a clue, most elimination is happening in a location I do not prefer.

   Comments:_____
   _____

2. How many litter boxes do you have and where are they located?_____
   _____

3. What is the size and type of litter boxes (covered, uncovered, automatic, oval, large rectangular, etc)?
   _____

4. What type of litter do you use and what brand? (scented or unscented, scoopable versus clay)
   _____

5. Does your cat like to play with toys? What type?
   _____

6. Does your cat use scratching posts?_____

7. If you have other pets in the household, describe the cat's relationship with them._____
   _____

8. _____

Canine and Feline Behavior for Veterinary Technicians and Nurses, First Edition. Edited by Julie K. Shaw and Debbie Martin.
© 2015 John Wiley & Sons, Inc. Published 2015 by John Wiley & Sons, Inc.
Companion Website: www.wiley.com/go/shaw/behavior

9. Has your cat ever shown any growling, hissing, or nipping/biting toward you or anyone else? If so, when?

    _____

    _____

10. Has your cat shown any of these signs; Any coughing, sneezing, itching, diarrhea, vomiting, or lack of appetite?

    _____

    _____

11. Any change in water or food consumption?

    _____

12. What type of food do you feed your cat and how often is he/she fed? Is food available all the time or at set "mealtimes"?

    _____

    _____

13. Any change in frequency of urination or defecation?

    _____

14. What, if any medications (over the counter or prescription) does your cat take or have applied routinely (at least monthly).

    _____

    _____

    _____

15. What are three things you enjoy about your cat?

    _____

    _____

    _____

16. Do you have any concerns or topics you would like to discuss?

    _____

    _____

    _____

Appendix 13
Juvenile/adolescent/adult dog (4 months to ~7 years) questionnaire

Owners name:_____ Today's date:_____

Dog's name:_____ Dog's age (DOB):_____

1. Where does your dog spend most of his/her day? (inside, outside, in a room, in a kennel, with you)?

    _____

2. Have you taken your dog to a training class? If so, where?_____

    _____

3. Do you train your dog? If so, how? (with treats, clicker training, etc)_____

    _____

4. Do you walk your dog? If so what type of collar does your dog wear for walks?_____

    If not, why?_____

5. Any problems with walking your dog?_____

6. How would you describe your dog's house training?
    - ❑ Great, not having any accidents
    - ❑ Good, a few accidents when I forget to take her/him out (less than once a month)
    - ❑ Could be better, numerous accidents a week
    - ❑ Not a clue, most elimination is happening in a location I do not prefer

    Comments:_____

    _____

7. If you have other pets in the household, describe the dog's relationship with them._____

    _____

    _____

Canine and Feline Behavior for Veterinary Technicians and Nurses, First Edition. Edited by Julie K. Shaw and Debbie Martin.
© 2015 John Wiley & Sons, Inc. Published 2015 by John Wiley & Sons, Inc.
Companion Website: www.wiley.com/go/shaw/behavior

8. Has your dog ever shown any growling, barking, snarling or nipping toward you or anyone else? If so, when?

    _____

    _____

9. Any coughing, sneezing, itching, diarrhea, vomiting, or lack of appetite?_____

    _____

10. Any change in water or food consumption?_____

    _____

11. What type of food do you feed your dog and how often is he/she fed? Is food available all the time or at set "mealtimes"?

    _____

12. Any change in frequency of urination or defecation?_____

    _____

13. What, if any medications (over the counter or prescription) does your dog take or have applied routinely (at least monthly including heartworm and flea/tick preventives)?

    _____

    _____

    _____

14. What are three things you enjoy about your dog?_____

    _____

    _____

    _____

15. Do you have any concerns or topics you would like to discuss?_____

    _____

    _____

    _____

    _____

Appendix 14
New kitten (less than 3 months) questionnaire

Owners name:_____ Today's date:_____

Cat's name:_____ Cat's age (DOB):_____

1. Where did you obtain your kitten from (breeder, petstore, friend, shelter, rescue, humane society, etc.)?

    _____

2. How long have you had your kitten?_____

3. How old was your kitten when you obtained him/her?_____

4. How many kittens were in the litter?_____

5. When were the kittens taken away from the mother?_____

6. Where does your kitten spend most of his/her day? (inside, outside, in a room, in a kennel, with you)?

    _____

7. How would you describe your kitten's litter box training?
    - ❏ Great, not having any accidents
    - ❏ Good, a few accidents have occurred
    - ❏ Not a clue, most elimination is happening in a location I do not prefer

    Comments:_____

8. How many litter boxes do you have and where are they located?_____

    _____

9. What is the size and type of litter boxes (covered, uncovered, automatic, oval, large rectangular, etc.)?

    _____

10. What type and brand of litter do you use? (scented or unscented, scoopable vs clay)

    _____

Canine and Feline Behavior for Veterinary Technicians and Nurses, First Edition. Edited by Julie K. Shaw and Debbie Martin.
© 2015 John Wiley & Sons, Inc. Published 2015 by John Wiley & Sons, Inc.
Companion Website: www.wiley.com/go/shaw/behavior

11. Does your kitten like to play with toys? What type?_____

12. Does your kitten use scratching posts?_____

13. Have your enrolled your kitten in a kitten class? If so, where?_____

14. If you have other pets in the household, describe the kitten's relationship with them._____

_____

15. Has your kitten ever shown any growling, hissing, or nipping/biting toward you or anyone else? If so, when?

_____

16. Has your kitten shown any of these signs: any coughing, sneezing, itching, diarrhea, vomiting, or lack of appetite?

_____

17. Any change in water or food consumption?_____

18. What type of food do you feed your kitten and how often is he/she fed? Is food available all the time or at set "mealtimes"?

_____

19. Any change in frequency of urination or defecation?_____

_____

20. What, if any medications (over the counter or prescription) does your kitten take or have applied routinely (at least monthly)_____

_____

21. What are three things you enjoy about your kitten?_____

_____

_____

_____

22. Do you have any concerns or topics you would like to discuss?_____

_____

_____

_____

Appendix 15
New puppy (less than 4 months) questionnaire

Owners name:_____ Today's date:_____

Dog's name:_____ Dog's age (DOB):_____

1. Where did you obtain your puppy from (breeder, petstore, friend, shelter, rescue, humane society, etc.)?

    _____

    _____

2. How long have you had your puppy?_____

3. How old was your puppy when you obtained him/her?_____

4. How many puppies were in the litter?_____

5. When were the puppies taken away from the mother?_____

    _____

6. Where does your puppy spend most of his/her day? (inside, outside, in a room, in a kennel, with you)?

    _____

    _____

7. How would you describe your puppy's house training?
    - ❏ Great, not having any accidents
    - ❏ Good, a few accidents when I forget to take her/him out
    - ❏ So-so, having several accidents a day
    - ❏ Not a clue, most elimination is happening in a location I do not prefer

    Comments:_____

8. Have your enrolled your puppy in a puppy socialization class? If so, where?_____

    _____

Canine and Feline Behavior for Veterinary Technicians and Nurses, First Edition. Edited by Julie K. Shaw and Debbie Martin.
© 2015 John Wiley & Sons, Inc. Published 2015 by John Wiley & Sons, Inc.
Companion Website: www.wiley.com/go/shaw/behavior

9. If you have other pets in the household, describe the puppy's relationship with them._____

    _____

10. Has your puppy ever shown any growling, barking, snarling or nipping toward you or anyone else? If so, when?

    _____

    _____

11. Has your puppy shown any of these signs; Any coughing, sneezing, itching, diarrhea, vomiting, or lack of appetite?

    _____

    _____

12. What type of food do you feed your puppy and how often is he/she fed? Is food available all the time or at set "mealtimes"?

    _____

    _____

13. Any change in water or food consumption?_____

14. Any change in frequency of urination or defecation?_____

15. What, if any medications (over the counter or prescription) does your puppy take or have applied routinely (at least monthly).

    _____

    _____

16. What are three things you enjoy about your puppy?

    _____

    _____

    _____

17. Do you have any concerns or topics you would like to discuss?

    _____

    _____

    _____

Appendix 16
Senior cat (greater ~12 years) questionnaire

Owners name:_____ Today's date:_____

Cat's name:_____ Cat's age (DOB):_____

1. How would you describe your cat's litter box training?
   - ❑ Great, not having any accidents
   - ❑ OK, a few accidents (less than once a month)
   - ❑ Could be better, several accidents a week
   - ❑ Not a clue, most elimination is happening in a location I do not prefer

   Comments:_____
   _____

2. How many litter boxes do you have and where are they located?_____
   _____

3. What is the size and type of litter boxes (covered, uncovered, automatic, oval, large rectangular, etc.)?
   _____
   _____

4. What type of litter do you use and what brand? (scented or unscented, scoopable versus clay)
   _____

5. Does your cat like to play with toys? What type?_____
   _____

6. Any changes in activity, such as being more active at night, or sleeping more during the day? Any increase in vocalization?
   _____

7. Does your cat seem disoriented at times or unable to recognize familiar people?_____
   _____

Canine and Feline Behavior for Veterinary Technicians and Nurses, First Edition. Edited by Julie K. Shaw and Debbie Martin.
© 2015 John Wiley & Sons, Inc. Published 2015 by John Wiley & Sons, Inc.
Companion Website: www.wiley.com/go/shaw/behavior

8. Has your cat ever shown any growling, hissing, or nipping/biting toward you or anyone else? If so, when?

    _____

9. Has your cat shown any of these signs; Any coughing, sneezing, itching, diarrhea, vomiting, or lack of appetite?

    _____

    _____

10. Any change in water or food consumption?_____

    _____

11. What type of food do you feed your cat and how often is he/she fed? Is food available all the time or at set "mealtimes"?

    _____

    _____

12. Any change in frequency of urination or defecation?_____

    _____

13. What, if any medications (over the counter or prescription) does your cat take or have applied routinely (at least monthly).

    _____

    _____

    _____

14. What are three things you enjoy about your cat?

    _____

    _____

    _____

15. Do you have any concerns or topics you would like to discuss?

    _____

    _____

    _____

Appendix 17
Senior dog (~7 + years) questionnaire

Owners name:_____ Today's date:_____

Dog's name:_____ Dog's age (DOB):_____

1. Where does your dog spend most of his/her day? (inside, outside, in a room, in a kennel, with you)?
    _____

2. Have you taken your dog to a training class? If so, where?_____
    _____

3. Do you train your dog? If so, how? (with treats, clicker training, etc.)_____
    _____

4. Do you walk your dog? If so what type of collar does your dog wear for walks?_____
    _____

5. If not, why?_____

6. Any problems with walking your dog?_____

7. Have you noticed any changes in your dog's personality or activity level?
    ❏ Less or more active
    ❏ Difficulty rising after resting or sitting
    ❏ Urine or stool accidents in the house
    ❏ More needy or anxious
    ❏ More standoffish
    ❏ Disoriented or failure to recognize familiar people

    Comments:_____
    _____

8. Has your dog ever shown any growling, barking, snarling or nipping toward you or anyone else? If so, when?
    _____
    _____

Canine and Feline Behavior for Veterinary Technicians and Nurses, First Edition. Edited by Julie K. Shaw and Debbie Martin.
© 2015 John Wiley & Sons, Inc. Published 2015 by John Wiley & Sons, Inc.
Companion Website: www.wiley.com/go/shaw/behavior

9. Any coughing, sneezing, itching, diarrhea, vomiting, or lack of appetite?_____

_____

10. Any change in water or food consumption?_____

_____

11. What type of food do you feed your dog and how often is he/she fed? Is food available all the time or at set "mealtimes"?

_____

_____

_____

12. Any change in frequency of urination or defecation?_____

_____

_____

13. What, if any medications (over the counter or prescription) does your dog take or have applied routinely (at least monthly including heartworm and flea/tick preventives)?

_____

_____

_____

_____

14. What are three things you enjoy about your dog?

_____

_____

_____

15. Do you have any concerns or topics you would like to discuss?

_____

_____

_____

Appendix 18
Pet selection counseling

Owner: _____ Email: _____
Address: _____
Home Phone: _____ Alt. Phone: _____

Pet Selection Counseling-Part 1: Lifestyle

1. Household members:

NAME	AGE	RELATIONSHIP

2. Current household pets:

NAME	AGE	SEX	SPECIES/BREED

3. Previous household pets

NAME	AGE	BREED

4. How often do adults visit?
☐ Daily
☐ Numerous times weekly
☐ 1-4 times monthly
☐ Infrequently

5. How often do children or teens visit?
☐ Daily
☐ Numerous times weekly
☐ 1-4 times monthly
☐ Infrequently

6. Would you say your current lifestyle is
☐ Very Hectic
☐ Moderately busy/controllable
☐ Calm / quiet

7. Does anyone in your family have special needs?
☐ Yes   ☐ No
If yes, please specify

8. Is anyone in your home allergic to animals?
☐ Yes   ☐ No
If yes, please specify:
_____

9. Are there any major family changes in your near future?
☐ Birth of a child
☐ Household move
☐ Schedule change
☐ Marital change
☐ Other: _____

Part 2: Care and Maintenance

10. You live
☐ In a house
☐ In an apartment
☐ On a farm
☐ Other:

11. What is your approximate yard size?
☐ Large (acre or more)
☐ Medium
☐ Small
☐ No yard to speak of

12. What type of fencing is around your yard?
☐ Chain-link
☐ Invisible Fence
☐ Privacy
☐ No fence

13. Where will your pet spend most of his time?
☐ Indoors
☐ Outdoors
☐ 50/50

14. How will a pet be managed in your back yard?
☐ Fence
☐ Tie-out
☐ Not sure

15. What will your pet's indoor areas include?
☐ Full access to rooms
☐ Limited access to rooms
☐ Allowed on furniture
☐ Allowed on some furniture

16. Where will your pet sleep?
☐ Crate
☐ Their own bed
☐ Family member's bed
☐ Outside
☐ Other

17. How long will your pet be left alone during the day?
☐ < 1hour
☐ 4 hours or less
☐ 8 hours or less
☐ > 8 hours
☐ Variable

18. Where will your pet be kept when you are not home?
☐ Crate
☐ Outside
☐ Free access to house
☐ Specific room

19. How much time do you plan on interacting with your dog daily?(training, playing, grooming, exercise, etc.)
☐ <1hour
☐ 1-2 hours
☐ > 3 hours

20. Prioritize 3 activities you would like to do with your pet (jogging, swimming, agility training, act):
1)
2)
3)

21. How often will you walk your pet off your property for mental stimulation?
☐ Twice a day
☐ Once daily
☐ Once weekly
☐ Less than once a week

22. Who will be in charge of feeding your pet?
☐ Family takes turns
☐ Mom/Dad
☐ Individual

23. Who will be In charge of cleaning up after the pet?
☐ Family takes turns
☐ Mom/Dad
☐ Individual

24. How often do you plan to train your pet?
☐ Multiple times a day
☐ Multiple times a week
☐ Occasionally
☐ As little as possible

25. If acquiring a puppy will you take it to socialization classes?
☐ Yes
☐ No
☐ Unsure, more information need

26. Do you plan on crate training your pet?
☐ Yes
☐ No
☐ Unsure, more information needed

27. Who will be responsible for administering your pet's medical care (medication, etc.)?
☐ Family takes turns
☐ Mom/Dad
☐ Individual:

28. Would you prefer to have your pet trained:
☐ Without assistance
☐ With the help of a private trainer
☐ Group training class
☐ Leave pet at a training facility
☐ Unsure, need more information

29. What will you do with your pet on occasions when you travel?
☐ Take pet on trip
☐ Board the pet
☐ Hire a pet sitter
☐ Other

Canine and Feline Behavior for Veterinary Technicians and Nurses, First Edition. Edited by Julie K. Shaw and Debbie Martin.
© 2015 John Wiley & Sons, Inc. Published 2015 by John Wiley & Sons, Inc.
Companion Website: www.wiley.com/go/shaw/behavior

Part 3: Financial Considerations

30. How much are you budgeting monthly for your pet's food?
□ $20 or less
□ $20-50
□ $100 or less

31. How much are willing to pay for your pet?
□ Free
□ Less than $50
□ Less than $100
□ Less than $500
□ Less than $1000
□ $1000 or more

32. Do you plan on spaying/ neutering your pet?
□ Yes
□ No
□ Unsure, need more information

33. How much are budgeting to spend **annually** on your pet's medical care?
□ Less than $200
□ $200 - $300
□ $301 - $400
□ More than $400
□ Whatever is necessary

34. Which of the following pet sources are you considering?
□ Reputable breeder
□ Animal shelter / humane society
□ Breed rescue organization
□ Pet store
□ Other

Part 4: Pet Characteristics

35. What other animals (not your own) will your pet interact with?
□ Dogs
□ Cats
□ Other
□ Often
□ Rarely
□ Never

36. Primary purpose for obtaining your pet?
□ Adult's pet
□ Family pet
□ Child's pet
□ Breeding
□ Show
□ Hunting
□ Protection
□ Farm / outside pet
□ Other

37. Breeds you are considering
1)

2)

3)

38. Has someone in your household owned a puppy less than 6 months of age?
□ Yes   □ No
How long ago?

39. What age would you like your pet to be when you acquire it?
□ As young as possible
□ 8 weeks
□ 6 months or older
□ Adult

40. Are you interested in training your pet?
□ Yes, I look forward to training my pet
□ No, I would like a pet that requires little training

41. House training problems
□ Could live with problem
□ Would do whatever it takes to correct the problem
□ Problem would prompt me to part with the pet

42. Shyness with people
□ Could live with problem
□ Would do whatever it takes to correct the problem
□ Problem would prompt me to part with the pet

43. Aloofness with family
□ Could live with problem
□ Would do whatever it takes to correct the problem
□ Problem would prompt me to part with the pet

44. Excitability
□ Could live with problem
□ Would do whatever it takes to correct the problem
□ Problem would prompt me to part with the pet

45. Demands attention
□ Could live with problem
□ Would do whatever it takes to correct the problem
□ Problem would prompt me to part with the pet

46. Jumping on people
□ Could live with problem
□ Would do whatever it takes to correct the problem
□ Problem would prompt me to part with the pet

47. Digging / yard destruction
□ Could live with problem
□ Would do whatever it takes to correct the problem
□ Problem would prompt me to part with the pet

48. Chewing / destruction
□ Could live with problem
□ Would do whatever it takes to correct the problem
□ Problem would prompt me to part with the pet

49. Excessive vocalization
□ Could live with problem
□ Would do whatever it takes to correct the problem
□ Problem would prompt me to part with the pet

50. How often do you plan to groom your pet at home?
□ Daily
□ Weekly
□ Monthly
□ As infrequently as possible

51. How important is it to you that your pet "guards your home"?
□ Very important
□ Important
□ Not important
□ Do not want a guard dog.

52. What size pet do you prefer?
□ Micro (less than 5 Ibs.)
□ Very small (less than 10 Ibs.)
□ Small (11-25Ibs.)
□ Medium (26-50 Ibs.)
□ Large (51-90 1b5+
□ Giant (greater than 90 Ibs.)
□ No preference

53. How important is it to you that your pet wants to sit in your lap, follow you around, etc.?
□ Very important
□ Important
□ Not important
□ I would rather have an independent dog.

54. Would you have your pet Professionally groomed?
□ Yes
□ No
□ Occasionally

55. How much does hair on your clothing or furniture bother you?
□ Can not tolerate
□ Can tolerate somewhat
□ Does not bother me

54. Please list any questions or concerns you may have:

_____
_____
_____
_____
_____

Appendix 19
Canine breeder interview questions

	Canine breeder interview questions
	What was this breed bred to do? (Lap dogs, guard dogs, etc.)
	Are the dogs from a working line or a show line?
	Will we be able to meet the parents of our puppy?
	What made you choose this sire?
	What made you decide to breed this particular bitch?
	How often do your breed your bitches?
	How many litters has this bitch had?
	What has been her history with litters? (Was she a good "Mom"?)
	How many puppies are in the litter?
	At what age do you allow the puppies to go to homes?
	What type of environment are the puppies kept? (Kennel, house, etc.)
	What type of environmental enrichment do you have for the puppies?
	How much exposure do the puppies have currently with people? How often are the puppies handled by people?
	Is this bitch good with children?

Canine and Feline Behavior for Veterinary Technicians and Nurses, First Edition. Edited by Julie K. Shaw and Debbie Martin.
© 2015 John Wiley & Sons, Inc. Published 2015 by John Wiley & Sons, Inc.
Companion Website: www.wiley.com/go/shaw/behavior

	Is the sire good with children?
	What behavior or temperament traits do you feel are most important in this breed?
	Are there any behavior or temperament traits you try to decrease in this breed when you considered which bitch and sire to use? What are those traits?
	Are there any common breed-specific behavior problems seen in this breed?
	Do you encourage deviations from breed standards? (i.e., Off colors, smaller than standard size)
	What health issues are common in this breed?
	What breed deviations, orthopedic issues, or other health problems have you seen in your particular line?
	Do you have your dogs OFA certified (or other breed specific health screens)?
	Are your dogs bred to be working dogs? (i.e., Do you have dogs that are service dogs, herding dogs, guard dogs, etc.)
	Who is the breeder's veterinarian and would it be OK for you to speak to the veterinarian?

General considerations

	Did the breeder "interview you" by asking you questions pertaining to your lifestyle and why you want this particular breed?
	Was the breeder open to your questions or defensive?

Appendix Section 2
Training exercises

The appendices can be downloaded and printed at www.wiley.com/go/shaw/behavior

Appendix 20
Acclimatizing a pet to a crate

1. The crate should be located in commonly used areas of the home.

2. Always give a treat for going in the crate.

3. A food stuffed storage device will entertain a pet for a longer period of time.

4. Hide treats daily in the confinement area. When the pet explores the area he will begin to believe in the crate fairy.

5. Going into the confinement area should always be fun. Use an upbeat tone and attitude rather than a threatening or scolding manner when confining a pet.

6. Never punish a pet by sending him to his crate.

7. Supply appropriate toys in the confinement area.

8. Feed the pet's meals in the crate with the door opened or closed.

9. Minimize the length of time the pet is in his confinement area by offering scheduled breaks. Excessive confinement will result in hyperactivity.

10. When first introducing the crate, the pet should be allowed to explore it his own pace. Reward the pet with readily consumed treats for showing interest in the crate.

11. Clicker training utilizing shaping can be an easy and fun way to teach a pet to enter a kennel on cue.

Canine and Feline Behavior for Veterinary Technicians and Nurses, First Edition. Edited by Julie K. Shaw and Debbie Martin.
© 2015 John Wiley & Sons, Inc. Published 2015 by John Wiley & Sons, Inc.
Companion Website: www.wiley.com/go/shaw/behavior

Appendix 21
Elimination training log

Time	Walking outside on leash in backyard, record urine/stool	Feed	Walk around the block	Train using small food treats
6 am				
7 am				
8 am				
9 am				
10 am				
11 am				
12 pm				
1 pm				
2 pm				
3 pm				
4 pm				
5 pm				
6 pm				
7 pm				
8 pm				
9 pm				
10 pm				

Walk outside every hour when home during the day, feed twice a day, walk around the block twice a day, train twice a day.

Canine and Feline Behavior for Veterinary Technicians and Nurses, First Edition. Edited by Julie K. Shaw and Debbie Martin.
© 2015 John Wiley & Sons, Inc. Published 2015 by John Wiley & Sons, Inc.
Companion Website: www.wiley.com/go/shaw/behavior

Appendix 22
Shaping plan for teaching a puppy to ring a bell to go outside to eliminate

Shaping plan for teaching a puppy to ring a bell to go outside to eliminate	
Hold a bell on a string directly in front of the puppy's nose	C/T head turn toward bell
	C/T nose touching bell
	C/T movement of the bell
Puppy may begin using paw to move bell	C/T slightest sound of bell
Before taking puppy outside to eliminate (may need to keep puppy on a leash to prevent wandering) hold the bell directly in front of him	Puppy touches bell, door opens as reward, outside to eliminate
Hang bell at door, before taking puppy outside (may need to keep puppy on leash at door) wait for puppy to orient to bell	Any orientation to bell and door opens as reward, outside to eliminate
	Continue raising criteria gradually for more movement of the bell before going outside
Puppy may begin ringing the bell any time he would like to go out to play.	Initially, take the puppy out every time he rings the bell, then begin only taking him out when you suspect he may have to eliminate, and ignore other times.

C/T, click and treat.

Canine and Feline Behavior for Veterinary Technicians and Nurses, First Edition. Edited by Julie K. Shaw and Debbie Martin.
© 2015 John Wiley & Sons, Inc. Published 2015 by John Wiley & Sons, Inc.
Companion Website: www.wiley.com/go/shaw/behavior

Appendix 23
Preventive handling and restraint exercises

Handling

1. The dog should be calm and relaxed before starting the exercise.

2. The dog should have previous clicker training experience and understand the association between the click and treat delivery.

3. Use small easily consumed treats and have your clicker ready.

4. Keep sessions short; 1–3 min.

5. Go slow and make it fun and positive (a negative experience could have a long lasting negative consequence).

6. Desensitization and counter conditioning will be utilized to facilitate relaxation with handling.

7. Begin by touching the dog gently in a specific spot for 1 s. Click while touching him. Remove your hand. Give the dog a treat.

    Body parts to touch include

head	mouth
ears	neck
nose	shoulders
back	flank
tail	elbows
chest	legs
belly	feet

8. After the dog is relaxed and comfortable with you gently touching him for 1 s on the various body parts, then increase to 2, 3, 4 s, and so on. Vary the length so it does not always get longer and longer.

9. Gradually increase the pressure of the touch and decrease the duration of contact. Reset duration to 1 s. Click while you are touching, then remove your hand, and offer a treat. Gradually increase the level of pressure.

10. Use one hand to touch and the other hand for the clicker. Avoid clicking near the dog's ears.

Canine and Feline Behavior for Veterinary Technicians and Nurses, First Edition. Edited by Julie K. Shaw and Debbie Martin.
© 2015 John Wiley & Sons, Inc. Published 2015 by John Wiley & Sons, Inc.
Companion Website: www.wiley.com/go/shaw/behavior

Restraint

1. The dog should be calm and relaxed before starting this exercise. Consider starting on the floor or you may use a table for a small dog.

2. Use special, readily-consumed treats such as canned cheese. Have your clicker ready

3. The dog should have previous clicker training experience and understand the association between the click and treat delivery.

4. Keep sessions short; 1–3 min.

5. Go slow and make it fun and positive (a negative experience could have long lasting negative consequences).

6. Gently place an arm around your dog and click. Release and offer a treat. Arm goes over his back and under the belly/chest.

7. Progress to cradling with one arm over his back and under his belly/chest and the other arm under his neck.

8. With each consecutive repetition, gradually increase the pressure and/or duration.

9. If while performing these exercises, your dog mildly struggles to get down:
   - Continue to hold him. (Note if the dog is panicking then it is best to release him rather than waiting)
   - Say nothing.
   - Wait until he calms down.
   - Give him a treat.
   - Put him down.

   Next time progress slower to avoid stress and struggling.

If your dog has shown aggression or extreme fear with restraint, do not attempt these exercises

Appendix 24
Preventive food bowl exercises

1. Other pets in the household should be out of sight or confined before implementing the exercise.

2. Place a few kibbles in the bowl and place the bowl on the ground. Allow the dog to eat **all** the food. Pick up the empty bowl and place a few more kibbles in the bowl. Repeat until the entire meal is fed. If the dog knows a "sit" cue you may ask him to sit prior to lowering the bowl.

3. Another variation: Start with a few kibbles in the bowl and as the dog is eating add a few more kibbles to the bowl until the entire meal is fed.

4. Toss a special treat in the bowl from a distance as you enter the room in which the dog is eating. This teaches the dog that human presence means something better will fall from the sky. It is a positive association with your presence.

    If a dog has shown aggression toward people over food in the past, do not attempt this preventive exercise.

Canine and Feline Behavior for Veterinary Technicians and Nurses, First Edition. Edited by Julie K. Shaw and Debbie Martin.
© 2015 John Wiley & Sons, Inc. Published 2015 by John Wiley & Sons, Inc.
Companion Website: www.wiley.com/go/shaw/behavior

Appendix 25
Teaching tug of war

1. The game should be initiated by bringing out a specific tug toy that is not always available to the dog. Using a 3–4 ft tug toy or a toy with a rope attached to it, allows the toy to be further from the person and helps prevent the dog accidently making contact with the person's hand while learning the game.

2. Give the verbal cue "take it" and present the tug toy. Move the tug toy slightly back and forth to foster interest or chase.

3. When the dog has the toy in his mouth, engage him in a gentle game of tug. Verbally reward his interest in the tug.

4. Freeze (stop tugging and any toy movement). Give the verbal cue "drop it" and prompt the release with a treat directly under the dog's nose. Reward with the treat for dropping the toy. Pick up the toy. If the dog is over aroused and unable to release the toy, calm down the level of tugging or verbal encouragement initially. Also consider a less exciting toy.

5. Add the cue, "sit" or "down," and reward the behavior with "take it" and presentation of the tug toy. This helps to control the dog's arousal.

6. Repeat the above steps. Eventually, you will delay your presentation of the treat after giving the "drop it" cue so that the treat does not need to prompt the behavior. Still reward dropping the item with a treat or the "take it" cue.

7. When the game is over, give the dog several treats and place the tug toy out of sight.

Canine and Feline Behavior for Veterinary Technicians and Nurses, First Edition. Edited by Julie K. Shaw and Debbie Martin.
© 2015 John Wiley & Sons, Inc. Published 2015 by John Wiley & Sons, Inc.
Companion Website: www.wiley.com/go/shaw/behavior

Appendix Section 3
Samples and letters

The appendices can be downloaded and printed at www.wiley.com/go/shaw/behavior

Appendix 26
Canine behavior plan of care sample

Consultation Date: 1-1-14

Client's Name: Mary and Betty Phone: 555-1212 Email: maryandbetty@happy.com
Address: 555 Happy Drive City: Happy town State: Oregon Zip: 55555
Dog's Name: Roo Age: 3 years Breed: Redtick M □ Mx□ F□ Fx■

Canine Behavioral Diagnosis

Aggression	Target of Aggression	
□ Conflict-induced	□	□
□ Possessive	□	**Ingestive**
□ Disease/Pain induced	□	□ Coprophagia
■ Fear/Defensive induced	□	□ Pica
□ Idiopathic	**Anxiety Disorders**	□ Predatory Behavior
■ IDA + Motivation	■ Generalized Anxiety	**Eliminative**
□ IDA-H + Motivation	□ Global fear	□ Housesoiling
□ Alliance induced	□ Separation Anxiety	□ Urine marking
□ Status induced	□ Sound/Thunderstorm phobia	□ Excitement urination
□ Learned	□ Specific fear or phobia	□ Extreme fear/appeasement urination
□ Maternal/hormonal induced	□ Acute conflict behaviors/stereotypy	**Other**
□ Play induced	□ Compulsive disorder	□ Cognitive dysfunction
□ Redirected	Specific fear(s) or phobia (s) noted:	□ Hyperexcitability
□ Territorial	■ strangers	□ Conditioned unwanted behavior
□	■ unknown dogs	□

Prescribed Treatment Plan (see back for details and further information)

Management	Training	□ Shape relaxation
■ Avoid triggers	■ Marker training	□ Leave it/ drop it
■ Ignore attention seeking behaviors	□ Lure reward training	□
□ Ignore at specific times	□ Other training	□
■ Cue➤response➤reward interactions	□ Agility training	□
□ Environmental modifications	□ Concept training	□
□	□ K9 Nose work® training	□
	□ Crate/confinement training	**Behavior Modification** (see back)
□ Crate confinement	□	■ Counter-Conditioning
□ Other confinement	□	■ On walks if needed
□	**Training Tools**	■ When other dogs are present
□ Umbilical cord	■ Head halter	□
□ Change primary caregiver	□ Basket muzzle	□
□ Increase mental stimulation	□ Other muzzle	□
■ Walk off property	□ Body harness	■ Response Substitution
□ Aerobic exercise	□ No pull harness	■ On walks if needed
□ Regular schedule	□ Anxiety clothing	□
□ Dietary change	□ Calming cap	□
□ Meal feed twice daily	□ Drag line	□
□	□ Tether	□
□	□ Interactive toys/puzzles	□ Systematic Desensitization
Other	□ Pheromones	□
□ Interruption of behavior	□ Remote Reward	□
□ Cease punishment	**Specific Behaviors to Train**	□
□ Remote punishment	■ Targeting	□
□ Grief counseling	■ Attention	□
□ Rehoming patient	□ "Look" and "Watch"	□ Other
□	■ Sit ■ Down □ Recall	□
□	■ Loose leash walking	□
□	■ Go to a place	□

Bite History				
Has the dog bitten? ■ yes □ no		Does the dog redirect aggression? □ yes		□ no
How severe were the bites?	Did not make contact ■	Did not break skin □	Puncture □	Medical care needed □
Does the dog give warning before biting? □ yes		□ no	□ unknown	
Note known triggers and other significant bite history:				

Very defensive warning, would prefer to run.

Medical Conditions and Medications

No known medical issues, normal blood chemistry profile and thyroid profile. We have started Roo on Fluoxetine 1 mg/kg SID (once daily). There may be a decrease in appetite short term. Please report back to me routinely with changes in behavior.

Comments and Treatment Details

Helix,
Thank you so much for assessing Roo for us. We agree with your assessment and feel very lucky to have your on our behavior team. My name is Nancy and I am Dr. Anderson's technician. I will be working to help coordinate communication and treatment.
From your astute observations and what history we were able to obtain we agree Roo seems to have poor social skills that are aggravated by her generalized anxiety. She will become aggressive but it certainly isn't her first choice for getting out of a situation.

1)Avoid triggers - this will be almost impossible to do until the medication begins to take effect
2)Marker training to build confidence (we are thrilled she is not afraid of the clicker)
3)We are going to ask Mary and Betty to ignore all 3 dogs unless they are interacting with them in a cue-response-reward format (please reinforce that behavior in Mary and Betty!) until their next appointment. There is tension between the dogs and we'd like to decrease any potential alliance that may be developing while Roo's medication takes effect.
4)They can train Roo and tether Cocoa and Misty in the room. Cocoa and Misty get tossed treats just for being in the room with Roo. (CC) Either have Roo on leash or the other dog's on the other side of a barrier to prevent Roo from running after a tossed treat intended for the other dogs.
5)On walks when another dog approaches use foundations skills and CC to turn away from the approaching dog. A head halter may be required. That is your choice.

We are intentionally keeping the treatment plan short at this time. We'd like to recheck Roo in one month to reassess how she is doing on the medication and then add further aspects to the treatment plan.

Please call anytime and we look forward to working with you on this and other behavior cases.
Dr. Happy and Nancy Happyday, RVT

Veterinarian Signature: *Dr. Happy*

Date: 1-1-14

Appendix 27
Sample field assessment

YOUR DOG'S
PERSONAL TRAINER

Mary - Owner, 60 year old, Female

Betty - Owner, 55 year old, Female, pending shoulder surgery

OWNER CONCERNS:

1. Aggression toward unknown dogs
2. Relationship with other dogs in the household
3. Aggression toward unknown people

SIGNALMENT and HISTORY : Roo (patient)

Roo is a 3 y.o. spayed female Redtick Coonhound adopted from a shelter at approximately 5 months of age. In her time following adoption, she experienced a number of aversive experiences regarding other dogs and people:

- approx 6 months of age – attacked by two Poodles
- approx 7 months of age – attacked by a dog being fostered by the household
- approx 9 months of age – attacked by a Pit Bull
- approx 2 years of age – attacked by a Boston Terrier who latched onto an ear
- whipped and beaten off in two separate incidents following Roo's charging at strangers
- almost two years of shock collar training regarding her triggers (bikers, joggers, skateboarders, other dogs, other people). Betty and Mary subsequently learned this made things worse for Roo and have stopped using the shock collar.

******Despite the above history, Roo has no bite history with humans or dogs.

HISTORY: Misty (Housemate)

Misty is a 4 y.o. spayed female (probably) Springer Spanel / Pointer mix. She was adopted from a shelter at approximately one year of age. Betty and Mary have worked hard to rehabilitate her and have had huge success in that endeavor.

HISTORY: Cocoa (Housemate)

Cocoa is a 2 y.o. neutered male Lab-Border Collie mix who was adopted from a shelter 11 months ago.

None of the dogs have been to formal training classes. Betty and Mary are seeking help at this time due to having to keep Roo away from people and other dogs, the possibility of serious altercations if they don't keep her away and the increasing difficulties with interactions among the dogs in the home. They feel there is a growing tension between the dogs within the household.

MEDICAL INFORMATION

It is reported that none of the dogs have any on-going medical issues at this time.

ASSESSMENT - MEETING OBSERVATIONS

We met for the assessment at their home. Betty and Mary have developed many routines for taking care of their dogs' physical needs, such as runs in a nearby field, leash walks, hide-it games and household "cuddle times".

ROO

Roo was reported to be the dog whose issues are a priority for them. Roo charged into the room to greet me with, at first, no barking. She was eagerly taking treats although she exhibited intense

---

1

helixfairweather@gmail.com   @2014 www.helixfairweather.com

Canine and Feline Behavior for Veterinary Technicians and Nurses, First Edition. Edited by Julie K. Shaw and Debbie Martin.
© 2015 John Wiley & Sons, Inc. Published 2015 by John Wiley & Sons, Inc.
Companion Website: www.wiley.com/go/shaw/behavior

FIELD ASSESSMENT
Betty, Mary - Roo

wrinkling of the forehead and a tightly pulled forward commissure. One of my movements startled her and she jumped back, weight shifted over her rear, barking with an almost closed mouth.

In subsequent barking at me, her body weight was shifted well forward with mouth puckered and wrinkled forehead. It was understandable that members of the public would feel threatened upon being rushed in this manner. Roo has been beaten in two incidents when she was off leash in public and charged at people barking in this manner.

As I worked with Roo doing some clicker training, I observed her easily startle with flicks of my hand to toss a treat. Each time she startled she would jump back with the above described body language and barking. Throughout my 2 hour assessment with her, she responded in this "never relaxed" fashion the entire time. She jumped at slight hand movements, my moving my head back (very small movement), to my lanyard dangling on the clicker, to my turning my body. She was NEVER relaxed. Betty and Mary report that Roo responds in this manner to many ordinary events that happen suddenly in her environment. In other words, there are multiple triggers for Roo's intense reactions and these are often events that cannot be controlled, prevented or managed.

I attempted a bit of impromptu counter-conditioning to the sight of my lanyard. With a dog who has a mild fear response to an item, one can expect to see forward progress in a trial session such as this. In the case of Roo, I observed signs that counter-conditioning to hanging straps would be possible. I believe she was reacting more to the quick movements than to the lanyard itself.

Throughout the two-hour assessment, Roo had moments of relaxed body features and facial features. She appeared to be a completely different dog at those times. However, those times did not last very long as another triggering event would occur.

I consider Roo to be exhibiting conflict-related responses. Because there are so many triggers, it's possible she is in a frequent state of anxiety and conflict (she wants to interact but her fear takes over).

In the course of my visit, we sat on living room furniture discussing the dogs while the dogs carried on their normal interactions. In observing Roo's interactions with her housemates, I observed that she does not give appropriate communication to the young dog, Cocoa. By observing Cocoa, I conclude he's not getting the information he needs from Roo as he persists in unacceptable behaviors until Roo suddenly has had enough and then attacks.

In my experience, I have observed other dog pairs with this type of interaction. Owners presume the issue is "dominance" or "bullying". I suspect that Roo's underlying anxiety and poor social skills lead to a much greater than necessary "correction" which then leads to an actual fight between the dogs.

FIELD ASSESSMENT
Betty, Mary - Roo

YOUR DOG'S
**PERSONAL
TRAINER**

MISTY

My observations of Misty were of a relaxed dog, eager to greet, eager to work with a stranger. She has certainly come a long way from her described fear issues of the past. Betty and Mary are doing "happy visits" to the veterinarian's office to help Misty learn to be more comfortable there. Clicker training will give them a big boost forward in that process. I observed ordinary self-control issues with Misty such as grabbing treats roughly and jumping on me excitedly. These can easily be smoothed out in training sessions focused on teaching her what TO do in given situations.

COCOA

Cocoa is just approaching the age of social maturity. Because none of the household dogs are effective communicators, there are no peace-keepers in the group. Cocoa, being the youngest, appears to me a bit adrift as a result. He continues to badger the other dogs to play with him. Misty can communicate to him with subtle head or body turns that she isn't interested and he does respond to those – IF the entire context is one of low stimulus. When there's too much arousal and activity, he loses the ability to pay attention to the subtleties of communication.

I am concerned about his being described as biting the throats of the other dogs. I did not observe an example of this at this time.

ASSESSMENT OF RESPONSES TO ANOTHER DOG WHEN ON LEASH

Roo was assessed on leash, starting at about a distance of 80 feet, with both a lifelike, stuffed dog on leash and a live Bearded Collie on leash. In both cases, Roo alerted to the other dog and gave off moderate excited barking indicating, to me, curiosity. We closed distance in both cases significantly without evoking her typical reactive response. Her typical response was not observed. However, using Betty and Mary's observations of Roo's responses to me in their home, I have a good sense of her reaction to certain dogs when spotted in public. I have enough information to know that she does have

a threshold distance we can work with and that there are low-level dogs we can use for establishing a baseline of acceptable responses.

3

helixfairweather@gmail.com   @2014 www.helixfairweather.com

FIELD ASSESSMENT
Betty, Mary - Roo

CURRENT PROBLEMS TO BE ADDRESSED

1. Roo's responses to triggers are frequent and they involve triggers that cannot be easily controlled. Addressing this underlying anxiety would be the first step.****SEE CONCERNS**

2. Roo's responses to her two major triggers – humans and dogs – when on leash and in public.

3. Building inter-dog communication skills.

CURRENT TRAINING AND MANAGEMENT PLAN

- **CLICKER TRAINING** (marker-based training) as a fast, efficient communication tool ("that's it, what you are doing right now is what I want")

- **FOUNDATION SKILLS**
  These are tools that will be used in the introductions to other people and to other dogs. These will also be used for teaching a household relaxation mode that will not only help Roo's anxiety and the other dogs' over-arousal, but will aid Betty in her recuperation from surgery. These will likely be a review for the dogs in some cases. Nevertheless, it's important to have a very large reinforcement history for these skills so that Betty & Mary can count on the dog being able to respond in real-life, arousal-packed situations. These foundation skills are:

  o **Relaxation on a mat** to be used as a safety zone and a signal that now it's time to bring down the arousal level and become calm again.
  o **Attention to the handler** under ever-increasing challenges, volunteered by each dog, until it becomes habit
  o **Leave It** – the ability to break off from that which the dog is about to do. This is very helpful in interrupting a reactive response before it even starts.
  o **Instant name response, sit, down, target to hand**

- **PUBLIC SKILLS**
  These are skills that will be used in behavior modification exercises involving other dogs. They are also the skills needed for navigating leash walks in the neighborhood. These skills are:

  o **Fast and fun about turn with loose leash walking**

  o **Learning to read the pre-cursor signs** that predict a reactive response is not far behind.

INTERACTIONS WITH BETTY AND MARY and CURRENT STATUS OF THE HUMAN ANIMAL BOND

All three dogs are well cared for and interacted with. It's obvious how much Betty and Mary care for their dogs and the time they put into giving them a good life. With Betty's increasing shoulder difficulties, culminating in surgery in December, there needs to be a more relaxed, calm nature to the household and that can be taught to the dogs rather than continual attempts to impose that by Betty and Mary. It is obvious Betty and Mary are deeply bonded to Roo.

Betty and Mary use food treats in training and the dogs respond to two or three trained cues when no triggering events are occurring. They are committed to improving the dog-dog interactions in their household.

***SPECIFIC CONCERNS

After observing Roo in her home environment, it is my profesional opinion that Roo's general anxiety is inhibiting her learning process and causing conflict and significant anxiety between her and the other dogs in the household. I am concerned that the stress could potentially lead to serious relationship issues down the road between the housemates. I am recommending Betty and Mary take Roo to their veterinarian for an examination, behavioral diagnosis and treatment plan that may or may not include anxiolytic medications.

 I would very much like to assist with helping Betty and Mary in the application of the prescribed treatment plan and look forward to working with the hospitals behavior team in Roo's follow up care.

Printed with permission:
Helix Fairweather, Karen Pryor Academy Certified Training Partner
Your Dog's Personal Trainer
helixfairweather@gmail.com

Appendix 28
Sample of a pet selection report

The husband of a family consisting of wife, 38 years old, husband, 49 years old, and 2 daughters, 8 and 11 years old, sought assistance with obtaining a dog for the family. This will be their first dog. The client was sent a pet selection questionnaire to be completed by the entire family.

Questionnaire results:

The financial consideration part of the questionnaire revealed the client was willing to spend $1000 or more on the purchase of a dog. They wanted to obtain a puppy from a reputable breeder. They were also willing to pay "whatever is necessary" on annual medical costs and would budget $100 or less monthly for food. They would like more information on neutering.

   The questions pertaining to pet characteristics revealed they were interested in a dog for the children, one that requires little training, and they would like to obtain the dog as young as possible. They would be willing to do "whatever it takes to correct the problem" should the dog develop house soiling issues, shyness with people, aloofness with family members, attention demanding behavior, jumping on people, digging, destructive chewing or excessive vocalization. They could live with a dog that is excitable. It was not important to them that the dog guard the house. They were planning to devote time to grooming the dog at home weekly and also have it professionally groomed routinely. They wanted a small dog less than 10 pounds. It was important to them that the dog would want to sit in their lap. They would not tolerate hair on clothing or furniture. Three breeds of dogs they were considering: Maltese, Cavalier King Charles Spaniel, and Mini-Havanese.

Consultation

A two hour in home appointment was performed and the following information was provided in writing and discussed with the entire family:

Recommendations:

❑ Suggested breed options:
- Miniature Poodle:
    - Pros: Small, lively, playful, bright, attentive, usually (should be) good with people and other animals, variety of colors, does not shed
    - Cons: Barking, joint or eye problems, grooming, may be difficult to find a good breeder
- Maltese:
    - Pros: Very small, bright, playful, usually (should be) good with people and other animals, does not shed
    - Cons: FRAGILE, difficult to house train, barking, grooming, medical concerns (orthopedic, liver)
- Havanese:
    - Pros: small but sturdy, playful, entertaining, does not shed
    - Cons: difficult to house train, barking, grooming, very expensive ($2500), not a large breeding stock (potential for genetic problems)

Canine and Feline Behavior for Veterinary Technicians and Nurses, First Edition. Edited by Julie K. Shaw and Debbie Martin.
© 2015 John Wiley & Sons, Inc. Published 2015 by John Wiley & Sons, Inc.
Companion Website: www.wiley.com/go/shaw/behavior

- Bichon Frise:
  - Pros: Small but sturdy, does not shed, does not require much exercise, usually (should be) good with people and other animals
  - Cons: difficult to house train, barking, grooming, skin problems
- Yorkie:
  - Pros: Small, lively, curious, does not need extensive exercise
  - Cons: FRAGILE, excitable (terrier), barking, difficult to house train, grooming
❑ Male versus female
❑ Choosing a breeder:
  - NEVER buy a puppy from a pet store! No reputable breeder will sell his/her puppies to a pet store.
  - Poor breeders:
    - Not interested in improving the breed and does not care about breed standards
    - AKC registration does not guarantee quality
    - Breeds 3+ different breeds
    - Dogs are kept or managed in kennels or in separate building
  - Good breeders:
    - Know and follow breed standards
    - Know health issue of the breed
    - They want to tell you everything about their dogs
    - Understand puppy development and puppies are properly socialized
    - Will not sell the puppy until it is at least 8 weeks old
    - Choose prospective owners carefully
    - Encourage you to meet the puppy's parents
    - Willing to give references
    - Have done medical testing and provide written proof that the sire and dam are free of potential genetic medical problems associated with the breed
  - Breeder quiz:
    - What are the breed standards?
    - What are the common health issues for the breed?
    - What testing has the breeder done with the Sire and Dam prior to breeding?
    - How old are the puppies' parents?
    - What made the breeder decide to breed these two dogs?
    - What is the history of the breed?
    - What environment are the puppies kept?
    - What is their socialization/enrichment/handling program for the puppies?
    - At what age are the puppies allowed to go to their new home?
    - Ask for references from the breeder's veterinarian and owners of dogs previously bred by the breeder
❑ Things to do before bringing the puppy home:
  - Set a routine or schedule for feeding and walking. A chart can be very helpful especially if multiple people will be sharing the responsibility.
  - Small breed dogs may need to be feed 3 times a day until 4 months old to avoid hypoglycemia
  - Purchase a crate and maybe also an exercise pen

- Purchase food (breeder should send some home with you)
- Purchase food and water bowls
- Purchase a collar and leash
- Purchase 2 or more Kong toys or other food storage toys
- *Puppy Start Right: Foundation Training for the Companion Dog* by Kenneth and Debbie Martin
- Decide and write down "Rules of the House"
- Have Karo syrup on hand in case of a hypoglycemic event
- Schedule an appointment with a veterinarian within a few days of obtaining the dog
- Consider using the Adaptil® Diffuser (Dog Appeasing Pheromone) near the kennel

❑ Things to look for in a puppy
  - Should be excited to meet new people
  - Should eagerly approach you, tail wagging, and curious
  - A shy or fearful puppy will become worse as it gets older
  - Hair coat should be shiny and clean
  - Eyes and nose should be clean and clear (no discharge)

❑ Problem prevention:
  - Socialization!!!!
  - Housetraining
  - Crate training
  - Play biting
  - Food bowl safety
  - Prevent fear of the Veterinary hospital/groomer

Resources:

Books:

Culture Clash by Jean Donaldson

Living with Kids and Dogs…Without Losing Your Mind by Colleen Pelar, CPDT

Puppy Start Right: Foundation Training for the Companion Dog by Kenneth and Debbie Martin

Puppy Training for Kids by Sarah Whitehead

On Talking Terms with Dogs: Calming Signals by Turid Rugaas

Websites:

Some websites for potential breeders in the geographical area of the client were provided.

Follow up

After the consultation, the client decided they would look for a female Maltese puppy. They were interested in obtaining a puppy in the next 2 to 3 months. It was stressed during the consultation that Maltese's can be difficult to house train due to their size. The owners understood this and were interested in pursuing the breed.

   The clients hired me to help them find a reputable breeder. I contacted a breeder that was within 1.5 hours of the client and engaged in actively showing their dogs in conformation. The owner of the kennel spoke with me for over 40 minutes. He was eager to discuss his dogs. He stated that in the past 15 years of breeding Maltese's, they had had one dog with a liver shunt and 10 patent ductus arteriosis. They screen for patella luxation. He gave me several veterinary references.

The breeder stated that they do not let their puppies leave until they are at least 12 weeks old. He felt they were able to provide better socialization than most pet owners and was also attempting to prevent separation anxiety. He allows the bitch to wean the puppies. Puppies and the bitch stay in the house and have exposure to people and household sounds. They are also taken outside in exercise pens on grass for short periods of time each day. They currently had four litters about 2–3 weeks apart. They would be ready to be adopted in about 2 months. The breeder was open to a visit from me or the family.

After talking with my client about the breeder, I recommended that I visit the breeder's home and meet some of their dogs. An hour visit in the breeder's home was performed. The puppies and bitches were very clean. The adult dogs were friendly and eagerly jumped into my lap. The breeder gave me a tour through the kennel area adjoining the home to allow me to meet the male dogs. Although they barked, they appeared friendly and outgoing. The facility was clean and the dogs were taken care of appropriately. They owned a total of 18 dogs. Some were old (16–18 years old) retired show dogs that were living as pets in the home. I was pleased with the visit and recommended the owners contact the breeder to obtain a puppy. The cost of the dog was more than what the owner anticipated, but the client was willing to pay the price.

The clients visited the breeder about 2 weeks later and were shown a 4 month old, Female that had been at a friend's house. I advised the client that I would be concerned about the socialization history, house training and why it was returned to the breeder. I contacted the breeder and determined the dog had been sold as the pick of the litter and was being co-owned by the breeder. However, she was "low in the legs." Her patellas were good but she was not going to be the correct proportion for conformation. She had been managed in the kitchen at the previous home and was trained to pee pads.

The breeder would have another 12 week old female available in the middle of May. I discussed the pros and cons of obtaining a 4 month old puppy. Although I encouraged the owner to wait for the younger puppy, I left the decision to the client. The client decided to obtain the 4 month old puppy.

Five training appointments were performed over a 1.5 month period. The entire family attended each appointment. The parents and girls were taught how to teach "Riley" to sit, down, come, leave it, drop it, place (go to bed), stay, and walk on a loose leash using lure reward and clicker training. The biggest challenge for the owner was the house training. Management and prevention options were discussed at each appointment. Two months after obtaining (the dog was now 6 months of age) "Riley", she was only having occasional urine accidents in the house (~3 times a week). Stool was always outside in the designated elimination area.

A follow up email from the owner nearly 2 years after obtaining the dog, revealed that the dog was completely house trained and a terrific companion for the family. The husband reported, "My 2 biggest concerns were sleeping through the night and pottying outside. She does great at both of these. She does seem to bark a lot but we were forewarned by you about this."

Discussion

Although a 4 month old Maltese would not have been my first pick for this family, they were educated on the pros and cons of a variety of small breed dogs that would fit their desires. Consequently, they were able to make an informed decision and set realistic expectations for their canine companion.

Provided courtesy of Debbie Martin, RVT, VTS (Behavior)

Appendix 29
Dr. Andrew Luescher's letter regarding puppy socialization

To Whom It May Concern:

This letter's purpose is to define Purdue University's recommendations for Puppy Class protocols.

The main objectives of puppy classes are exposure and desensitization to potentially frightening stimuli, socialization, and the teaching of appropriate dog-owner interaction. Although simple commands are trained as well, obedience training is not a main objective of puppy classes.

Puppies go through well-defined developmental stages. Puppy classes are designed to utilize the sociability of young puppies. **However, the socialization period of dogs ends at around 12–14 weeks of age.** Up to that age, puppies can readily learn not to fear new things, and to develop appropriate social behavior. If this opportunity to shape puppy behavior is missed, the puppies are likely to show behavior disturbances later in life. **Therefore, in order to maximize the benefits of puppy classes, puppies should be enrolled at 7-10 weeks of age if possible, the sooner the better.**

The puppy classes at Purdue University's Animal Behavior Clinic start any time between 7 and 14 weeks of age *and* **at least 10 days after initial vaccination for the Distemper/Parvo combination and Bordatella.** We encourage the use of an intranasal Bordatella/Parainfluenza (+/− Adeno) combination and the use of a high-titer, low-passage Parvo vaccination. These should be vaccinations administered after a thorough veterinary exam. Several vaccines are currently on the market, which meet these requirements.

Trainers and veterinarians have had concerns about placing puppies at risk in an environment where they may pick up an infectious disease. As with anything, one must always weigh the risks and benefits. "Puppy cuteness" only lasts so long and many more puppies currently lose their homes due to behavior reasons than die of viral diseases.

We are aware of only one Parvo problem in a puppy preschool class in Minnesota in the early 90's and none since high titer Parvo vaccines gained mainstream use in 1995. There have been no Puppy Class participants infected with Parvo virus in any puppy classes offered at Ohio State or Purdue University. These are both facilities that treat high humane society caseloads and numerous Parvo cases annually.

Preliminary investigations underway at the University of Pennsylvania suggest that low-level exposure to pathogens, like what might occur in a clean although not completely sterile environment, may actually promote a "stronger" or more responsive immune system. (verbal communication with Dr. Karen Overall, dipl ACVB 1998)

Let's welcome new puppies into our society by showing them what we expect, not dispose of them because we failed to communicate our expectations at a time when the puppies are most impressionable.

Sincerely,

Andrew Luescher, DVM, PhD., Diplomate ACVB
Director, Animal Behavior Clinic, Purdue University

Steve Thompson, DVM, Diplomate ABVP,
Certified in Canine/Feline Practice
Director, The Pet Wellness Clinic, Purdue University

Canine and Feline Behavior for Veterinary Technicians and Nurses, First Edition. Edited by Julie K. Shaw and Debbie Martin.
© 2015 John Wiley & Sons, Inc. Published 2015 by John Wiley & Sons, Inc.
Companion Website: www.wiley.com/go/shaw/behavior

Appendix 30

Dr. RK Anderson's letter regarding puppy socialization

TO: My Colleagues in Veterinary Medicine:

Common questions I receive from puppy owners, dog trainers and veterinarians concern: 1) what is the most favorable age or period of time when puppies learn best? 2) what are the health implications of my advice that veterinarians and trainers should offer socialization programs for puppies starting at 8 to 9 weeks of age.

Puppies begin learning at birth and their brains appear to be particularly responsive to learning and retaining experiences that are encountered during the first 13 to 16 weeks after birth [Dr. Anderson is saying that the prime time for puppy socialization stops somewhere between 13 and 16 weeks, although more socialization occurs after that time]. This means that breeders, new puppy owners, veterinarians, trainers and behaviorists have a responsibility to assist in providing these learning/socialization experiences with other puppies/dogs, with children/adults and with various environmental situations during this optimal period from birth to 16 weeks.

Many veterinarians are making this early socialization and learning program part of a total wellness plan for breeders and new owners of puppies during the first 16 weeks of a puppy's life -- the first 7-8 weeks with the breeder and the next 8 weeks with the new owners. This socialization program should enroll puppies from 8 to 12 weeks of age as a key part of any preventive medicine program to improve the bond between pets and their people and keep dogs as valued members of the family for 12 to 18 years.

To take full advantage of this early special learning period, many veterinarians recommend that new owners take their puppies to puppy socialization classes, beginning at 8 to 9 weeks of age. At this age they should have (and can be required to have) received a minimum of their first series of vaccines for protection against infectious diseases. This provides the basis for increasing immunity by further repeated exposure to these antigens either through natural exposure in small doses or artificial exposure with vaccines during the next 8 to 12 weeks. In addition the owner and people offering puppy socialization should take precautions to have the environment and the participating puppies as free of natural exposure as possible by good hygiene and caring by careful instructors and owners.

Experience and epidemiologic data support the relative safety and lack of transmission of disease in these puppy socialization classes over the past 10 years in many parts of the United States. In fact; the risk of a dog dying because of infection with distemper or parvo disease is far less than the much higher risk of a dog dying (euthanasia) because of a behavior problem. Many veterinarians are now offering new puppy owners puppy socialization classes in their hospitals or nearby training facilities in conjunction with

Canine and Feline Behavior for Veterinary Technicians and Nurses, First Edition. Edited by Julie K. Shaw and Debbie Martin.
© 2015 John Wiley & Sons, Inc. Published 2015 by John Wiley & Sons, Inc.
Companion Website: www.wiley.com/go/shaw/behavior

trainers and behaviorists because they want socialization and training to be very important parts of a wellness plan for every puppy. We need to recognize that this special sensitive period for learning is the best opportunity we have to influence behavior for dogs and the most important and longest lasting part of a total wellness plan.

Are there risks? Yes. But 10 years of good experience and data, with few exceptions, offers veterinarians the opportunity to generally recommend early socialization and training classes, beginning when puppies are 8 to 9 weeks of age. However, we always follow a veterinarian's professional judgment, in individual cases or situations, where special circumstances warrant further immunization for a special puppy before starting such classes. During any period of delay for puppy classes, owners should begin a program of socialization with children and adults, outside their family, to take advantage of this special period in a puppy's life.

If there are further questions, veterinarians may call me at 651-644-7400 for discussion and clarification.

Appendix 31
Sample puppy socialization class curriculum*

* With permission from Kenneth and Debbie Martin from Puppy Start Right for Instructors online course via www.karenpryoracademy.com

All classes are approximately 1 h in length and meet once a week. After completing orientation, owners then complete four classes with their puppy.

Orientation presentation

Orientation allows for the human participates to learn about what to expect in puppy class and is a prerequisite to attending class with a puppy. Ideally orientation should be offered weekly in order to enroll new puppies immediately.

Orientation covers
- class format and what to expect;
- socialization defined;
- introduction to clicker training;
  - begin to teach attention and targeting at home;
- positive proactive socialization;
- body language and signs of fear;
- what to do if my puppy is afraid;
- successful canine parenting;
- positive problem solving;
- what to bring to class.

Health and handling class

Health and handling class includes the following topics:
- Training topic: Sit
- Problem prevention and solving topics
  - Crate/confinement training
  - Handling and restraint
  - Muzzle training
  - Elimination training

Canine and Feline Behavior for Veterinary Technicians and Nurses, First Edition. Edited by Julie K. Shaw and Debbie Martin.
© 2015 John Wiley & Sons, Inc. Published 2015 by John Wiley & Sons, Inc.
Companion Website: www.wiley.com/go/shaw/behavior

Wheels and children's toys class

Wheels and children's toys class includes the following topics:

- Training topic: Loose Leash Walking
- Problem prevention and solving topics
  - Counter surfing and stealing objects
  - Digging
  - Independence training
  - Hide and seek or Find it game

Obstacles and sounds class

Obstacles and sounds class includes the following topics:

- Training topic: Leave it and drop it
- Problem prevention and solving topics
  - Play biting/mouthing
  - Gotcha game (collar grab)
  - Food bowl exercise

Costumes and appearances class

Costumes and appearances class includes the following topics:

- Training topic: Recall/come
- Problem prevention and solving topics
  - Chewing
  - Jumping
  - Spay and Neuter

Appendix 32
Sample kitten class curriculum

Each class is approximately 1 h in length. Kittens should be less than 14 weeks of age when starting class.

Week 1 Topics

Feline communication and body language

Appropriate owner–kitten play with toys

Litter box preferences and recommendations

Environmental enrichment

Handling for routine at home medical care

Teaching a come when called

Week 2 Topics

Importance of daily routine

Acclimating a kitten to a harness and leash

Scratching

Multi cat household recommendations

Reintroduction of cats after a vet visit

Handling for routine at home medical care AGAIN!

Teaching sit and high five

Canine and Feline Behavior for Veterinary Technicians and Nurses, First Edition. Edited by Julie K. Shaw and Debbie Martin.
© 2015 John Wiley & Sons, Inc. Published 2015 by John Wiley & Sons, Inc.
Companion Website: www.wiley.com/go/shaw/behavior

Index

A

ABC *see* antecedent–behavior–consequence
acceptance, 107
acepromazine, 291, 292
acetylcholine, 287
acknowledging, 86
active defense, 118
active listening, 87
activity levels, 62
acute conflict behaviors, 215
acute hepatic necrosis, 294
adolescent period
    behavior wellness examination, 201
    canine behavior and development, 48
    feline behavior and development, 67
    juvenile/adolescent/adult dog classes, 196–198
    juvenile/adolescent/adult dog questionnaire, 337–338
adult period
    adult cat questionnaire, 335–336
    behavior wellness examination, 202
    canine behavior and development, 48
    feline behavior and development, 67
    juvenile/adolescent/adult dog classes, 196–198
    juvenile/adolescent/adult dog questionnaire, 337–338
aerobic exercise, 221
affective conditioning, 138
affordances, 119
aggression
    alliance-induced aggression, 211
    body postures, 32–33
    communication, 90, 91, 98–99, 105–106
    conflict behavior, 36–37
    conflict-induced aggression, 207–209
    diagnosis and descriptions of behavior disorders, 206–214
    disease- or pain-induced aggression, 210
    fear/defensive aggression, 55–57, 207, 210–211
    feline behavior and development, 55–57, 58, 60
    grief counseling, 105–106
    human–animal bond, 81
    idiopathic aggression, 211
    inter-cat aggression, 211
    inter-dog aggression, 211
    learned aggression, 212
    learning, 127
    maternal/hormonal induced aggression, 212
    medical differentials, 3, 4, 5, 13
    muzzles, 233
    pain-induced aggression, 210
    petting-induced aggression, 209–210
    play-induced aggression, 212
    possessive aggression, 209
    preventive care, 147, 150, 169–171, 200
    psychopharmacology, 294, 299
    redirected aggression, 212
    status-induced aggression, 211, 212
    territorial aggression, 212–213
    treatment plan, 220
    veterinary behavior consultation, 13, 16–17
agility training, 228
allelic differences, 116–117
alliance-induced aggression, 211
allorubbing, 58, 115
alpha-2 agonists, 293, 298–299
alprazolam, 292, 294–295
American Animal Hospital Association (AAHA), 101
Americans with Disabilities Act (ADA), 72–73
American Veterinary Society of Animal Behavior (AVSAB), 7–9, 221–222, 224
amitripytline, 293, 295
amygdala, 286
anal licking, 4
anger, 105–106
animal-assisted therapy (AAT), 71–72
animal behavioralists, 6–8
Animal Behavior Society (ABS), 7
animal cruelty/abuse, 73–74
animal hoarders, 75–76
animal shelters, 186, 187–188
antecedent–behavior–consequence (ABC), 172, 175–176, 179–180
anthropomorphic interpretations, 89–90
anticipated responsibilities, 186
anticipatory grief, 107
antidepressants, 292–293, 295–297
antipsychotics, 291–294
anxiety and fear
    acute conflict behaviors, 215
    behavior modification, 260–262
    canine behavior and development, 40
    classical conditioning, 137
    communication, 85
    compulsive disorder, 215
    diagnosis and descriptions of behavior disorders, 207, 210–211, 214–215
    feline behavior and development, 55–57, 58
    generalized anxiety, 214
    global fear, 214
    greeting a fearful patient, 277–279
    human–animal bond, 77

Canine and Feline Behavior for Veterinary Technicians and Nurses, First Edition. Edited by Julie K. Shaw and Debbie Martin.
© 2015 John Wiley & Sons, Inc. Published 2015 by John Wiley & Sons, Inc.
Companion Website: www.wiley.com/go/shaw/behavior

Harquin
watched
the hunt
leave.

He made quite sure they had gone before he ventured out, taking with him, as a souvenir, the squire's hat which he found in the marsh. His family was very pleased to see him returning home safe and sound, and came out to meet him.

And so the foxes were able to live in peace and wander freely in the valley, since nobody ever went there to hunt again. As for the gamekeeper, he no longer works for the squire.

Now Harquin has children of his own and they still live in the same home. Often before they go to sleep, he tells them about the famous hunt. They all listen intently to his stories, except for one of his sons, who is bored. He wants to go beyond the valley.